Periodontology at a Glance

Periodontology at a Glance

Valerie Clerehugh
BDS, PhD, FDS RCS (Ed)
Professor of Periodontology, Leeds Dental Institute
Leeds, UK

Aradhna Tugnait
BChD, MDentSci, PhD, FDS RCS (Ed)
Lecturer in Restorative Dentistry, Leeds Dental Institute
Leeds, UK

Robert J. Genco
DDS, PhD
Distinguished Professor of Oral Biology and Microbiology
School of Dental Medicine and School of Medicine and
Biomedical Sciences
State University of New York at Buffalo, USA

WILEY-BLACKWELL
A John Wiley & Sons, Ltd., Publication

This edition first published 2009

Blackwell Publishing was acquired by John Wiley & Sons in February 2007. Blackwell's publishing programme has been merged with Wiley's global Scientific, Technical, and Medical business to form Wiley-Blackwell.

Registered office
John Wiley & Sons Ltd, The Atrium, Southern Gate, Chichester, West Sussex, PO19 8SQ, United Kingdom

Editorial offices
9600 Garsington Road, Oxford, OX4 2DQ, United Kingdom
2121 State Avenue, Ames, Iowa 50014-8300, USA

For details of our global editorial offices, for customer services and for information about how to apply for permission to reuse the copyright material in this book please see our website at www.wiley.com/wiley-blackwell.

Library of Congress Cataloging-in-Publication Data
Clerehugh, Valerie.
Periodontology at a glance / Valerie Clerehugh, Aradhna Tugnait, Robert Genco.
p. ; cm. – (At a glance)
Includes bibliographical references and index.
ISBN 978-1-4051-2383-9 (pbk. : alk. paper) 1. Periodontics. I. Tugnait, Aradhna. II. Genco, Robert J. III. Title. IV. Series: At a glance series (Oxford, England)
[DNLM: 1. Periodontal Diseases–Handbooks. WU 49 C629p 2009]

RK361.C537 2009
617.6′32–dc22

2008053123

A catalogue record for this book is available from the British Library.

Set in 9/11.5pt Times by Graphicraft Limited, Hong Kong
Printed and bound in Singapore by Ho Printing Singapore Pte Ltd

5 2014

Contents

Preface

Periodontology is the specialty of dentistry concerned with diseases of the supporting tissues of the teeth. Periodontal disease in its most severe forms affects between 5% and 15% of the population in industrialised countries, while disease presenting at the early and intermediate stages is widespread, as is the reversible condition of gingivitis. As such any practitioner of dentistry or dental hygiene will be confronted with patients presenting with periodontal problems on a daily basis. Current research suggests that periodontal disease is also linked to other general health problems including diabetes, cardiovascular disease and strokes. Thus periodontal diseases and their management may have effects beyond that of the oral cavity.

In the UK and USA, as in other countries, periodontal care is delivered in general dental practice, specialist periodontal practice and the dental hospital setting. Perhaps more than any other area of dentistry at the time of writing, the management of periodontal patients is often achieved by an integrated dental team. The continuing development of the roles of professions complementary to dentistry can only enhance the scope for the delivery of effective patient care.

Periodontology at a Glance is the latest title in the widely known At a Glance series. It is designed to provide a concise review of the field of periodontology and includes the underpinning principles of the subject and their clinical applications. It is designed as a study aid and revision guide for students of dentistry, hygiene and therapy. It is also a useful tool for dental practitioners, hygienists and therapists to update their knowledge of this continually developing subject.

In the typical visual At a Glance style, this book uses a double-page spread for each topic. Salient information has been distilled from the literature and presented in easy to read notes, tables, diagrams and figures. Where teeth are referred to in the text and figures the following notation is used: UR, upper right quadrant; UL, upper left quadrant; LR, lower right quadrant; and LL, lower left quadrant. The permanent teeth are referred to as '1' (indicating central incisor) to '8' (indicating third molar), to give UR1 as the upper right permanent central incisor and UR8 as the upper right permanent third molar.

The chapters are self-contained and can therefore be read in any order. Cross referencing will direct the reader to additional relevant chapters in the book. Each chapter ends with a box of key points to present the reader with the essential take-home messages for a particular topic. References and further reading for each chapter are provided in the Appendix at the end of the book.

We hope you enjoy using this book.

Acknowledgements and dedications

Professor Iain L. C. Chapple, Professor of Periodontology, University of Birmingham is credited with writing Chapter 31, 'Non-plaque-induced gingival conditions and lesions'. We are very grateful to him for his contribution to our book and for the figures he provided in other chapters: Figs 38.5 and 40.9. Thanks are due to Quintessence for permission to publish images in the following Figures in Chapter 31: Fig 31.3b, Fig 31.4, Fig 31.5, Fig 31.7, Fig 31.8 and Fig 31.9.

We thank Quintessence for permission to publish Figs 35.5 (b), (d) and 35.6 (c), and Wiley-Blackwell for permission to use Fig 5.5.

We extend our thanks to the Photography Department at Leeds Dental Institute for their expertise in the clinical photographs they supplied. We would also like to acknowledge the following colleagues for providing the figures listed:

- Mr Paul Gregory: Fig. 37.7.
- Dr Margaret Kellett: Fig. 41.1.
- Dr Susan Kindelan: Figs 40.7 and 40.8.
- Professor Phil Marsh: Fig. 4.3.
- Mr Peter Nixon: Figs 25.4c, 26.5, 27.3, 28.3, 28.7, 30.10 and 32.5.
- Mr Adam Steel for the artwork in Fig. 7.4.
- Dr Bob Turner: Fig. 5.1.
- Dr Simon Wood: Fig. 4.4.
- Ms Victoria Yorke: Fig. 18.6
- Mr Paul Franklin: Fig. 14.9.

This book was originally inspired in collaboration with Caroline Connelly. We are very grateful to the Wiley-Blackwell team for bringing this book to fruition, and Katrina Chandler deserves a particular mention in this regard. More recently we have enjoyed working with Sophia Joyce, Mirjana Misina and Jane Andrew, amongst others. A huge amount of hard work has gone into the preparation of *Periodontology at a Glance* and we acknowledge the dedication and craftsmanship of all involved.

Dedications

Professor Val Clerehugh wishes to thank her husband, Tony, daughter, Mary, and parents, Mary and Bas, for their unconditional love and support in the preparation of this book and dedicates this book to them.

Dr Aradhna Tugnait would like to dedicate this book to Keith, Adella, Torrin and Anuja whose dependable love gives purpose to every endeavour.

Professor Robert Genco wishes to thank Rose Parkhill for her excellent assistance with the book, and his wife Frances, for her support and encouragement.

1 Anatomy of the periodontium

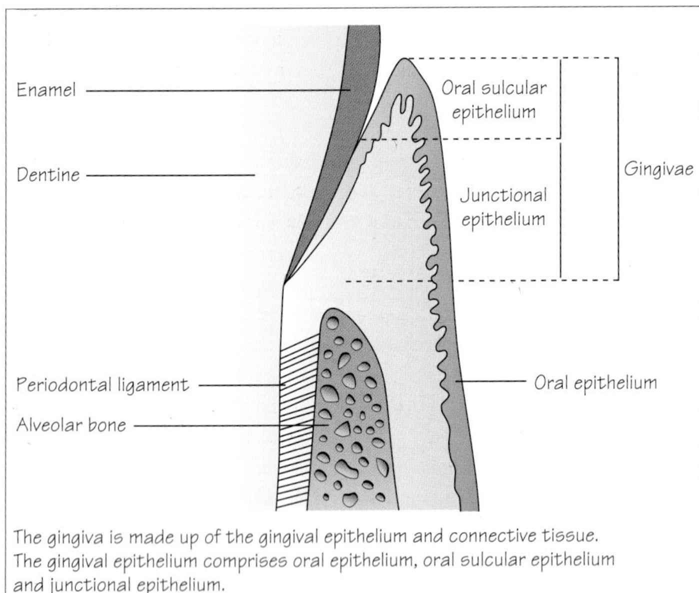

Figure 1.1 Longitudinal section through part of a tooth showing healthy periodontal tissues.

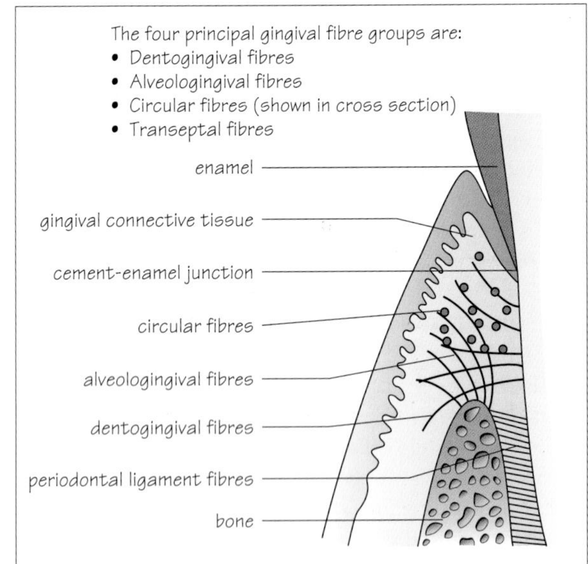

Figure 1.2 Dentogingival fibres, alveolar crest fibres and circular fibres in the gingival connective tissue.

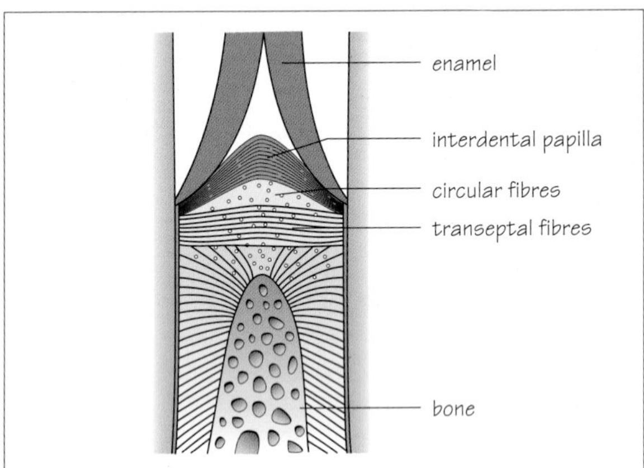

Figure 1.3 Interdental area showing transeptal and circular fibre groups in the gingival connective tissue.

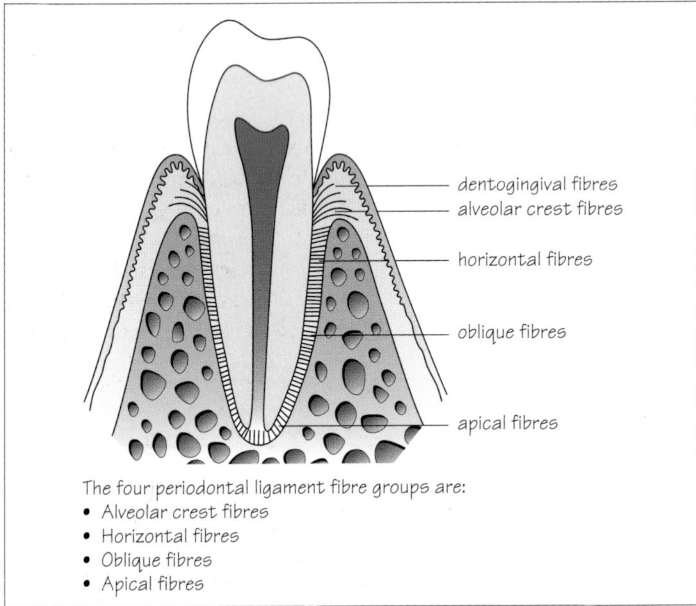

Figure 1.4 The periodontal ligament.

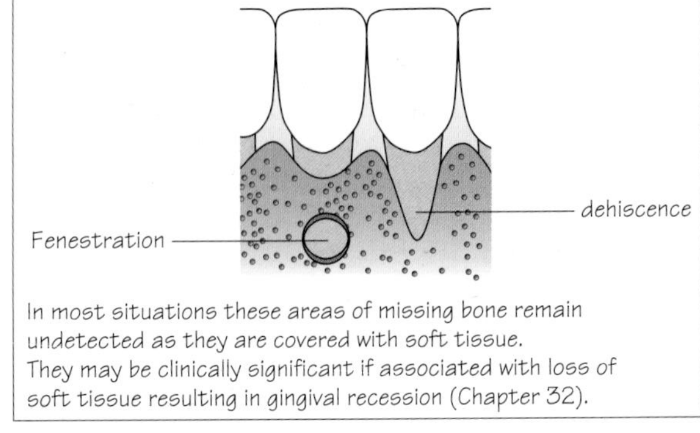

Figure 1.5 Bony fenestration and dehiscence.

The periodontal tissues form the supporting structures of the teeth. The principal components of the periodontium are shown in Fig. 1.1:

- Gingivae (including epithelium and connective tissue).
- Periodontal ligament.
- Cementum.
- Alveolar bone.

Gingivae

The gingivae in health are pink and firm with a knife-edge appearance, scalloped around the teeth. In certain ethnic groups the gingivae may be pigmented. In health, the gingival margin is a few millimetres coronal to the cement–enamel junction. The gingival sulcus (or crevice) is a shallow groove which may be between 0.5 and 3 mm in depth around a fully erupted tooth. The gingival tissues are keratinised and appear paler pink than sites of non-keratinised oral epithelium.

Gingival epithelium

The gingival epithelium comprises (Fig. 1.1):

- Oral epithelium (OE).
- Oral sulcular epithelium (SE).
- Junctional epithelium (JE).

The gingival sulcus is lined by SE and JE.

Oral epithelium

- The OE is an orthokeratinised, stratified, squamous epithelium.
- Surface cells lose their nuclei and are packed with the protein keratin.
- It presents an impermeable physical barrier to oral bacteria.

The basal layer of epithelial cells is thrown up into folds overlying the supporting connective tissue. These folds increase the surface area of contact between the epithelium and connective tissue and are known as rete ridges or rete pegs.

Oral sulcular epithelium

- There are no rete ridges.
- Cells are keratinised but still have nuclei (parakeratinised).

Junctional epithelium

- The JE forms a specialised attachment to the tooth via:
  - a hemidesmosomal layer within the JE cells;
  - a basal lamina produced by the epithelial cells.
- The JE is non-keratinised and has a very fast turnover of cells (2–6 days compared to 1 month for OE).
- The most apical part of the JE lies at the cement-enamel junction in health.
- The JE at its widest point is 20–30 cells thick coronally.
- The JE tapers until it is only one cell in width apically.
- The JE is permeable with wide intercellular spaces through which cells and substances can migrate (such as bacterial toxins or host defence cells).
- Migration of the JE from its position in health apically onto the root cementum indicates a loss of periodontal attachment and progression to the disease state of periodontitis.

Gingival connective tissue

The gingival connective tissue (or lamina propria) is made up of collagen fibre bundles called gingival fibres, around which lie ground substance, fibroblasts, blood and lymph vessels and neural tissues. The four fibre groups are shown in Figs 1.2 and 1.3.

Periodontal ligament

The periodontal ligament forms the attachment between the cementum and alveolar bone. It is a richly vascular connective tissue within which lie bundles of collagen fibres; these are divided into four groups based on their position (Fig. 1.4).

Within the ligament are mechanoreceptors that provide sensory input for jaw reflexes. Cells from the periodontal ligament are involved in the formation and remodelling of alveolar bone and cementum. The periodontal ligament acts to dissipate masticatory forces to the supporting alveolar bone and its width, height and quality determine a tooth's mobility.

Cementum

Cementum is a mineralised tissue overlying the root dentine. It does not undergo physiological remodelling but is continuously deposited throughout life. Cementum is classified into two types:

- Acellular.
- Cellular.

Acellular cementum

Acellular cementum forms on root dentine during root formation and tooth eruption. Fibres inserted from the periodontal ligament are mineralised within the cementum and are known as Sharpey's fibres and are abundant in acellular cementum.

Cellular cementum

Cellular cementum lies over the acellular cementum. It contains cells called cementocytes which lie in lacunae. The cellular cementum layer is thicker in the apical region of the root where it is between 0.2 and 1 mm thick.

Alveolar bone

- The walls of the sockets are lined with a layer of dense bone called compact bone, which also forms the buccal and lingual/palatal plates of the jaw bones.
- In between the sockets and the compact jaw bone walls lies cancellous bone that is made up of bony trabeculae.
- The compact bone plates of the jaws are thicker on the buccal aspect of the mandibular molars and thinnest on the labial surface of the mandibular incisors.

The thickness of the compact bone layer is relevant to the choice of local analgesia techniques as the anaesthetic solution passes through bone to reach the nerve supply. The thin bone, particularly in the lower incisor region, can manifest as incomplete bony coverage in the form of fenestrations and dehiscences (Fig. 1.5).

The tooth sockets are lined with compact bone within which the principal fibres of the periodontal ligament are inserted. This area of bone can appear as a dense white line called the lamina dura on a radiograph.

Key points

- Gingivae
  - JE forms the specialised attachment to the tooth
  - The most apical part of JE lies at the cement–enamel junction in health
  - Supported by connective tissue containing collagen fibre bundles
- Periodontal ligament
  - Forms attachment between the cementum and bone
- Cementum
  - Mineralised and deposited continuously
- Alveolar bone
  - Compact and cancellous bone
  - Periodontal ligament fibres inserted into compact bone lining the tooth sockets

2 Classification of periodontal diseases

A. Dental plaque-induced gingival diseases*

1. Gingivitis associated with dental plaque only
   a. Without other local contributing factors
   b. With other local contributing factors
2. Gingival diseases modified by systemic factors
   a. Associated with the endocrine system
      1) puberty-associated gingivitis
      2) menstrual cycle-associated gingivitis
      3) pregnancy-associated
         a) gingivitis
         b) pyogenic granuloma
      4) diabetes mellitus-associated gingivitis
   b. Associated with blood dyscrasias
      1) leukaemia-associated gingivitis
      2) other
3. Gingival diseases modified by medications
   a. Drug-influenced gingival diseases
      1) drug-influenced gingival enlargements
      2) drug-influenced gingivitis
         a) oral contraceptive-associated gingivitis
         b) other
4. Gingival diseases modified by malnutrition
   a. Ascorbic acid-deficiency gingivitis
   b. Other

*Can occur on a periodontium with no attachment loss or on a periodontium with attachment loss that is not progressing

B. Non-plaque-induced gingival lesions

1. Gingival diseases of specific bacterial origin
   a. *Neisseria gonorrhoea*-associated lesions
   b. *Treponema pallidum*-associated lesions
   c. Streptococcal species-associated lesions
   d. Other
2. Gingival diseases of viral origin
   a. Herpes virus infections
      1) primary herpetic gingivostomatitis
      2) recurrent oral herpes
      3) varicella-zoster infections
   b. Other
3. Gingival diseases of fungal origin
   a. *Candida* species infections
      1) generalised gingival candidosis
   b. Linear gingival erythema
   c. Histoplasmosis
   d. Other
4. Gingival lesions of genetic origin
   a. Hereditary gingival fibromatosis
   b. Other
5. Gingival manifestations of systemic conditions
   a. Mucocutaneous disorders
      1) lichen planus
      2) pemphigoid
      3) pemphigus vulgaris
      4) erythema multiforme
      5) lupus erythematosus
      6) drug-induced lesions
      7) other
   b. Allergic reactions
      1) dental restorative materials
         a) mercury
         b) nickel
         c) acrylic
         d) other
      2) reactions attributable to
         a) toothpastes/dentifrices
         b) mouthrinses/mouthwashes
         c) chewing gum additives
         d) foods and additives
      3) other
6. Traumatic lesions (factitious, iatrogenic, accidental)
   a. Chemical injury
   b. Physical injury
   c. Thermal injury
7. Foreign body reactions
8. Not otherwise specified (NOS)

Figure 2.1 Classification of gingival diseases.

Classification

- An up-to-date classification:
  - allows the clinician to be aware of the full range of periodontal diseases and conditions that can affect the patient
  - provides a basis for the diagnosis and subsequent management of the patient
- The classification in Figs 2.1–2.8 derives from the 1999 International Workshop for the Classification of Periodontal Diseases and Conditions, which was convened to reclassify these diseases and conditions due to a previous lack of consensus
- The new categories added to the 1999 classification were:
  - gingival diseases
  - necrotising periodontal diseases
  - abscesses
  - periodontitis associated with endodontic lesions
  - developmental or acquired deformities and conditions

A. Localised
B. Generalised

Figure 2.2 Classification of chronic periodontitis.

A. Localised
B. Generalised

Figure 2.3 Classification of aggressive periodontitis.

A. Associated with haematological disorders
 1. Acquired neutropenia
 2. Leukaemias
 3. Other
B. Associated with genetic disorders
 1. Familial and cyclic neutropenia
 2. Down syndrome
 3. Leukocyte adhesion deficiency syndromes
 4. Papillon–Lefèvre syndrome
 5. Chediak–Higashi syndrome
 6. Histiocytosis syndromes
 7. Glycogen storage disease
 8. Infantile genetic agranulocytosis
 9. Cohen syndrome
 10. Ehlers–Danlos syndrome (types IV and VIII)
 11. Hypophosphatasia
 12. Other
C. Not otherwise specified (NOS)

Figure 2.4 Classification of periodontitis as a manifestation of systemic diseases.

A. Necrotising ulcerative gingivitis (NUG)
B. Necrotising ulcerative periodontitis (NUP)

Figure 2.5 Classification of necrotising periodontal diseases.

A. Gingival abscess
B. Periodontal abscess
C. Pericoronal abscess

Figure 2.6 Classification of abscesses of the periodontium.

A. Combined periodontic–endodontic lesions

Figure 2.7 Classification of periodontitis associated with endodontic lesions.

A. Localised tooth-related factors that modify or predispose to plaque–induced gingival diseases/periodontitis
 1. Tooth anatomical factors
 2. Dental restorations/appliances
 3. Root fractures
 4. Cervical root resorption and cemental tears
B. Mucogingival deformities and conditions around teeth, including gingival recession and gingival overgrowth
 1. Gingival/soft tissue recession
  a. Buccal or lingual recession
  b. Interproximal (papillary)
 2. Lack of keratinised gingiva
 3. Decreased vestibular depth
 4. Aberrant frenum/muscle position
 5. Gingival excess
  a. Pseudopocket
  b. Inconsistent gingival margin
  c. Excessive gingival display
  d. Gingival enlargement
 6. Abnormal colour
C. Mucogingival deformities and conditions on edentulous ridges
D. Occlusal trauma
 1. Primary occlusal trauma
 2. Secondary occlusal trauma

Figure 2.8 Classification of developmental or acquired deformities and conditions.

Changes in classification categories in 1999

- Chronic periodontitis:
  - change in terminology from 'adult periodontitis' to 'chronic periodontitis'
  - additional descriptors according to extent and severity
- Aggressive periodontitis:
  - replacement of previous term 'early onset periodontitis' by 'aggressive periodontitis'
  - distinct and separate entity from chronic periodontitis and must be managed accordingly
  - specific features delineate the localised form from the generalised form
- Refractory periodontitis:
  - no longer considered a separate disease entity and has been excluded from the classification
  - refractory can be a descriptor applied to any disease that proves non-responsive to treatment
- Recurrent periodontitis:
  - denotes the return of the disease and is not a separate disease entity
- Poorly controlled diabetes and tobacco smoking:
  - were excluded from the section on periodontitis as a manifestation of systemic diseases since both can be significant modifiers of all forms of periodontitis

Key point

- Knowledge of current classification provides a basis for subsequent diagnosis and management

Periodontal epidemiology

(a)

Epidemiology is the study of the distribution and determinants of health-related states or events in specified populations, and the application of this study to the control of health problems

(b)

Study	includes	Surveillance, observation, hypothesis testing, analytical research and experiments
Distribution	refers to	Analysis by time, place and classes of persons affected
Determinants	are the	Physical, biological, social, cultural and behavioural factors that influence (periodontal) health
Health-related states or events	include	(Periodontal) diseases, causes of morbidity, behaviour such as tobacco use, reactions to preventive regimes, and provision and use of health services
Specified populations	are	Those with identifiable characteristics
Application of this study to the control of health problems	makes explicit	The aim of epidemiology is to promote, protect, and restore (periodontal) health

Figure 3.1 (a) Definition of epidemiology (Last, 2001). (b) Definitions of epidemiological terms (Last, 2001).

Prevalence	Number or % of affected subjects in population with disease at defined threshold
Extent	Number or % of affected teeth or sites with disease at defined threshold
Severity	How advanced disease is May be bands of severity, e.g. 1–2 mm clinical attachment loss (CAL) is slight; 3–4 mm is moderate; 5+ mm is severe May be mean mouth data, e.g. mean severity of CAL = 3.4 mm
Incidence	Number of new cases of disease at a defined threshold that appear in a population over a predetermined period of time
Threshold of disease	Level of disease being studied, e.g. clinical attachment loss of 2 mm; e.g. probing depths of 6 mm or more

Figure 3.3 Common terms in epidemiology.

(a)

TYPES OF PERIODONTAL EPIDEMIOLOGY

- OBSERVATIONAL STUDIES
  - Descriptive / Analytical / Pragmatic
  - Cross-sectional / Longitudinal / Case–control / Case–cohort
- Local / Regional / National / International
- EXPERIMENTAL STUDIES
  - Clinical trial
    - Phase 0
    - Phase I
    - Phase II
    - Phase III
    - Phase IV
  - Randomised controlled trial
  - Crossover trial
  - Split-mouth trial
  - Community trial

(b)

- Descriptive study
  - Describes existing distribution of variables without regard to causal or other hypotheses
- Analytical study
  - Examines associations, causal relationships, tests hypotheses
- Pragmatic study
  - Aim is to improve health status or care of a specified population, provide a basis for decisions about health care, or evaluate previous actions

(c)

- Cross-sectional study
  - Study conducted at one particular time
  - Temporal relationships cannot be explored
- Longitudinal study (cohort study)
  - Study extends over a period of time
  - Temporal relationships can be explored

(d)

- Case–control study
  - Observational study of group of subjects with disease (cases) and group of subjects without disease (controls)
    - Both groups examined for history of exposure of interest or presence of putative risk factors; statistical comparison of frequency of exposure to see if associations between exposure and disease
    - No intervention; often retrospective
- Case–cohort study
  - Analytical study of group of subjects without disease who are classified according to presence of exposure of interest
    - Subjects followed longitudinally; controls drawn from same cohort as cases regardless of disease status
    - If incidence of disease is greater in subjects exposed to a factor of interest, the factor is considered predictive of disease
      - e.g. patients who smoke more cigarette packs (i.e. greater pack years) develop more periodontitis than non-smokers over same time

(e)

- Phase 0
  - First in-human clinical studies,
  - Exploratory, microdoses of drug, very few participants
- Phase I
  - Safety and pharmacological profile of drug/treatment
  - Few healthy volunteer participants (< 100)
- Phase II
  - Pilot studies to assess efficacy of drug/treatment – does it work?
- Phase III
  - Extensive clinical trials to determine safety and efficacy
- Phase IV
  - Final phase conducted after approval of drug by national drug registration authority, e.g. Food and Drug Administration in USA; Medicines and Healthcare products Regulatory Agency in UK
  - Post-marketing surveillance

(f)

- Randomised controlled trial (RCT) – gold standard
  - Subjects randomly allocated to test or control treatment group and followed, in parallel, longitudinally
- Cross-over trial
  - Tests effects of therapies that are fully reversible with no lasting effect
  - 3 phases: first experimental therapy; washout; second experimental therapy
- Split-mouth trial
  - Subject receives 2 or more different types of therapy, mouth split (usually at random) so each section receives one type of therapy
- Community trial
  - Unit of allocation to receive a preventive or therapeutic regime is the whole community

Figure 3.2 (a) Types of periodontal epidemiology. (b) Descriptive, analytical and pragmatic studies. (c) Cross-sectional and longitudinal studies. (d) Case–control and case–cohort studies. (e) Clinical trial phases. (f) Types of trial.

Attributes of a good index are that it should be:
- Valid (i.e. measures what it purports to measure)
- Reliable (i.e. can be reproduced if re-measured)
- Quick
- Simple
- Acceptable to the examiner and subject and use minimum equipment
- Amenable to statistical analysis

Figure 3.4 Attributes of a good periodontal index.

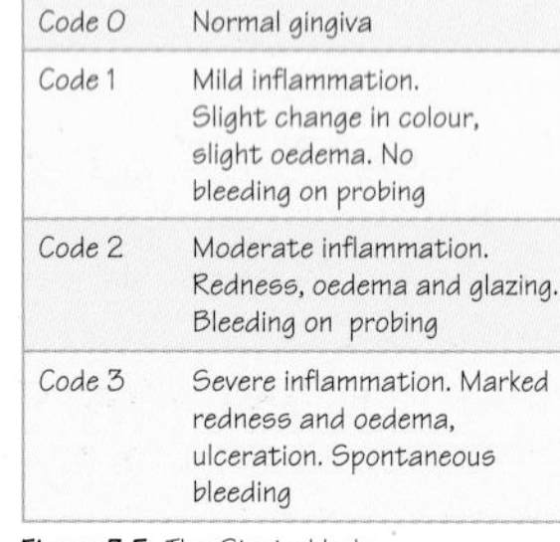

Code 0	Normal gingiva
Code 1	Mild inflammation. Slight change in colour, slight oedema. No bleeding on probing
Code 2	Moderate inflammation. Redness, oedema and glazing. Bleeding on probing
Code 3	Severe inflammation. Marked redness and oedema, ulceration. Spontaneous bleeding

Figure 3.5 The Gingival Index (Löe & Silness, 1967).

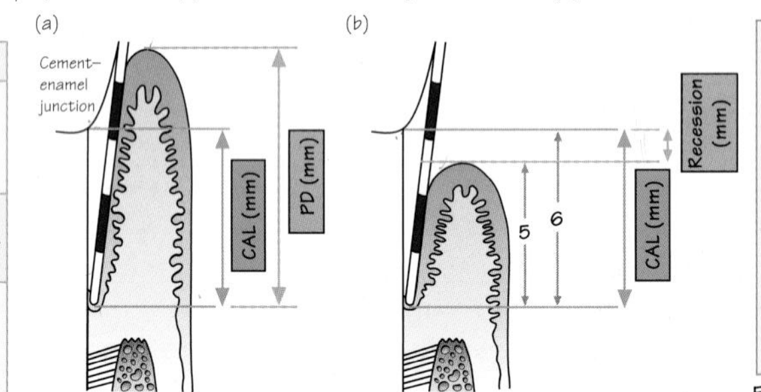

Figure 3.6 (a) Clinical attachment loss (CAL) and probing depth (PD). (b) CAL and recession.

- Probing force
- Probe angulation
- Thickness of probe (thick tip diameter of probe will underestimate compared with thin probe)
- Accuracy of probe markings
- Examiner experience
- Degree of inflammation of tissues (tendency to overestimate if inflamed)
- Presence of subgingival calculus or anatomical feature (may impede probing)
- Location of probing (anterior easier than posterior, buccal more reproducible than palatal/lingual sites)

Figure 3.7 Factors influencing probing accuracy.

Record CPITN epidemiology teeth in adults:

UR7, UR6	UR1	UL6, UL7
LR7, LR6	LL1	LL6, LL7

USA notation	2, 3 / 31, 30	8 / 24	14, 15 / 19, 18

CPITN codes
0 = Healthy
1 = Bleeding on probing
2 = Calculus or plaque retention factor
3 = Shallow pocket 4 or 5 mm
4 = Deep pocket 6 mm or more

Record index teeth in adolescents:

UR6	UR1	UL6
LR6	LL1	LL6

USA notation	3 / 30	8 / 24	14 / 19

Age 7–11 years, only use codes 0–2 to avoid false pockets

Figure 3.8 Community Periodontal Index of Treatment Needs (CPITN).

(a)

Pockets
- 3507 adults: CPITN-based methodology
- 54% had shallow pockets 4 or 5 mm
- 1% youngest (16–24 years) had deep pockets ≥ 6 mm
- 5% overall sample had deep pockets ≥ 6 mm

(b)

Clinical attachment loss
- CAL measured for first time using CPI-C probe (*n* = 3507)
- 43% had CAL ≥ 4 mm on at least one tooth
- 14% youngest (16–24 years) and 85% oldest had CAL ≥ 4 mm
- None of youngest had CAL ≥ 6 mm
- 31% oldest (65 years and over) had CAL ≥ 6 mm

Figure 3.9 UK national survey (representing population) data, 1998, on the prevalence of: (a) pockets, and (b) clinical attachment loss (CAL).

(a)

- 15 132 adults: CAL methodology
- 99% youngest (18–24 years) had CAL ≥ 1 mm on at least 1 tooth and 32.8% of sites
- 1.9% of youngest and 35% of oldest (55–64 years) had more severe CAL ≥ 5 mm
- 5.7% youngest and 18.1% oldest had pockets 4–6 mm
- < 0.1% youngest and 1.1% oldest had pockets ≥ 7 mm
- More disease in blacks; low education status

(b)

NHANES 1988–94 (*n* = 26 852) and 1999–2004 (*n* = 25 336)
- Nationally representative samples
- Two randomly selected quadrants, mesio-buccal and mid-buccal sites
  - Pocket depths
  - Attachment loss
  - Recession
- Improvement in periodontal health for adults and seniors

Prevalence of periodontal disease* *at least 1 site with CAL ≥ 3 mm and 1 site with pocket ≥ 4 mm		
Age (years)	1988–1994 (%)	1999–2004 (%)
20–34	8.48	3.84
35–49	15.73	10.41
50–64	21.87	11.88

Figure 3.10 The prevalence of periodontitis based on: (a) US national survey (representing population) data, 1985–86, and (b) US National Health and Nutrition Examination Surveys (NHANES) data, 1988–94 and 1999–2004.

Epidemiology is the study of the distribution and determinants of health-related states or events in specified populations, and the application of this study to the control of health problems (Fig. 3.1).

Types of periodontal epidemiology

There are different types of periodontal epidemiology (Fig. 3.2). Periodontal epidemiological studies seek to understand the natural course of the different periodontal diseases and the factors that influence their distribution (Fig. 3.3). Causative and risk factors (Chapters 10, 11) need to be established in order to determine the aetiology and determinants of disease development. Evidence-based research is important to establish the effectiveness of treatment methods and products and preventive regimes for periodontal diseases at a population level.

Ultimately, the particular research question and the aims and objectives of the study determine the type, design, size and duration of the epidemiological study.

Methodology

Periodontal indices

Measuring periodontal disease involves the use of a periodontal index (Fig. 3.4). There is no single periodontal index that satisfies all the desirable requirements in every type of study and many exist (Barnes *et al.*, 1986).

Gingival indices

In the 1960s the Gingival Index was introduced in which the codes used mixtures of signs of inflammation: colour change, oedema, bleeding on probing and ulcerations (Fig. 3.5) – it is a compound index. Although widely used, assigning a code is difficult if not all signs are present or if signs from two codes occur. Dichotomous indices (presence or absence of condition) are alternatives, e.g. bleeding on probing.

Plaque indices

Plaque indices have faced similar problems. The Plaque Index (Löe & Silness, 1967) assesses plaque thickness at the gingival margin. Other indices use disclosing solutions and measure plaque area (e.g. the Turesky modification of the Quigley–Hein Index), while yet others, like the O'Leary Plaque Index, simply record presence or absence but count the per cent of sites affected (Barnes *et al.*, 1986).

Periodontal indices

Russell's Periodontal Index was reported in 1956 and was the first index to be used widely. This was followed by Ramfjord's Periodontal Disease Index in 1959, which introduced the method for measuring the clinical attachment level. This has been the gold standard and basis of epidemiological clinical recording ever since (Fig. 3.6).

Other recordings may involve probing depths and recession. Ethical issues around limiting radiation doses can restrict the use of radiographic measurements. Technological advances enable digital manipulation of images; subtraction radiography allows detection and measurement of small bone changes.

Recording

Full mouth recording of data provides the most information, but some partial recording systems – although generally underestimating disease levels – have been incorporated into large-scale epidemiological studies in order to increase the sample size whilst retaining key information. UK and US national surveys have used this approach.

Other recording issues relate to operator measurement errors – many factors influence probing accuracy (Fig. 3.7). Also, it is important to remember that the periodontal tissues themselves are biologically active and therefore subject to change!

Statistical management

It is essential to distinguish between association and causation. Confounding variables also need to be taken into account, i.e. when the variable is not of primary interest but may affect the study results anyway. Due to measurements of multiple sites within the mouth and repeated recordings over time in some types of study, careful appraisal of data management options is necessary. In addition to the more conventional tests, multilevel modelling and structural equation modelling offer useful approaches for periodontal epidemiology (Tu et al., 2008).

CPITN: global data bank

Use of the Community Periodontal Index of Treatment Needs (CPITN) for screening (Fig. 3.8) in many different countries and populations has yielded a global data bank. Summary findings include:

- 15–19 years: bleeding and calculus are prevalent.
- 35–44 years: calculus and shallow pockets are most prevalent; uncommon to find healthy tissues.
- Deep pocketing is not prevalent.
- Differences are present according to age, ethnic status, developing/developed countries, social class and various risk factors.

Global epidemiology

Population studies confirm the link between plaque and gingivitis. Over 82% of US adolescents have overt gingivitis and UK national data also show a majority of those aged 8 years or more with gingival inflammation – similar global trends have been reported (Albander & Rams, 2002). Incipient chronic peridontitis can begin in adolescents. Adults worldwide exhibit gingival bleeding and inflammation. Gingivitis precedes periodontitis, and there are no data to suggest that periodontitis develops in the absence of gingival inflammation.

- Slight to moderate periodontitis is widespread (Figs 3.9, 3.10).
- Severe periodontitis affects a relatively small subset of populations in the UK, rest of Europe, USA, Central and South America, Africa and Asia/Oceana.
- Greatest prevalence of periodontitis has been found in Africans, Hispanics and Asians.
- Certain risk factors have been identified, including smoking and poorly controlled diabetes (Chapters 10, 11, 36, 37).
- Localised aggressive periodontitis affects <0.1–0.2% caucasian and <2.6% black Africans; the generalised form probably affects <5%.
- More, and better, longitudinal analytical studies are needed (Borrell & Papapanou, 2005).
- Definitions of what constitutes a 'case' of periodontitis are needed (Borrell & Papapanou, 2005) (Chapter 9).

Key points

- There are different types of epidemiological study
- There is no single ideal periodontal index
- The type of study and index depend on the study aims and objectives
- CPITN and other epidemiological data have highlighted differences in global disease prevalence and severity

4 Role of plaque in the aetiology of periodontal diseases

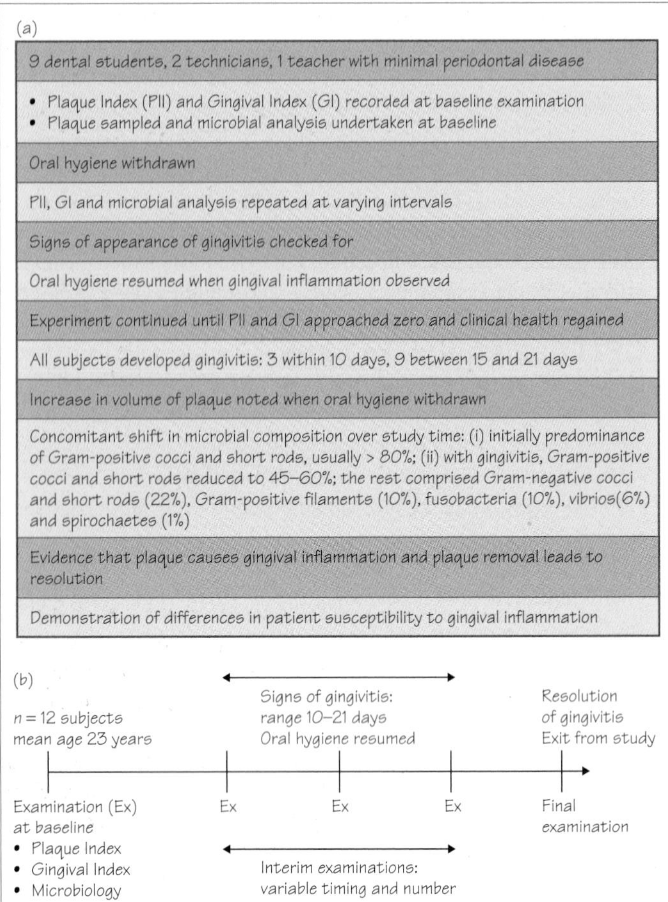

Figure 4.1 (a) Stages and (b) design of a classic study on experimental gingivitis in humans.

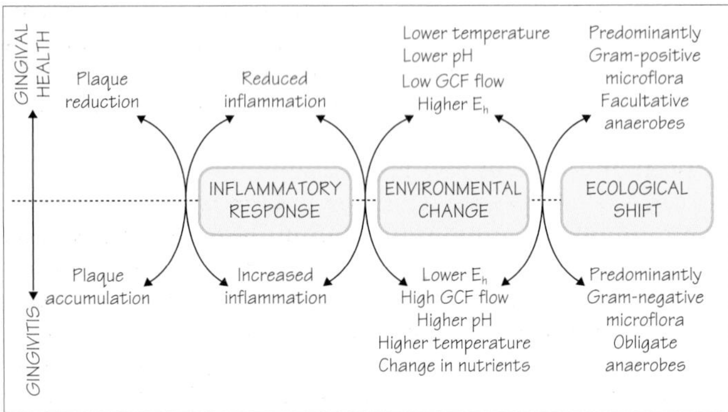

Figure 4.5 Schematic diagram of the ecological plaque hypothesis (Marsh 1991, 1994). GCF, gingival crevicular fluid.

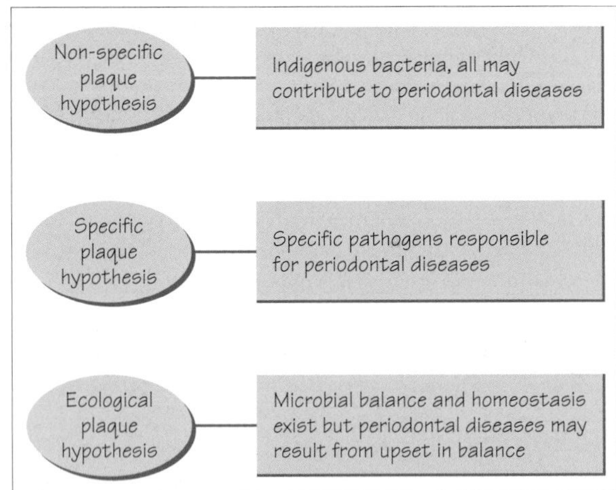

Figure 4.2 Non-specific, specific and ecological plaque hypotheses.

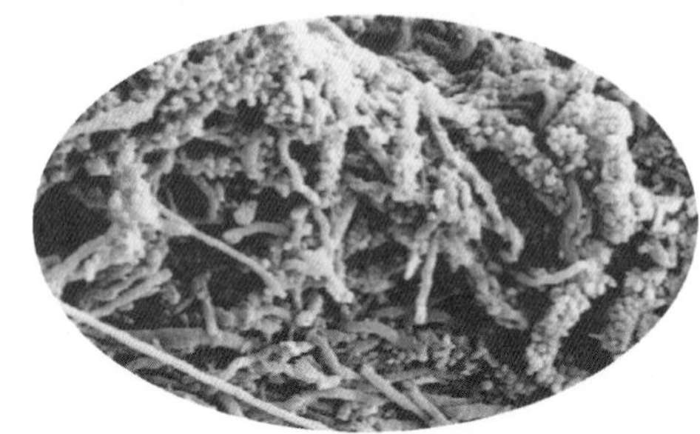

Figure 4.3 Climax microbial community in plaque biofilm showing the diverse range of microbial forms. Courtesy of Professor P. Marsh.

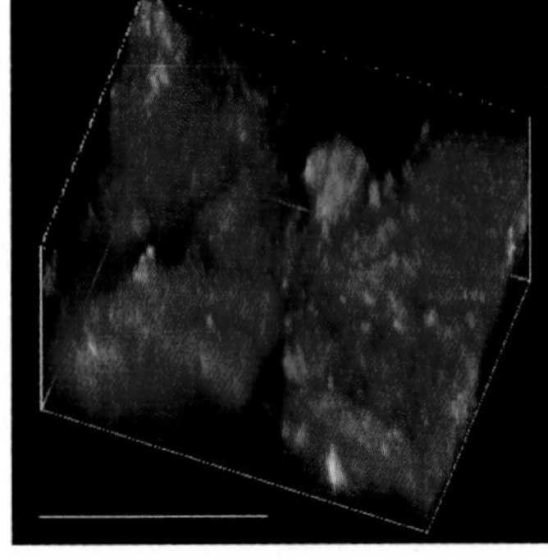

Figure 4.4 Noran Odyssey confocal laser scanning microscope image of an intact 1-week-old plaque biofilm formed *in vivo* using the Leeds *in situ* device. The image shows the three-dimensional structure and variations in plaque biofilm density: pink areas are biomasses of bacteria; dark areas are voids, channels or spaces. The image was achieved by volume rendering of a series of x–y (horizontal) sections. Scale bar = 50 µm. Courtesy of Dr S. Wood (Wood et al., 2002).

Since the classic experimental gingivitis study in 1965 (Loë *et al.*, 1965), the aetiological role of dental plaque as the key agent in gingivitis has been acknowledged (Fig. 4.1). Nowadays, plaque is considered a good example of a biofilm (Marsh, 2005) and there are three different but interrelated hypotheses of its role in the aetiology of periodontal dieases (Loesche, 1976, 1979; Theilade, 1986; Marsh, 1991, 1994) (Fig. 4.2).

Plaque as a biofilm

Dental plaque has been defined as a diverse community of microorganisms found on the tooth surface as a biofilm, embedded in an extracellular matrix of polymers of host and microbial origin. Biofilms are defined as matrix-embedded microbial populations, adhering to each other and/or to surfaces or interfaces (Marsh, 2005). The production of extracellular polymers forms a functional matrix.

Table 4.1 Stages of plaque biofilm formation.

Stage	Plaque biofilm formation
1 Pellicle formation	Host and bacterial molecules, salivary glycoproteins, are adsorbed onto the tooth surface leading to acquired pellicle formation
2 Transport	Transport of bacteria to the pellicle occurs via natural salivary flow, Brownian movement or chemotaxis. Adsorption of coccal bacteria onto pellicle occurs within 2 hours – pioneer species include *Neisseria, Streptococcus sanguis, S. oralis* and *S. mitis*, also Gram positive rods, mainly *Actinomyces*
3 Long-range interactions	Long-range physicochemical interactions leading to reversible adhesion between the microbial cell surface and the pellicle involving van der Waal's attractive forces and electrostatic repulsion
4 Short-range interactions	Short-range stereochemical interactions between adhesions on microbial cell surface and receptors on acquired pellicle lead to irreversible adhesion
5 Co-aggregation	Co-aggregation (co-adhesion) of new bacteria to the already attached bacteria results in an increasingly diverse microflora
6 Multiplication	Multiplication of attached organisms leads to confluent growth and biofilm formation. Adherent bacteria synthesise extracellular polymers
7 Detachment	Detachment of bacteria allows colonisation at new sites

Formation and properties

Biofilm formation involves several stages (Table 4.1) before the diverse climax community is derived (Fig. 4.3). Microbial homeostasis is critical and can protect against colonisation by exogenous species. Breakdown may occur due to host defence, local, systemic or other factors.

Plaque as a biofilm has various properties:

- It is spatially organised in a complex three-dimensional structure with pores and channels running through it (Fig. 4.4).
- The physical architecture protects it from desiccation and phagocytosis.
- It is less susceptible to antibiotics, e.g. a neutralising enzyme such as β-lactamase in the gingival crevicular fluid can inactivate antibiotics introduced to the site.
- Novel gene expression, novel proteins expressed. Growth in biofilms can have a direct effect on gene expression – many organisms have a radically different phenotype following attachment to a surface or host receptor, co-adhesion with other organisms or binding to a host protein. Indirect effects on gene expression may be due to an altered environment (e.g. pH, sugar concentration). Altered gene expression can also reduce the sensitivity of the biofilm to antibiotics.
- Cell–cell communication, which can take place in various ways, for example via:

  (i) horizontal gene transfer; (ii) small diffusible peptides; (iii) quorum sensing, using signalling compounds to regulate gene expression; (iv) autoinducer 2, which mediates messages between Gram-positive and Gram-negative species in a mixed species community; (v) cross-talk between host cells and bacteria.
- Physiological heterogeneity: microorganisms of the same microbial species can exhibit different physiological states in a biofilm, even if in very close proximity to each other.
- Spatial and environmental heterogeneity: bacterial metabolism in the plaque leads to varying gradients that are crucial to microbial growth, and these varying environments for pH, oxygen tension, redox potential and nutrients give sufficient heterogeneity for diverse organisms with different metabolic and growth needs to coexist at the same site.
- Community life style supports a wider habitat range for growth and synergistic properties. The early colonisers alter the local environment and facilitate attachment and growth of later, sometimes more fastidious, microorganisms, which leads to microbial succession and increased diversity. This produces more metabolic diversity and efficiency. Nearby cells can produce neutralising enzymes (β-lactamase) that protect susceptible microorganisms against antimicrobials or environmental stress. The properties of the plaque biofilm community are greater than the individual components of the biofilm.
- Pathogenic synergism: the remit of a pathogen is to damage the host tissue and the benefit of being in a biofilm community is the synergist enhancement of the virulence potential of individual subgingival microbes. There are various points along the way when the pathogenic potential can be influenced: microbial adherence, acquisition of nutrients from the host, multiplication, overcoming or evasion of the host defences, tissue invasion and finally tissue damage.

Plaque hypotheses

Non-specific plaque hypothesis

This plaque hypothesis (Theilade, 1986) embraces the notion that if plaque develops undisturbed, it will grow in volume and change in composition from essentially aerobic Gram-positive cocci and rods located supragingivally to Gram-negative cocci and rods that are increasingly anaerobic as plaque extends subgingivally; filaments, fusobacteria, spirils and spirochaetes are also found. The microflora produce virulence factors that lead to tissue inflammation/destruction. Plaque removal by effective toothbrushing following oral hygiene advice, or control by pharmacological agents, restores the original supragingival flora and influences the subgingival domain as well.

Specific plaque hypothesis

The specific hypothesis (Loesche, 1976, 1979) centres around the periodontal diseases which have a specific microflora associated with them, such as necrotising ulcerative gingivitis (see Chapter 38) and localised aggressive periodontitis (*Aggregatibacter actinomycetemcomitans*). For these conditions, elimination of the specific bacteria leads to resolution of the disease, usually with the adjunctive use of systemic antibiotics.

Ecological plaque hypothesis

More than 700 different types of oral microflora have been recognised. For disease to occur, the organisms need to increase in number until they reach a level where they can damage the host. According to this hypothesis (Marsh, 1991, 1994), in gingivitis when plaque accumulates there is a stress to the system, inflammation develops and this causes environmental changes leading to an ecological shift in the microflora that is likely to provoke more inflammation. The philosophy is that disease can be prevented by targeting the causative agents and the driving forces behind their selection (Fig. 4.5). If unsuccessful, gingivitis can progress to periodontitis (Chapters 8, 9).

Key points

- Plaque is a biofilm and key in the aetiology of periodontal diseases
- Biofilm forms in stages and has various properties
- There are three different but interrelated plaque hypotheses: non-specific; specific; ecological

5 Plaque microbiology

Table 5.1 Different methods of examining plaque microbial composition.

Method	Advantages	Disadvantages
Microscopy	Recognition of morphological types Determine spatial arrangements of organisms Recent novel, sophisticated applications, e.g. atomic force microscopy gives very high image resolution	Slow and labour intensive Precise speciation using immunological or hybridisation methods only possible for a few species in sample
Culture – predominant	Can detect unrecognised species Provides cultures for further analysis	Very labour intensive Expensive Some uncultivable species Difficult to culture spirochaetes
Culture – selective media	Can detect specific species	As above Need to know which species to investigate Few suitable media Limited species identification
Immuno-fluorescence, ELISA	Quite specific Rapid Cheaper than culture Can distinguish species Can provide counts or proportions of specific species	Limited numbers of monoclonal or polyclonal antisera available Takes time to develop Relatively small numbers can be run
PCR	Reasonable sensitivity Quite specific With appropriate primers can detect very small numbers of species present Rapid	Dichotomous (i.e. detects presence/absence not quantities) Expensive Depends on amplification Not suitable for large numbers of species in large numbers of samples
Real-time PCR	Quantitative Sensitivity* Specificity†	Relatively slow As above, limited numbers can be processed
DNA–DNA hybridisation	Quantitative Sensitivity* Specificity† Low likelihood of cross-reactions with other species	Only detects species for which probes are available Modest numbers of species for modest number of samples
Checkerboard DNA–DNA hybridisation	Quantitative Sensitivity* Specificity† Can use whole sample without dilution or amplification by PCR Large numbers of species and samples Inexpensive Rapid	Only detects species for which probes are available Samples must be of appropriate size Possible cross-reactions if inappropriate sample size
16S rDNA amplification cloning	Detection of cultivable and uncultivable species Phylogenetic positioning of taxa	Very expensive Small numbers of samples

* Sensitivity is ability to correctly identify presence of organism(s).
† Specificity is ability to correctly determine absence of organism(s).

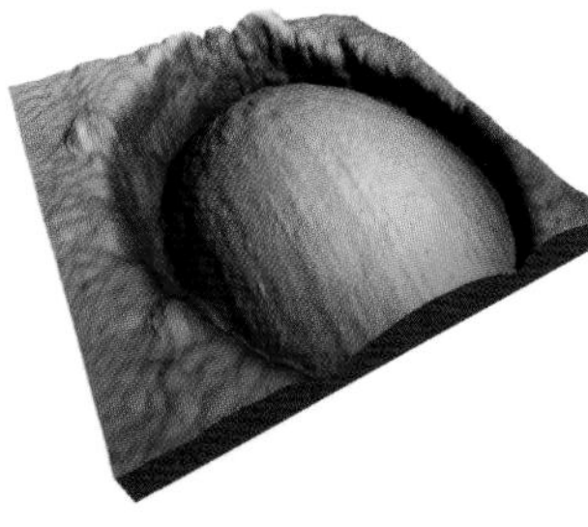

Figure 5.1 Atomic force microscope image of live *Streptococcus salivarius* (NCTC 8618) trapped in a pore in a track-etched polycarbonate membrane under phosphate-buffered saline. x–y dimensions = 774 nm. Work funded by the Medical Research Council, UK. Courtesy of Dr R. Turner.

Designated periodontal pathogens:
- *Aggregatibacter actinomycetemcomitans*
- *Porphyromonas gingivalis*
- *Tannerella forsythia*

Suspected periodontal pathogens include:
- *Prevotella intermedia*
  - Split into two distinct species *Prevotella intermedia* and *Prevotella nigrescens* in 1992
- *Fusobacterium nucleatum*
- *Campylobacter rectus*
- *Eikenella corrodens*
- *Peptostreptococcus micros*
- *Selenomonas* species
- *Eubacterium* species
- Spirochaetes
  - Only 10 cultivated so far

Figure 5.2 Designated and suspected periodontal pathogens.

- According to Koch's postulates for a pathogen to cause disease, it must:
  - Be isolated from every case of disease
  - Not be recovered from cases of other types of disease, or non-pathogenically
  - Induce disease in experimental animals after isolation and repeated growth in pure culture

Figure 5.3 Koch's postulates.

Virulence factors include:
- Fimbriae for adherence to host tissue, invasion
- Proteases–break down host proteins, deregulate host defences
- Bone resorbing factors
- Cytotoxic metabolites
- Leukotoxin–kills neutrophils
- Toxin e.g. cytolethal distending toxin
- Capsule
- Induction of inflammatory response, modulation of cytokines/chemokines

Figure 5.4 Pathogenic virulence factors.

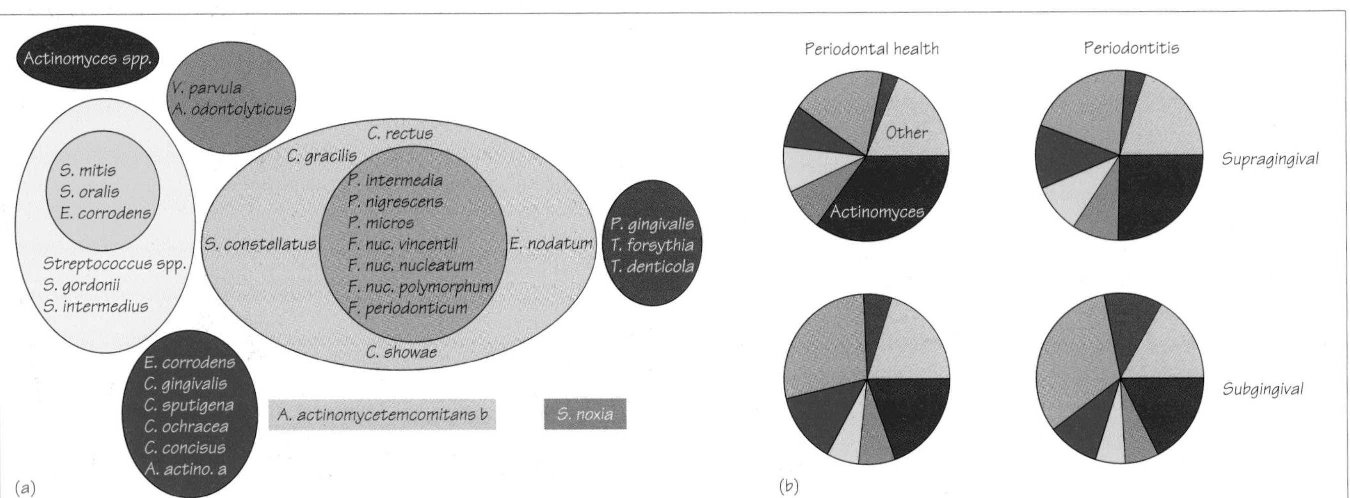

Figure 5.5 (a) Microbial complexes. From Socransky *et al.* (1998). (b) Mean % DNA probe count proportions in health and periodontitis. From Socransky and Haffajee (2008).

Over 700 different microbial species have been found in the oral cavity, although only half have been cultivated. Usually 100–200 species will colonise an individual's mouth, reflecting great diversity. More than 400 species may be found in periodontal pockets, of which over 250 have been isolated, characterised and named.

Plaque bacteria can attach to: tooth surfaces (either crown or root), periodontal tissues (either sulcular, junctional or pocket epithelium lining), connective tissues (if access is gained via ulcerated pocket epithelium) or other bacteria already attached to these surfaces. Hence there are many pathways for the oral bacteria to exert their effects. The fact that teeth, unlike many other body surfaces, are solid, non-shedding structures, predisposes them to microbial accumulation.

Microbiological techniques

Many different ways of investigating the microbial composition of plaque have been used, each with advantages and disadvantages (Socransky & Haffajee, 2005; Teles *et al.*, 2006) (Table 5.1):

- Microscopy (Fig. 5.1).
- Culture.
- Immunofluorescence: enzyme-linked immunofluorescence assay (ELISA) uses specific antibody to detect bacterial antigens (i.e. it is species specific).
- Polymerase chain reaction (PCR):
  - this uses a DNA polymerase to amplify a piece of DNA by *in vitro* enzymatic replication rather than in living cells like *Escherichia coli*;
  - PCR can amplify a single or a few copies of a piece of DNA and generate millions of copies of the DNA piece quickly.
- Real-time PCR: this can view the increase in amount of DNA as it is amplified.
- DNA–DNA hybridisation:
  - this measures the degree of genetic similarity between pools of DNA sequences;
  - it is usually used to determine the genetic distance between two species;
  - it allows the species to be arranged in a phylogenetic tree.
- Checkerboard DNA–DNA hybridisation: this provides a simultaneous quantitative analysis of 40 microbial species against up to 28 mixed samples on a single membrane.
- 16S rDNA amplification cloning: 16S rDNA sequences contain hypervariable regions that can provide species-specific signature sequences which are useful for bacterial identification to species level.

Microbial composition of plaque in health and disease

In health, the bacteria are predominantly Gram positive and include: streptococci (with *Streptococcus sanguis*, *S. oralis* and *S. mitis* being pioneer species), *Neisseria*, *Nocardia* and *Actinomyces*. 'Milleri' streptococci (*S. anginosus*, *S. constellatus* and *S. intermedius*) are believed to contribute to disease progression. Gingivitis develops as the amount of plaque increases. The proportion of capnophylic (especially *Capnocytophaga* spp.) and obligately anaerobic Gram-negative bacteria rises; *Fusobacteria* are common and there is an increased proportion of *Actinomyces*. Periodontitis is associated with a diverse subgingival microflora and a large number of obligately anaerobic Gram-negative rods and filament-shaped bacteria, many of which are asaccharolytic but proteolytic. Three bacterial species were designated as periodontal pathogens at the 1996 World Workshop in Periodontology and several other bacteria are suspected periodontal pathogens (Fig. 5.2).

Mechanisms of pathogenicity

It is difficult to translate the original, classic Koch's postulates of causation of disease by a pathogen (Fig. 5.3) to periodontal diseases. However, in general, for a periodontal pathogen to cause disease (Fig. 5.4), it must be able to do the following three things.

1 Colonise, achieved by:

- Attaching to one or more surfaces: (i) adhesins enable binding to host tissue, and (ii) co-aggregation to bacteria attached to surface.
- Multiplying using available nutrients.
- Competing successfully against other species trying to inhabit the site.
- Defending itself from host defences.

2 Produce factors that damage the host tissue directly or indirectly (by causing host tissue to damage itself).

3 Release and spread.

Complexes

Plaque ecology is fascinating. It has been observed that certain groups of organisms coexist in a rather structured way. Using whole genomic DNA probes and checkerboard DNA–DNA hybridisation on 13 261 plaque samples from 185 subjects, Socransky et al (1998) identified five complexes of bacteria to which they assigned colours red, orange, green, yellow and purple (Fig. 5.5a). There was an outlier group comprising *Actinomyces naeslundii* genospecies 2 (*A. viscosus*; shown in deep purple in Fig. 5.5a), which sometimes joined the purple complex, and another comprising *Selenomonas noxia* and *Aggregatibacter actinomycetemcomitans* serotype b (shown in grey in Fig. 5.5a)

- The red complex is associated with periodontitis, deeper pockets and bleeding on probing; it is reduced by root surface debridement.
- Red complex species are generally found with orange complex species.
- Orange complex species are closely associated with each other.
- *Actinomyces* (dark purple) and streptococci (yellow) are early colonisers, followed by the green complex.
- Purple complex species are closely associated with each other, and may act as a bridge to the orange, then red complex.

Proportions

The relative amount of plaque in periodontitis patients exceeds that in healthy patients, and the relative proportions of the different complexes are also seen to change (Fig. 5.5b). The numbers of organisms found supragingivally on a tooth surface may exceed 10^9, while individual subgingival sites can harbour numbers ranging from a thousand in a healthy crevice to hundreds of millions ($>10^8$) in a deep pocket.

Whether or not periodontal diseases develop depends on a complex interplay between the microbial challenge, ecology and host defences.

Key points

- There are over 700 species in the oral cavity and 400 species in the periodontal pocket, only half of which have been cultivated
- Various microbiological techniques have been developed to identify bacteria, each with advantages and disadvantages
- Microbial composition alters from health to disease
- A few bacteria have been designated as periodontal pathogens
- Pathogens use a variety of mechanisms to exert damage
- Microbial complexes have been identified

6 Calculus

Table 6.1 Differences between supragingival and subgingival calculus.

	Supragingival calculus	Subgingival calculus
Location	Coronal to gingival margin	Apical to gingival margin within gingival sulcus or periodontal pocket
Distribution	Adjacent to openings of salivary ducts: • lingual of mandibular incisors (sublingual duct) • buccal maxillary second molar (parotid duct)	No predilection for particular parts of mouth Approximal and lingual sites more affected than buccal sites
Appearance	Creamy-white colour May become nicotine-stained in smoker	Brownish-black due to haemorrhagic elements from gingival crevicular fluid and black pigments from calcified anaerobic rods
Morphology	Undifferentiated morphology – amorphous deposit	Variable: • ledges or rings around tooth, especially on the cement-enamel junction • on root surface(s) as crusty, spiny, nodular formations, thin veneers, fern-like arrangements, individual islands. • supragingival on subgingival deposits
Detection	Visible clinically Detection enhanced by air drying, which gives chalky appearance	By probing – tactile sensation enhanced by using ball end of WHO 621 probe. If deposit is located at entrance to pocket: • it may be visible as dark shadow under the gingival margin; • by directing air jet from three-in-one syringe at entrance to pocket it may be possible to retract the gingiva and see deposit directly. Following gingival recession, subgingival deposit may become located supragingivally and be easily visible Radio-opaque calculus 'wings' may be visible on approximal sites on radiographs
Formation	Nucleation and crystal growth are heterogeneous Calcification is heterogeneous Deposit builds up in layers with variable mineral content in the layers	Nucleation and crystal growth are heterogeneous Calcification is more homogeneous (uniform) than supragingival calculus Deposit builds up in layers, each with similarly high mineral density
Mineral content and source	Mean of 37% by volume (range 16–51% in the different layers) Derived from saliva	Mean of 58% by volume (range 32–78% in the different layers) Derived from gingival crevicular fluid
Composition	70–80% inorganic salts Mainly calcium, phosphate (lower ratio than subgingival calculus) Small amounts of magnesium, sodium, carbonate and fluoride. Regular distribution of fluoride Traces of other elements Organic matrix constitutes 15–20% of dry weight: protein (55%), lipid (10%) and carbohydrate	Greater concentration of calcium, magnesium and fluoride than in supragingival calculus Higher calcium to phosphorus ratio than in supragingival calculus Irregular distribution of fluoride
Crystal type	Mostly octacalcium phosphate and hydroxyapatite Some whitlockite Only a little brushite In the presence of low pH and high calcium to phosphorus ratio, brushite appears first in newly formed calculus; but as it matures it transforms to hydroxyapatite or whitlockite and is therefore rarely seen	Whitlockite is the major constituent; it develops under anaerobic, alkaline conditions in the presence of magnesium, zinc and carbonate and contains small amounts magnesium (3%) Hydroxyapapatite is also present Octacalcium phosphate present in the ledge/ring formations of subgingival calculus typically found just under the gingival margin No brushite

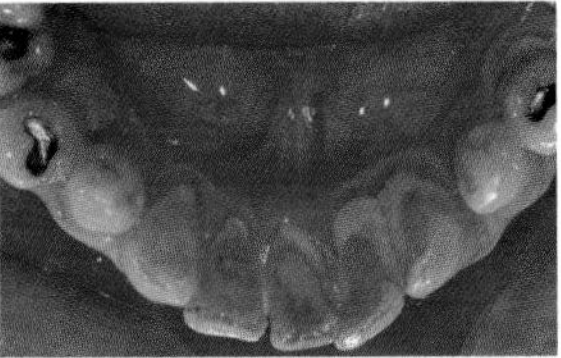

Figure 6.1 Supragingival calculus on the lingual of the mandibular anteriors and premolars, near the opening of the sublingual (Bartholin's) duct, showing nicotine stains from tobacco smoking.

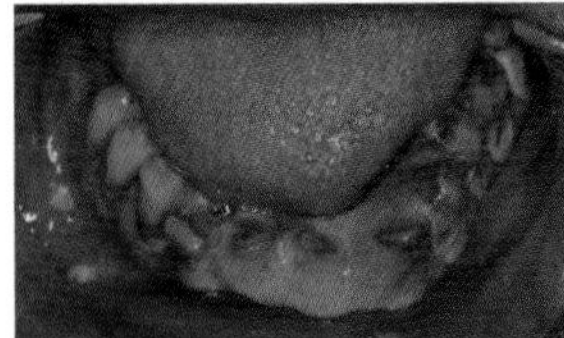

Figure 6.2 Gross deposits of supragingival calculus in an Asian man.

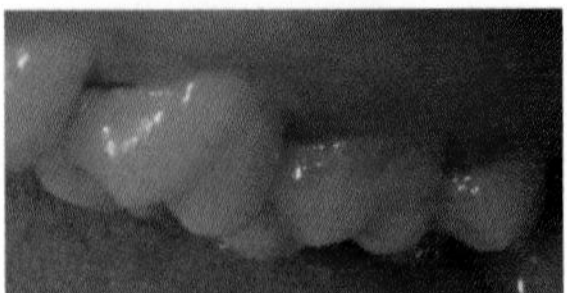

Figure 6.3 Supragingival calculus on the buccal of the maxillary second molar opposite the opening of the parotid (Stensen's) duct.

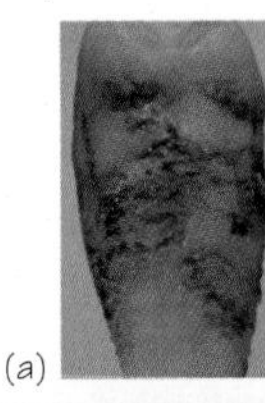

(a)

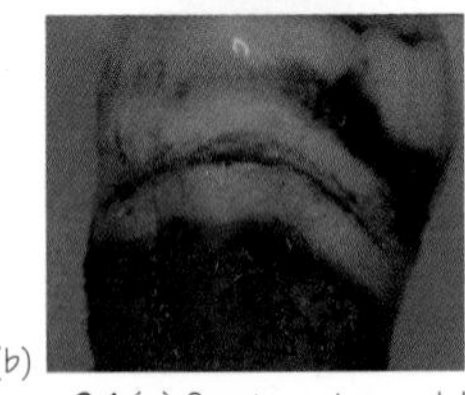

(b)

Figure 6.4 (a) Crusty, spiny, nodular deposits of subgingival calculus on an extracted tooth root. (b) Ring (ledge) formation of subgingival calculus around the cement–enamel junction on an extracted molar stained with Gomori's stain. The periodontal fibres are stained turquoise.

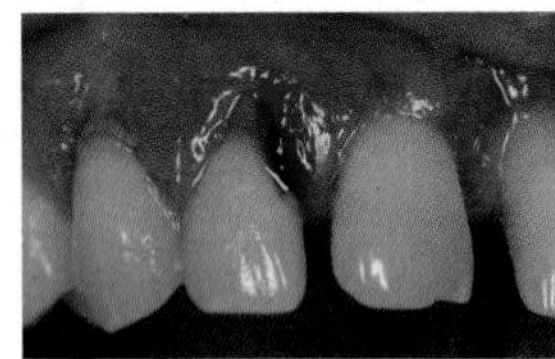

Figure 6.5 Ring (ledge) formation of subgingival calculus visible on the cement–enamel junction of UR3 and UR2 in a 35-year-old Asian female with aggressive periodontitis following loss of attachment; dark shadows of calculus are visible on the distal of UR1 and mesial of UL1.

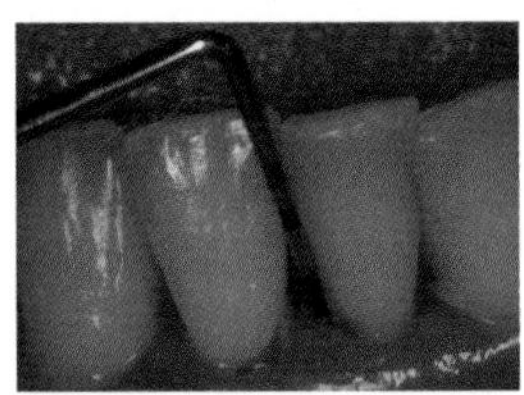

Figure 6.6 Thin veneers of subgingival calculus exposed on the labial of LR2 and distobuccal of LR1 following reduction in oedema and inflammation after commencing non-surgical therapy in a 28-year-old female. The oral hygiene still needs improving.

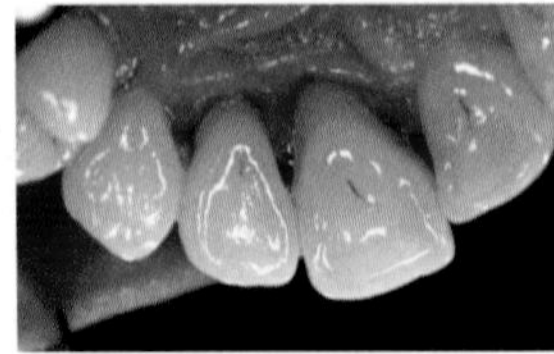

Figure 6.7 Ledges of subgingival calculus exposed at the palatal gingival margin of UR1 and UR2 following reduction in oedema and inflammation after instigating oral hygiene and interdental brushing, but prior to root surface instrumentation.

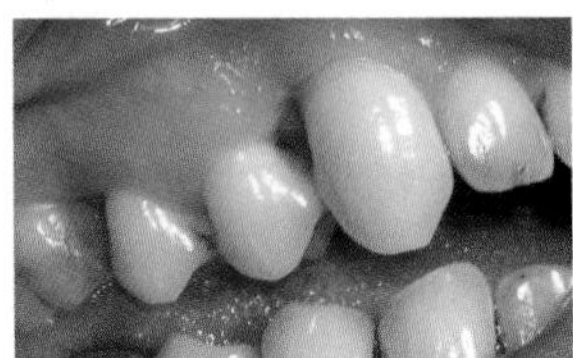

Figure 6.8 Subgingival calculus exposed on the mesial of UR4 following reduction in oedema and inflammation after instigating oral hygiene and interdental brushing, but prior to root surface instrumentation.

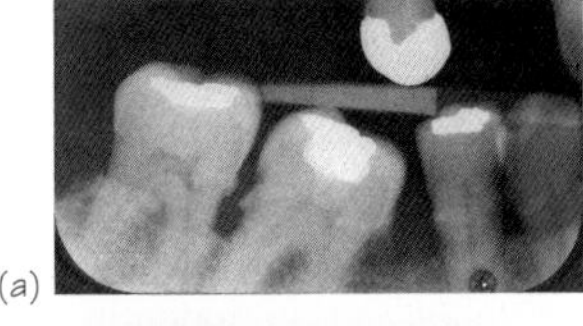

(a)

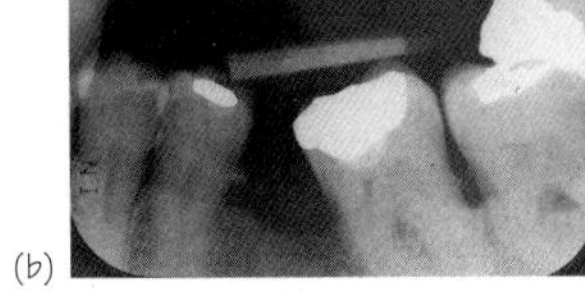

(b)

Figure 6.9 (a, b) Calculus 'wings' are visible on the approximal surfaces of most teeth on bitewing radiographs of this patient with chronic periodontitis.

Dental calculus is defined as the calcified or calcifying deposits that are found attached to the surfaces of teeth and other solid structures in the oral cavity. Supragingival calculus has been extensively studied, particularly in the 1960s and 1970s, whilst subgingival calculus and its formation and composition have been studied much less. There are many differences between the two types (Roberts-Harry & Clerehugh, 2000; Jin & Yip, 2002) (Table 6.1).

Formation of calculus

Calculus formation is always preceded by plaque formation. Initially, pellicle forms on the tooth surface or irregular root cementum and, when this calcifies, the calcified crystals create a strong bond to the surface affected, especially on the cementum at the sites of previous insertions of Sharpey's fibres. Implant surfaces tend to be smoother, therefore calculus may be less adherent.

The plaque accumulations become the organic matrix for the subsequent mineralization of the deposit. Small crystals appear in the intermicrobial matrix between the bacteria; first the matrix becomes calcified and then the bacteria become mineralised. Supragingival calculus formation can occur within 12 days of a scale and polish, by which time up to 80% of the inorganic content may be present. However, the development and maturation of the crystal composition can take place over a long period.

Mineralisation requires nucleation of crystal seeds then crystal growth. The ions for supragingival calculus derive from saliva. Plaque forms the environment for the heterogeneous nucleation of calcium and phosphate crystals, which occurs even with a transient supersaturation of the ions. A rise in pH and salivary flow rate influence the supersaturation of saliva and are therefore instrumental in calculus formation. Other ions may be incorporated into the structure depending on the conditions. Acidic phospholipids and specific proteolipids in cell membranes have a role in microbial mineralization. Gingival crevicular fluid yields the calcium, phosphate and proteins for subgingival calculus to form. Nucleation inhibitors (e.g. magnesium) and crystal growth inhibitors present in some salivary proteins or dentifrices can influence calculus formation.

Crystal types

There are four different crystal types of calcium phosphate, which are found in differing proportions in supragingival and subgingival calculus (Table 6.1):

- Octacalcium phosphate: $Ca_8H_2(PO_4)_6{\cdot}5H_2O$.
- Hydroxyapatite: $Ca_{10}(PO_4)_6(OH)_2$:
  - where other cations capable of substituting for calcium Ca^{2+} are strontium Sr^{2+}, lead Pb^{2+}, potassium K^+ and sodium Na^+;
  - where carbonate CO_3^- or hydrogen phosphate HPO_4^- can replace phosphate ions PO_4^-;
  - where chloride Cl^- or fluoride F^- can replace the hydroxyl ion OH^-.
- Whitlockite: β-$Ca_3(PO_4)_2$. This is sometimes called magnesium-containing beta-tricalcium phosphate as magnesium can substitute for calcium.
- Brushite (dicalcium phosphate dihydrate): $CaHPO_4{\cdot}2H_2O$.

Morphology

Supragingival calculus

Supragingival calculus forms as an amorphous, creamy coloured mass building up in layers on the buccal of the maxillary molars or the lingual of the mandibular anterior teeth. It can readily become stained, e.g. by nicotine (Figs 6.1–6.3).

Subgingival calculus

Crusty, spiny, nodular deposits and ledge- or ring-type deposits are common (Roberts-Harry *et al.*, 2000) (Table 6.1; Figs 6.4, 6.5). At a microscopic level, well-aligned ribbon-shaped octacalcium phosphate crystals are probably formed by filamentous organisms and account for the formation of ledge-type deposits. They may represent a transitional calculus between supragingival and subgingival deposits as they are exposed to both saliva and gingival crevicular fluid.

Individual islands of calculus are thought to represent nucleation sites in early calculus formation. Superficially located deposits, including thin, smooth veneers, which are more difficult to detect by tactile sensation, can become visible near the gingival margin following reduction in gingival oedema and inflammation once plaque control improves or treatment is underway – this makes their subsequent removal easier (Figs 6.6–6.8). Radiographs should be routinely checked for calculus deposits that appear like radio-opaque 'wings' on proximal surfaces – small deposits will not be visible (Fig. 6.9).

Pathogenicity

Plaque always forms on top of calculus. The plaque biofilm that forms over the smooth crystalline surface of supragingival calculus contains filamentous organisms. Supragingival calculus is often associated with gingivitis and gingival recession. Subgingival calculus has an irregular, porous surface covered by a plaque biofilm that contains cocci, rods and filaments and which can act as a reservoir for periodontal pathogens and endotoxin. The presence of subgingival calculus and its plaque layer have been associated with the subsequent development of periodontitis and higher rates of disease progression in adolescents and adults.

Subgingival calculus composition and ethnicity

Studies have shown that the prevalence of subgingival calculus is greater in certain ethnic groups, including Asians. It has been found that Indo-Pakistani subjects have significantly less magnesium in apical deposits of subgingival calculus than white caucasians (Roberts-Harry *et al.*, 2000). It is hypothesised this makes their calculus more insoluble and helps explain the tenacious nature of the calculus and its greater accretion.

Anti-calculus dentifrices

Anti-calculus dentifrices work on the principle of crystal growth inhibition to prevent the formation of supragingival calculus and have not been shown to be effective against subgingival deposits, e.g., triclosan with pyrophosphate and co-polymer; zinc citrate.

Key points

- Calculus is always covered by a plaque biofilm
- Supragingival calculus:
  - forms near the openings of the salivary ducts
  - its mineral content is derived from saliva
  - is associated with gingivitis and recession
- Subgingival calculus:
  - has no predilection for particular parts of the mouth
  - its mineral content is derived from gingival crevicular fluid
  - is detected by probing, direct vision or on radiographs
  - there are different morphological types
  - there is ethnic variation in prevalence and composition
  - is associated with subsequent periodontitis

7 Host defences

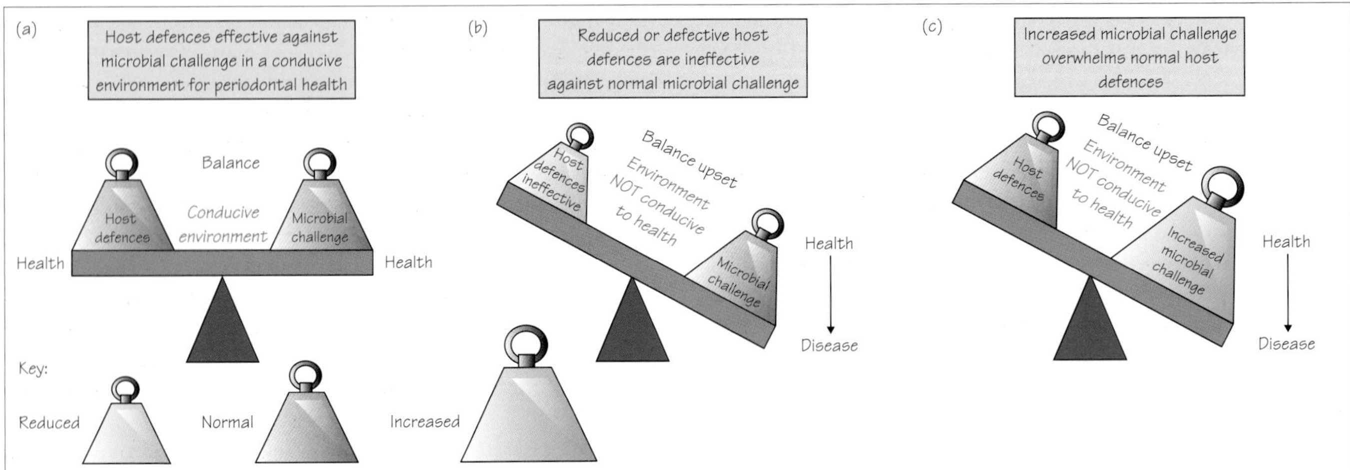

Figure 7.1 Concept of balance between host defences, microbial challenge and environment. (a) Balance and periodontal health. (b) Host defences have a defect or are ineffective against microbial challenge, tipping the balance to periodontal destruction. (c) Microbial challenge overwhelms the host defences leading to an upset balance and periodontal destruction – this may relate to the environment not being conducive and/or changes in quality, quantity or virulence of microorganisms.

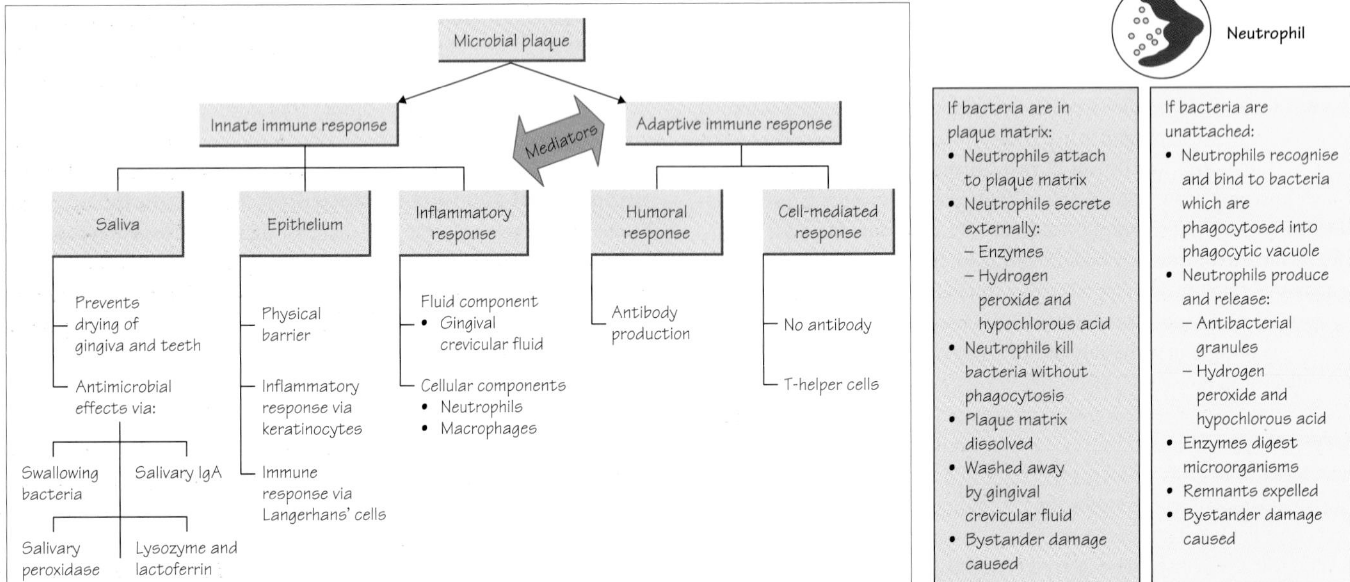

Figure 7.2 Host defences against microbial plaque.

Figure 7.3 The role of neutrophils in phagocytosis or the killing of microorganisms.

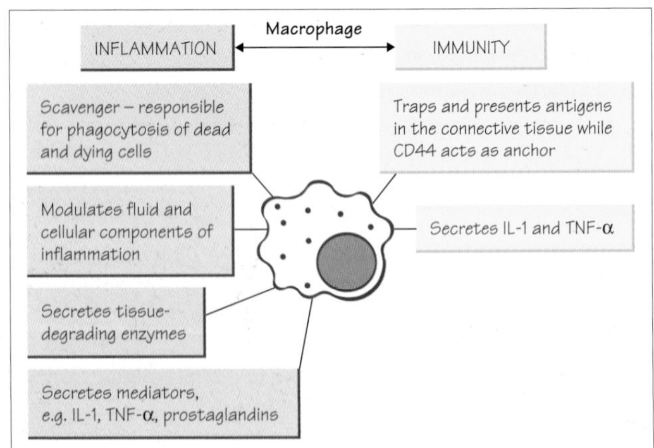

Figure 7.4 The role of macrophages in inflammation and immunity.

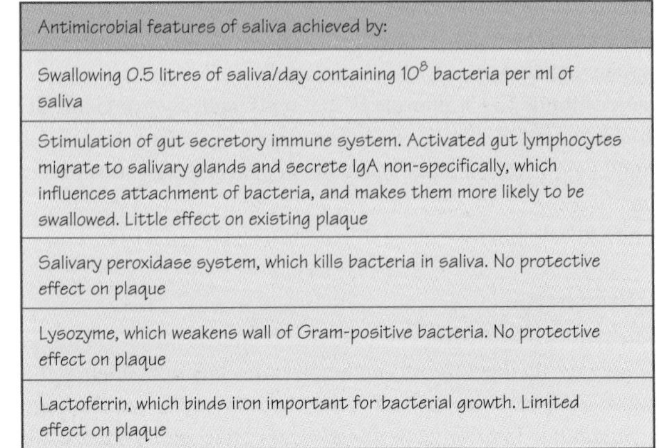

Antimicrobial features of saliva achieved by:
Swallowing 0.5 litres of saliva/day containing 10^8 bacteria per ml of saliva
Stimulation of gut secretory immune system. Activated gut lymphocytes migrate to salivary glands and secrete IgA non-specifically, which influences attachment of bacteria, and makes them more likely to be swallowed. Little effect on existing plaque
Salivary peroxidase system, which kills bacteria in saliva. No protective effect on plaque
Lysozyme, which weakens wall of Gram-positive bacteria. No protective effect on plaque
Lactoferrin, which binds iron important for bacterial growth. Limited effect on plaque

Figure 7.5 Some of the antimicrobial features of saliva.

Nature of host defences

The host defences are like a two-edged sword, since although they are meant to be protective, bystander damage to the periodontal tissues may also occur. A delicate balance exists between the host defences, microbial challenge and ecological environment within the periodontal tissues, such that any upset can tip the balance and lead to periodontal destruction (Fig. 7.1).

Microbial plaque is the primary aetiological agent in the development of periodontal diseases, however patient susceptibility is strongly influenced by the patient's host defences (Fig. 7.2), as well as genetic factors. Plaque in the gingival crevice initiates an inflammatory response. Innate immunity is inbuilt and requires no prior experience or exposure. Adaptive immunity is stimulus specific, and uses recognition, memory and binding to help in the elimination of the infecting agents, either by the humoral immune response or the cell-mediated response. Mediators link inflammation and immunity.

Key components of the host defences

Inflammatory response

This provides a rapid response of the tissues to injury. Its functions are to dilute/wall off damaging microorganisms, kill them and protect the host from bacterial invasion. It is relatively non-specific, although current evidence suggests there are some specific aspects (e.g. bacterial lipopolysaccharide from the cell wall of Gram-negative bacteria is specifically recognised by host receptors such as toll-like receptors). Bystander damage can occur.

The fluid component, gingival crevicular fluid, forms as a result of acute inflammation and it: washes non-adherent bacteria out of the crevice; increases in volume with increasing inflammation; contains mediators of inflammation and antibacterial agents (e.g. complement, antibody and breakdown products, which are nutrients for plaque).

The cellular response involves neutrophils, which form the first line of defence (Fig. 7.3), and macrophages, which have important functions in both the inflammatory and immune responses (Fig. 7.4). Neutrophil defects are associated with increased periodontal destruction in various disorders, including: Chediak–Higashi syndrome, Papillon–Lefèvre syndrome, leukocyte adhesion deficiency, some cases of localised aggressive periodontitis, and poorly controlled diabetes.

Epithelium

Intact epithelium provides a physical barrier to plaque microorganisms, and is achieved by: epithelial cells being tightly attached to each other; keratinisation; the presence of a permeability barrier, although once the junctional epithelium has transformed into pocket-lining epithelium, with microulcerations and a leaky structure, the protective function is compromised.

The inflammatory response is due to:

- cells of the junctional epithelium, which release cytokines, especially interleukin-8 (IL-8), IL-1, tumour necrosis factor-α (TNF-α) and cytokine-induced neutrophil chemoattractant-2;
- expression of host-defence peptides, such as α- and β-defensins.

The immune response occurs as a result of Langerhans' cells (tissue macrophages) in the gingival epithelium.

Saliva

Saliva prevents drying of the teeth, gingival and oral tissues. It has antimicrobial effects (Fig. 7.5). The effects of saliva are supragingival, with no direct effects subgingivally. A lack of saliva (xerostomia) predisposes to the development of supragingival plaque, gingivitis and cervical caries. This may be a feature of certain drugs (e.g. tricyclic antidepressants, antipsychotics, antimuscarinics), mouth breathing or following irradiation/surgery involving the salivary glands.

Humoral immune response

This is directed towards antibody production.

- Epithelial Langerhans' cells take antigenic material from microorganisms to lymph nodes and present it to the circulating lymphocytes, which recognise specific antigen and undergo clonal expansion.
- B-lymphocytes differentiate into plasma cells that secrete antibody against specific antigen under the control of T-helper lymphocytes.
- Antibody production is thought to be protective, particularly IgG and IgA, although precise mechanisms are unknown.
- Antibody may be produced systemically or locally to: aggregate microorganisms; stop them from adhering to epithelium; work with complement to lyse bacteria; work with neutrophils for opsonisation and phagocytosis.
- Titres of antibody vary between individuals and also before and after treatment; in general they rise after therapy.
- High levels may indicate either a positive immune response or an inability of the body to eliminate the pathogen.
- Antibody avidity is a measure of effective immune function.

Cell-mediated response

This does not need antibody as the T-cell has its own T-cell receptor. Following presentation of antigen, T-helper lymphocytes: produce cytokines; assist differentiation of B-cells into plasma cells; activate neutrophils and macrophages (Figs 7.3, 7.4).

The histological picture of gingivitis is consistent with a Th1 response. There is a shift from predominantly T-cell to B-cell lesions as gingivitis progresses to periodontitis, with T-cells having an immunoregulatory role. The relative importance of T-helper subsets (Th1, Th2) is poorly understood, but Th2 cells appear to outnumber Th1 cells in periodontitis. The notable exception is *Aggregatibacter actinomycetemcomitans*, which induces high levels of IgG2 that are dependent on Th1 for their production.

Mediators

Mediators are soluble, chemical messengers that regulate/provide a link between the inflammatory response, the immune response and tissue damage. Their actions are short-lived, potent and subject to rapid inactivation, and include:

(i) Cytokines, e.g. pro-inflammatory IL-1, IL-6 and TNF-α; anti-inflammatory IL-4 and IL-10; and transforming growth factor-β (both pro- and anti-inflammatory). (ii) Prostaglandins, e.g. PGE-2 (responsible for bone resorption, neutrophil chemotaxis, vascular permeability and dilation). (iii) Matrix metalloproteinases (pro-inflammatory, degrade connective tissue).

Key points

- A delicate balance exists between microbial plaque, host defences and the ecological environment
- Innate and adaptive immune responses are intended to be protective against plaque but bystander damage can occur
- Innate immunity involves the inflammatory response, saliva and intact epithelium
- Adaptive immunity comprises the humoral (most important) and cell-mediated responses
- Mediators link the inflammatory and immune responses

8 Development of periodontal diseases

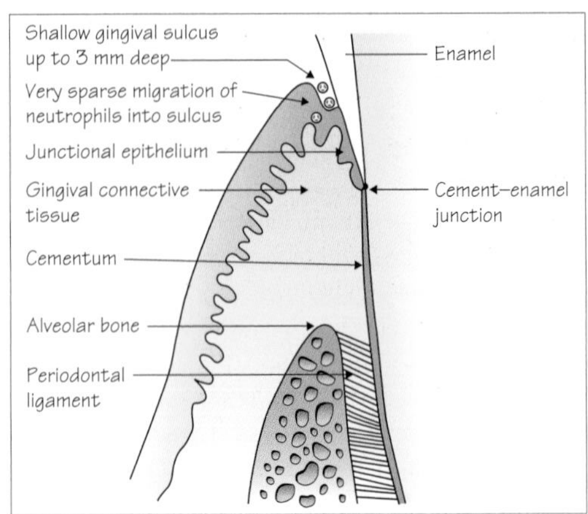

Figure 8.1 Pristine gingiva. This state of fastidious oral hygiene is rarely achieved clinically. There is very sparse neutrophil migration into the sulcus and no inflammatory response.

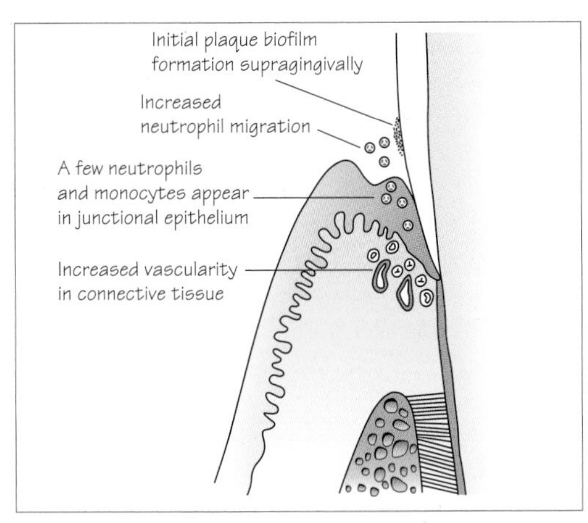

Figure 8.2 An initial lesion.

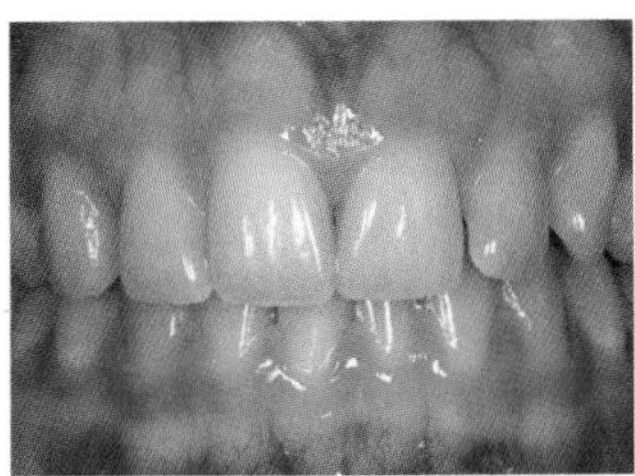

Figure 8.3 Clinically healthy gingiva in a 19-year-old female.

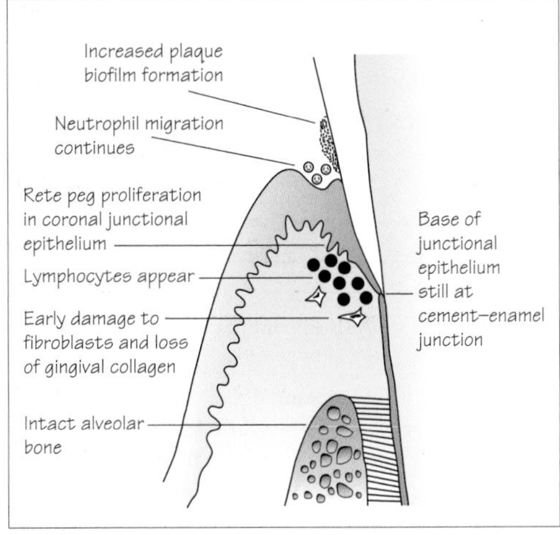

Figure 8.4 An early lesion.

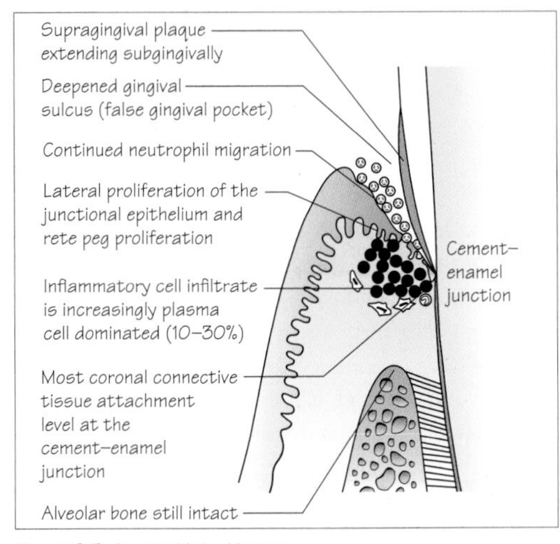

Figure 8.5 An established lesion.

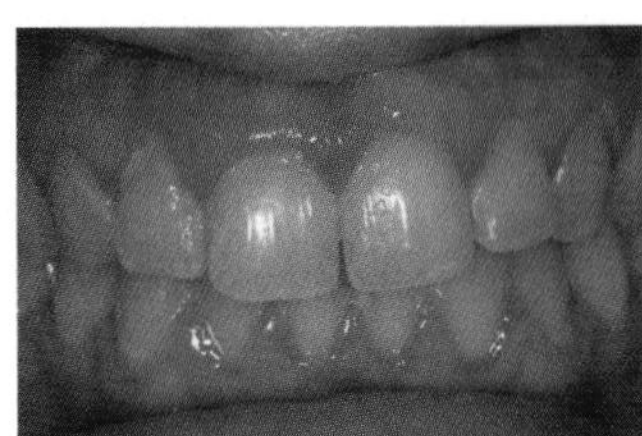

Figure 8.6 Clinical plaque-induced gingivitis. There is visible plaque, blunted interdental papillae, and the marginal gingiva are red, slightly swollen and inflamed.

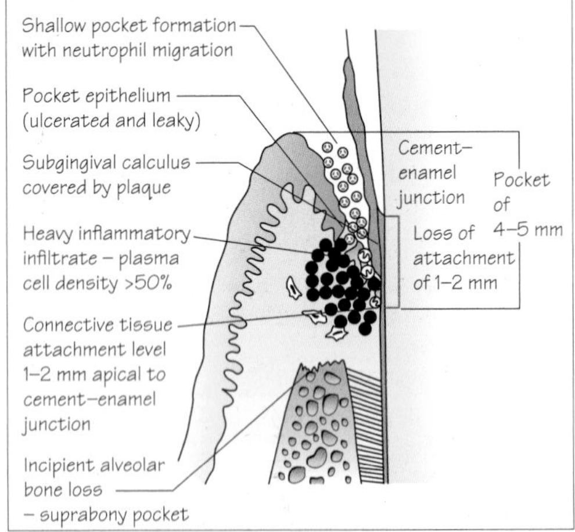

Figure 8.7 An 'advanced' lesion (note 'advanced' here is a descriptor of the stage of histological lesion not a descriptor of clinical severity) showing incipient periodontitis: true shallow periodontal pockets (4–5 mm); CAL of 1–2 mm; and incipient alveolar bone loss (horizontal), with the formation of a suprabony pocket.

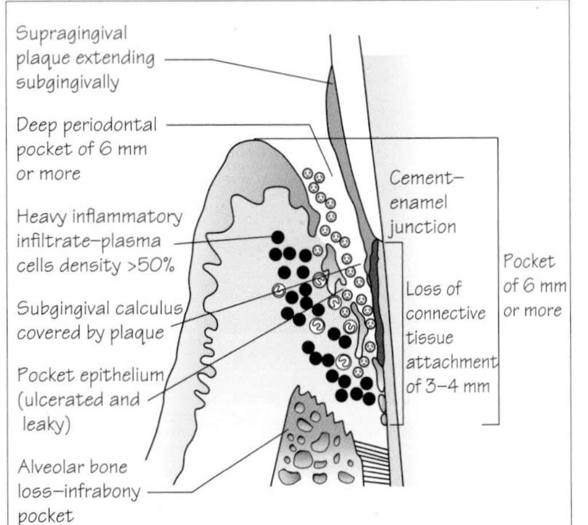

Figure 8.8 An 'advanced' lesion (note 'advanced' here is a descriptor of the stage of histological lesion not a descriptor of clinical severity) showing moderate periodontitis: typically, true deep periodontal pockets (6 mm or more) and CAL of 3–4 mm are present; alveolar bone loss may be vertical, rather than horizontal, with the formation of an infrabony pocket. Note that 5 mm or more of CAL is considered to be severe.

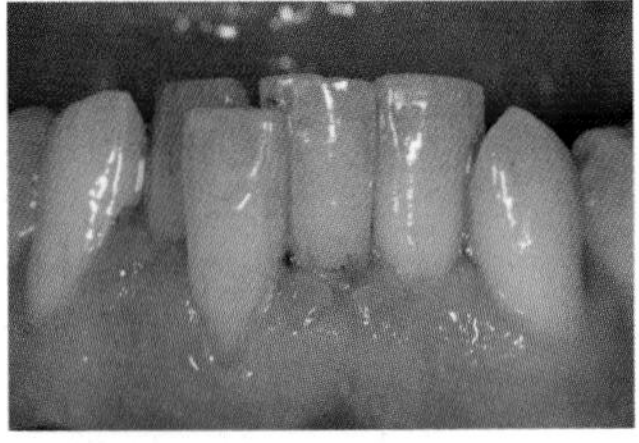

Figure 8.9 Patient with moderate chronic periodontitis showing swollen, inflamed gingivae and recession/clinical attachment loss. The gingival margins are blunted and there is loss of contour.

Following the fifth European Workshop on Periodontology in 2005, the consensus view was that gingivitis and periodontitis are a continuum of the same chronic inflammatory condition that affects the supporting structures of the teeth. It was concluded that: (i) gingivitis may be more important than previously thought; (ii) prevention of gingivitis is the primary preventive measure for preventing periodontitis; and (iii) susceptibility to gingivitis and periodontitis is very variable.

The well-documented model of transition from health to periodontitis by Page and Schroeder in 1976 has been re-visited more recently in the light of current research (Kinane *et al.*, 2008).

Stages of development from health to gingivitis to periodontitis

Pristine gingiva versus clinically healthy gingiva

Pristine gingivae (Fig. 8.1) free from any histological inflammation are extremely difficult to achieve without extreme measures of fastidious plaque control. 'Clinically healthy gingiva' is a term used to describe the level of gingival health attained by patients practising a meticulous standard of oral hygiene. Nevertheless, an initial inflammatory lesion can form at a histological level following plaque biofilm formation even in such motivated patients (Figs 8.2, 8.3).

Initial lesion

- Inflammation begins within 24 hours of plaque accumulation, leading to vasodilation of the various arterioles, capillaries and venules in the dentogingival plexus, and an increase in gingival crevicular fluid (GCF).
- Inflammatory infiltrate increases:
  - neutrophils (i.e. polymorphonuclear leucocytes) migrate into the gingival sulcus with the aid of adhesion molecules: (i) intercellular adhesion molecule 1 (ICAM-1), and (ii) endothelial leukocyte adhesion molecule 1 (ELAM-1);
  - a few lymphocytes and macrophages appear;
  - most lymphocytes have the capability to produce cluster determinant 44 (CD44) receptors on their surfaces, which allows binding to connective tissue.
- The cellular response develops in 2–4 days and is maintained by chemotactic substances from plaque, host defence cells and secretions.
- Gingiva appear clinically healthy.

Early gingival lesion

After about 1 week of plaque accumulation, the early lesion develops (Fig. 8.4):

- Inflammatory infiltrate increases.
- Vessels remain dilated, and more vessels appear, thereby contributing to the redness of the gingiva and clinical signs of inflammation.
- An increase in lymphocytes and neutrophils occurs, and are the predominant cells in the infiltrate. There are very few plasma cells.
- Fibroblasts start to show signs of cell damage.
- Early loss of gingival collagen is seen in the infiltrated area. This allows space for infiltrating cells.
- Basal cells of the junctional and sulcular epithelium proliferate, serving to enhance the mechanical barrier.
- Rete peg proliferation occurs to try and maintain the epithelial barrier function.
- Some coronal epithelium is lost and, consequently the plaque biofilm begins to extend subgingivally.
- The early lesion can persist without shifting to established gingivitis.

Established lesion

It is difficult to predict when this stage of the lesion will develop (Fig. 8.5); it involves the following:

- Increased GCF.
- Increased inflammatory infiltrate.
- Neutrophils predominate, with greatly increased migration.
- Plasma cells form 10–30% of the infiltrate.
- Fibroblasts continue to show signs of cell damage.
- Loss of gingival collagen continues laterally and apically, allowing more space for the infiltrating cells.
- Rete pegs extend further into the connective tissue.
- The junctional epithelium is no longer attached closely to the tooth and has transformed into a pocket epithelium (gingival 'false' pocket):
  - this allows the subgingival plaque to extend more apically;
  - the pocket epithelium is leaky, and may be ulcerated.
- Clinical features of gingivitis are seen – redness, swelling and bleeding (Fig. 8.6).
- Established lesion may remain stable or may become active and progress to periodontitis.

'Advanced' lesion

As the gingival pocket deepens, probably due to the epithelium spreading apically in response to the effects of the plaque constituents, the plaque extends more and more subgingivally (Figs 8.7, 8.8):

- Inflammatory infiltrate extends apically and laterally into the connective tissues of the attachment process.
- Plasma cells dominate and constitute >50% of the cell types.
- Irrespective of type of periodontitis classification, the following irreversible changes occur:
  - loss of periodontal connective tissue attachment;
  - apical migration of the junctional epithelium and the formation of a true periodontal pocket, lined with pocket epithelium;
  - alveolar bone loss.

In the initial stages, the pockets will be shallow (4–5 mm) and an incipient clinical attachment loss (CAL) of 1–2 mm will occur. Bone loss is likely to be horizontal with suprabony pockets (i.e. base of pocket coronal to crest of alveolar bone) (Fig. 8.7).

As the disease develops, the pockets become deep (6 mm or more), clinical attachment loss increases (moderate CAL is 3–4 mm, severe CAL is 5 mm or more) and bone loss occurs, possibly vertical with infrabony pockets (i.e. base of pocket apical to crest of alveolar bone) (Figs 8.8, 8.9).

The transition between the stages from health to gingivitis to periodontitis is difficult to predict and some patients and sites within a patient's mouth are more susceptible than others, reflecting the importance of the oral environment and the balance between the microbial challenge, host defences and various risk factors.

Key points

- Initial, early and established lesions are different stages of gingivitis
- An advanced lesion represents the stage of irreversible clinical attachment loss, apical migration of junctional (pocket) epithelium to form a true pocket, and alveolar bone loss
- Susceptibility to gingivitis and periodontitis varies between patients and sites
- The time scale for transition between stages is unpredictable and variable

9 Progression of periodontal diseases

Matrix metalloproteinase (MMP) activity is controlled by four mechanisms:

1. MMPs are synthesised and secreted as inactive precursors; conversion to active forms requires activation by proteinases like plasmin and trypsin
2. Growth factors and cytokines regulate production of MMP especially Il-1 and transforming growth factor-β
3. Serum and tissue inhibitors can neutralise the activity of MMP
4. Tissue inhibitors of MMP (TIMP) prevent conversion of precursors of MMPs to their active forms

Figure 9.1 Matrix metalloproteinase activity.

- Sites are categorised as active or inactive
- Active sites break down at a constant rate
- Fluctuations in the rate of progression at an active site are possible

(a)

UR1: Slight 'linear' CAL from 1 to 2 mm between 15 and 80 years
LL6: Moderate 'linear' CAL from 2 to 4 mm between 15 and 80 years
UR6: Severe 'linear' CAL from 2 to 10 mm between 15 and 50 years when tooth is extracted

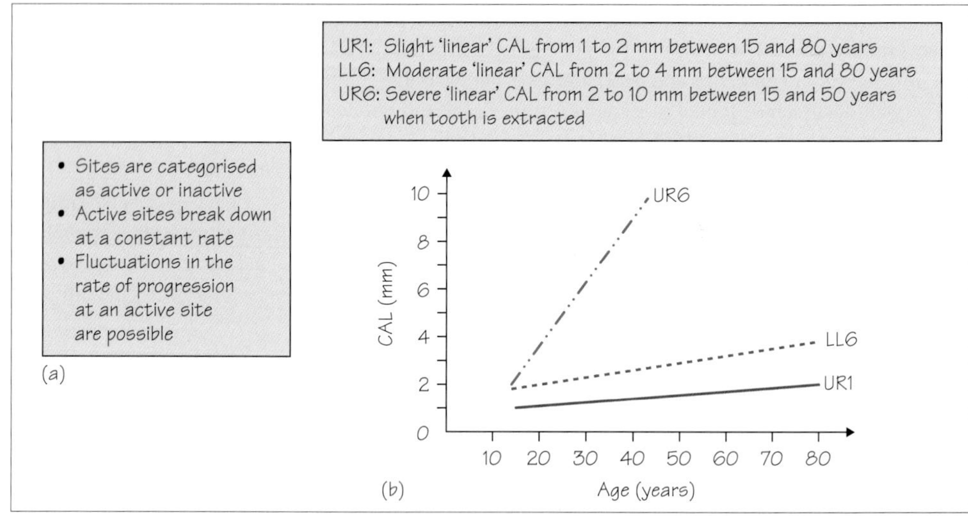

Figure 9.2 (a) Continuous rate model of clinical attachment loss (CAL). (b) Examples of three sites showing different rates of continuous 'linear' CAL over the patient's lifetime.

- Sites are categorised as active or inactive
- Bursts of activity are short – a few days or weeks
- One or more bursts can occur at each active site
- Occurrence of bursts is independent of the previous burst history

(a)

UR1: Slight CAL in random burst from 1 to 2 mm between 15 and 80 years
LL6: Moderate CAL in random bursts from 2 to 4 mm between 15 and 80 years
UR6: Severe CAL in random bursts from 2 to 10 mm between 15 and 50 years when tooth is extracted

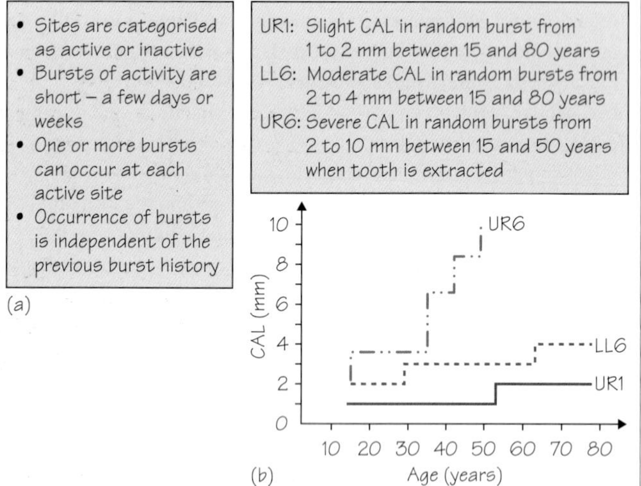

Figure 9.3 (a) Random burst model of clinical attachment loss (CAL). (b) Examples of the same three sites as in Fig. 9.2b showing random bursts of CAL over the patient's lifetime but with the same clinical outcome.

- Multiple active sites break down within a relatively short period of time, with long periods of quiescence which can last months or years
  - periods of activity may be clustered around particular phases in a patient's life perhaps when stress, illness or some other periodontal risk factor comes into effect (i.e. transient)

(a)

UR1: Slight CAL in burst from 1 to 2 mm around 50 years
LL6: Moderate CAL in bursts from 2 to 4 mm around 50 years
UR6: Severe CAL in bursts from 2 to 10 mm mainly around 50 years when tooth is extracted

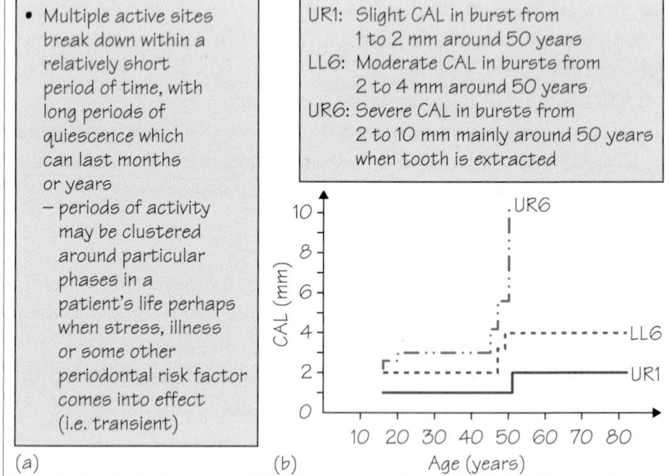

Figure 9.4 (a) Asynchronous multiple burst model of clinical attachment loss (CAL). (b) Examples of the same three sites as in Figs 9.2b and 9.3b showing asynchronous bursts of CAL over the patient's lifetime but with the same clinical outcome.

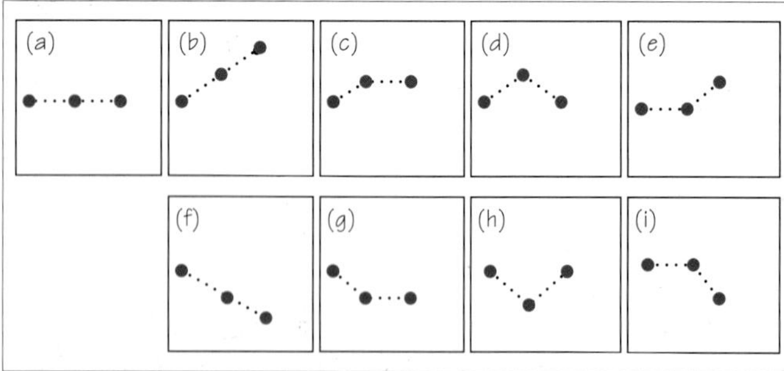

Figure 9.5 Possible patterns of clinical attachment loss at an individual site between three time points: (a) no change; (b) loss then loss again; (c) loss then plateau; (d) loss then gain with a net result of no change; (e) no change, then loss, leading to net loss; (f) gain then gain; (g) gain then plateau, leading to net gain; (h) gain then loss with a net result of no change; and (i) no change then gain, leading to net gain in attachment.

Proposed criteria for a two-level definition of a periodontitis case:

- Presence of proximal attachment loss ≥ 3 mm in ≥ 2 non-adjacent teeth
- Presence of proximal attachment loss ≥ 5 mm in ≥ 30% teeth present

(a)

Proposed criteria for a definition of periodontitis progression

- Presence of ≥ 2 teeth demonstrating a longitudinal loss of proximal attachment of ≥ 3 mm
- Longitudinal radiographic bone loss of ≥ 2 mm at ≥ 2 teeth may be substituted where no serial clinical measures

(b)

Figure 9.6 Proposed criteria for: (a) periodontitis, and (b) periodontitis progression.

Periodontal diseases can progress in individuals and at various sites within the mouth at different times and rates, and the extent and severity of the resulting disease can be variable and unpredictable. Relevant to progression are: changes in the connective tissues during progression; susceptibility; models of progression.

Changes in the connective tissues during progression

Building on what was covered in Chapters 7 and 8, periodontal disease progression involves complex inflammatory and immune responses, affecting epithelial and connective tissue turnover and activity associated with the infiltrating inflammatory cells. Great numbers of B- and T-cells accumulate in the tissues, although their role has not been fully elucidated. During the transition from gingivitis to periodontitis there is a shift from T- to B-cell lesion.

As the initial inflammatory response to plaque develops adjacent to the gingival margin, connective tissue destruction begins and can result in up to 70% loss of collagen within the foci of inflammation.

With further development, the destruction expands deeper towards the periodontal ligament and alveolar bone. Simultaneously, a form of frustrated repair is initiated with fibrosis and scarring coexisting at the foci of inflammation. At this stage a combination of factors, including the connective tissue response together with inflammatory cell regulation, can result in the lesion being contained with no further development of bone loss and attachment loss.

However, if the lesion does progress from contained gingivitis to more progressive periodontitis, then biochemical analyses have shown numerous quantitative and qualitative changes occur to the fibrous and non-fibrous components of the gingival connective tissues. The changes to the periodontal ligament, bone and cementum have been less well characterised. Apical migration of the junctional epithelium requires coordinated cell proliferation and migration of the cells over the connective tissue substratum, which has been modified by the inflammatory process. These events are likely to be regulated by variable expression of integrands and other adhesion molecules at the epithelial–connective tissue interface. Anti-inflammatory drugs, tissue growth factors or host modulating chemotherapeutic agents may influence progression.

Various interrelated pathways and mechanisms are involved in the destruction of the extracellular matrix, including activity of the matrix metalloproteinases (MMPs) (Fig. 9.1), reactive oxygen species and phagocytosis of matrix components.

There are also many cytokines and growth factors (in particular platelet-derived growth factor, insulin-like growth factor, interleukin-1 (IL-1), transforming growth factor-β, prostaglandin E2 and interferon-γ) that have a direct influence on connective tissue cellular activities and result in the activation of cell migration, cell attachment, DNA synthesis and matrix synthesis.

Susceptibility

An individual's susceptibility to the periodontal diseases depends on the interplay between a number of factors including the nature and virulence of the microbial challenge, their own oral ecology, the robustness of their host defences, their own genetic make up and the presence of risk factors including: smoking, poorly controlled diabetes, specific bacteria, gene polymorphisms, race/ethnicity, obesity, osteoporosis/osteopenia and stress (Chapters 10–13).

Models of progression

Measurement

Periodontal disease progression is traditionally measured by clinical attachment loss (CAL) or probing pocket depth recordings, or by radiographic methods at several sites per tooth. Clinical measurements with manual probes to the nearest millimetre are quite crude, although some electronic probes allow readings to 0.1 mm. However, many factors influence the accuracy of such measurements, e.g. degree of inflammation, tooth location and obstruction by subgingival calculus (see also Fig. 3.7). Radiographic methods include simple measurements direct from films or more sophisticated methods such as subtraction radiography.

Models of periodontal disease progression

Various models of periodontal disease progression were proposed by Socransky *et al.* in 1984:

- Linear or continuous rate theory of progression (Fig. 9.2).
- Random burst model (Fig. 9.3).
- Asynchronous multiple burst theory (Fig. 9.4).

The implication of the linear theory is that once a site has lost attachment it will continue to get worse and thus treatment is essential. If the burst concept is correct it implies that the aetiological factors are not continuously present but rather are only present prior to and during the bursts – with a possible interpretation that treatment may not be indicated for inactive sites. The inherent difficulty is in trying to detect and predict 'bursts'.

Patterns of progression at a site

A further consideration is what can happen at an individual site. It is possible for the site to stay the same, consistently lose attachment, consistently gain attachment, or to have mixed patterns of loss and gain (Fig. 9.5). The outcome over a period of time may be net gain (Fig. 9.5f, g, i), net loss (Fig. 9.5b, c, e) or no change of attachment level (Fig. 9.5a, d, h).

Definition of progression

It was concluded at the fifth European Workshop on Periodontology in 2005 that studies of risk factors and progression should use a consistent definition for 'periodontitis case' and 'periodontitis progression' to improve consistency in data interpretation globally (Tonetti & Claffey, 2005) (Fig. 9.6).

Statistical modelling

Socransky did not favour the notion of the constant rate hypothesis. However, various statistical models have since been applied (DeRouen *et al.*, 1995) and it has not been possible to exclude either the continuous rate theory or the burst theory. Using multilevel modelling, Gilthorpe and colleagues (2003) concluded that the linear and burst theories are a manifestation of the same phenomenon, namely that loss of attachment progresses in some sites, while other sites improve, in a cyclical manner.

Key points

- Complex changes occur in the connective tissues during the transition from gingivitis to periodontitis
- Susceptibility to progression depends: on several factors
- Linear and burst models for progression have been proposed
- Statistical models including multilevel modelling suggest that the theories are a manifestation of the same phenomenon: some sites progress, some improve in a cyclical manner

10 Risk and periodontal diseases

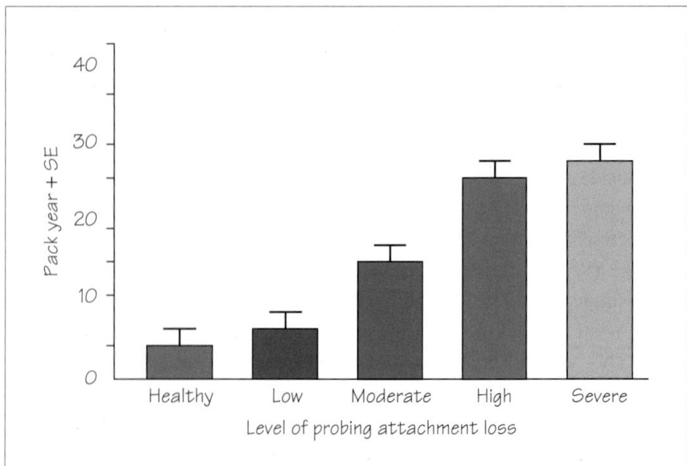

Figure 10.1 Pack years of cigarette smoking and clinical attachment loss.

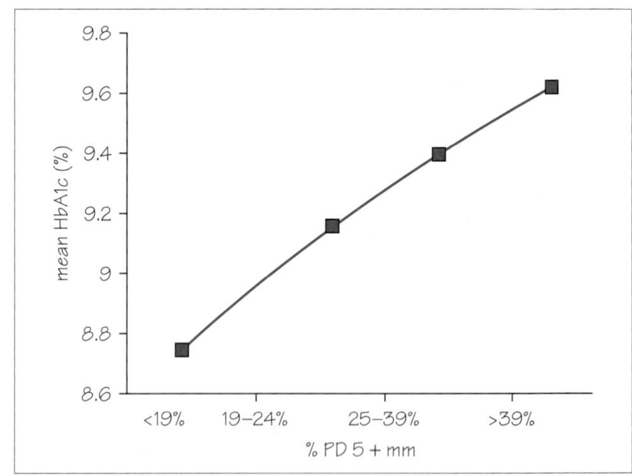

Figure 10.2 Periodontal disease and glycaemic control: cause or effect?

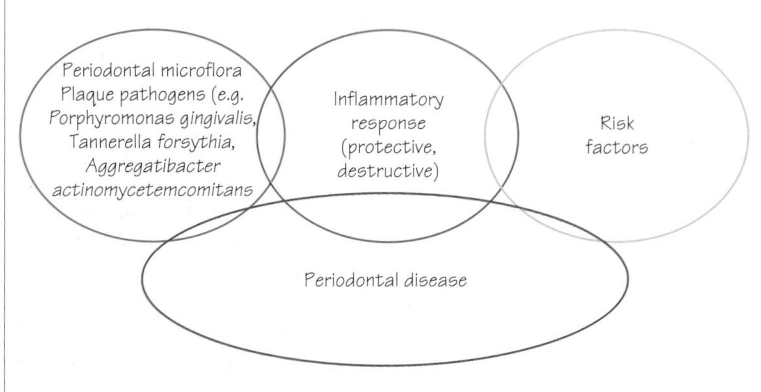

Figure 10.3 Interaction of periodontal microflora, the inflammatory response and risk factors.

Table 10.1 Levels of evidence for risk determinants in chronic diseases and characteristics of these studies which make the factors more convincing, and not likely to be spurious associations.

Type of study	Study characteristics
Cross-sectional or case–control studies	Confounding factors are eliminated or adjusted for in the analysis
Longitudinal epidemiological studies (establish temporality and evidence for effects in causal pathway)	Dose–response effects
Mechanism studies	Study results are consistent among various independent studies
Intervention studies	Effects are clinically meaningful
	Relationship is biologically plausible

Table 10.2 Systemic risk determinants for periodontal disease.

Systemic risk factors	Systemic risk indicators
Smoking	Low dietary calcium
Diabetes mellitus type 1 and 2	Postmenopausal osteoporosis and osteopenia
Race	Visceral obesity
Genetics	Stress and inadequate coping
Male gender	
Polymorphonuclear leukocyte (neutrophil) function	
Socioeconomic status (low educational level)	
Acquired systemic infections (e.g. human immunodeficiency virus (HIV))	
Severe malnutrition (cancrum oris)	

Table 10.3 Modification of risk factors for periodontal disease.

Risk factor/indicator	Modification
Risk factor	
Smoking	Smoking cessation
Diabetes	Improve glycaemic control
Risk indicator	
Low dietary calcium	Calcium supplementation
Osteoporosis or osteopenia	Bone-sparing agents, calcium, and vitamin D supplementation
Visceral obesity	Diet and exercise
Stress and inadequate coping	Stress reduction measures

Although dental plaque accumulation is a cause of periodontal disease, it may not be a sufficient cause since some individuals have large accumulations of dental plaque and suffer little periodontal disease, while others have very little plaque accumulation and suffer severe periodontal disease. It appears then that risk factors are important in periodontal disease; determining who develops the disease, the severity of the disease the individual develops, which sites in the dentition are affected, the rate of progression of the disease, the response to therapy, and the recurrence rate. In assessing risk, the probability that a disease outcome will occur following a particular exposure is estimated (Last, 2001).

What is a risk factor?

A risk factor can be an aspect of personal behaviour or life style, an environmental exposure, or an inborn or inherited characteristic that changes the susceptibility to periodontal disease. It can also be a local factor which increases the infection of a site.

- On the basis of epidemiological evidence, at first usually cross-sectional studies, putative risk factors are associated with disease after accounting for possible confounding factors (Last, 2001).
- Longitudinal studies can help determine if the presence of the factor precedes the onset of disease, which strengthens the evidence that the factor is truly related to the disease, and not just a chance association.
- True risk factors are part of the causal chain or expose the host to the causal chain (Beck, 1998) and evidence for causality usually comes from animal and *in vitro* studies of mechanism of action (Fig. 10.3).
- Finally, true risk factors will most often affect disease outcome if removed or moderated. This can be determined by randomized controlled trials where the risk factor is removed or reduced and the disease outcome is measured.

Different terms are used for factors associated with disease risk. Risk indicators are associated with increased probability of disease, based upon cross-sectional studies carefully designed to eliminate those confounders that may result in spurious associations. A risk indicator may be a probable or putative risk factor. If confirmed in a longitudinal study and determined to be in the causal pathway, they would be called risk factors. There are other terms used, such as risk markers, which are attributes or exposures associated with an increased probability of the disease. Risk markers are not usually factors or in the causal pathway, but are somehow associated with the true risk factor. An example of a risk marker is increased waist circumference in adults, which is a measure of excess abdominal adiposity. The abdominal or visceral adipose tissue is a true risk factor since it contributes to the causal pathway of diabetes.

Briefly, true risk factors are not only associated with the disease and precede the development of disease or worsen disease progression, but are shown to be in the causal pathway by studies of mechanism. If risk factors are reduced, this often will result in less disease. Proof of the effect of reduction or modification of risk factors on the disease comes from randomized controlled trials (Table 10.1).

Types of risk factors for periodontal disease

There are two major classes of risk factors for periodontal disease.

1 *Local factors* such as overhanging restorations and root caries that tend to allow for plaque accumulation and hence result in more periodontal disease. Other local risk factors for periodontal disease include pocket depth, intrabony pockets especially involving furcations, and root canal infections.

2 *Systemic factors* that affect the entire body, such as cigarette smoking, diabetes mellitus and genetic factors (Table 10.2).

Are risk factors modifiable?

Many risk factors are modifiable, including local factors such as overhanging restorations and systemic factors such as smoking. An overhanging restoration can be removed, and smoking can be eliminated by engaging in a smoking cessation programme. Other risk factors are non-modifiable, such as genetic factors.

Levels of exposure to risk factors

Often risk factors have a clear dose response, i.e. the more exposure to the risk factor, the greater the susceptibility to the disease. This is the case for cigarette smoking, for example. There is a direct linear relationship between the exposure to smoking estimated by the number of pack years of cigarette smoking and the amount of alveolar bone loss, as seen in periodontal patients (Fig. 10.1). Also, there is a direct linear relationship between the level of glucose control in patients with diabetes and the severity of periodontal disease (Fig. 10.2).

These observations bring up the concept of a threshold. For many risk factors, it is believed that there is a threshold below which the risk factor has a negligible clinical effect on the disease. For example, blood cholesterol levels below 200 mg/dl are thought to be normal, but levels above this are considered to increase the risk for heart disease.

Modification of risk factors is part of the management of periodontal disease

It has been shown that glycaemic control in patients with diabetes and smoking cessation enhance the prognosis of treatment for periodontal disease and are important measures in the prevention of recurrence of periodontal disease. Weight control, calcium supplementation, control of stress and enhancement of coping skills may also prove important in the management of periodontal disease in high risk individuals (Table 10.3). Definitive proof, however, of the effects of their intervention is not yet available.

It is also clear that the removal of local risk factors such as overhanging restorations, restoration of root caries, and reduction of periodontal pockets all are important in the management of periodontal disease and particularly in preventing recurrence.

Key points

- Overgrowth of dental plaque may be a necessary, but not sufficient, cause of periodontal disease
- Risk factors work to change the susceptibility or resistance of individuals to the disease-causing effects of dental plaque
- Risk factors can be local or systemic
- Risk factors are in the causal pathway and, if altered, will alter the course of periodontal disease
- Other factors called risk markers may be associated with periodontal disease, but are not in the causal pathway and, if altered, may not affect the disease
- Evidence to establish true risk factors can come from population-based epidemiological studies – studies of causality evaluating the risk factor to the disease causal pathways. Evidence can also be sought in intervention studies, which help establish whether or not risk modification will contribute to disease reduction.

Systemic risk factors for periodontal diseases

Table 11.1 Systemic risk determinants for periodontal disease.

Systemic risk factors	Systemic risk indicators (potential risk factors)
Smoking	Low dietary calcium
Diabetes mellitus type 1 and type 2	Postmenopausal osteoporosis and osteopenia
Race	Visceral obesity
Genetics	Stress and inadequate coping
Male gender	
PMN function	
SES (low educational level)	
Acquired systemic infections (e.g. HIV)	
Severe malnutrition (cancrum oris)	

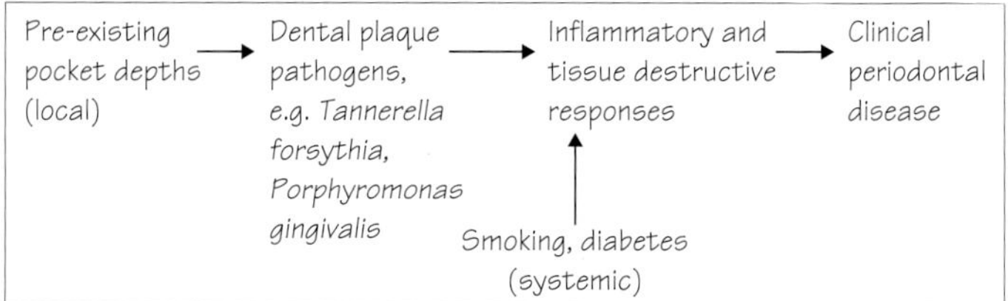

Figure 11.1 Local and systemic risk factors affecting the oral causal microbiota pathways and infection in periodontal disease.

Systemic risk factors for periodontal disease are those conditions that affect most, if not all, tissues of the body. They are in contrast to the local risk factors described in Chapters 10 and 14 that influence periodontal tissues at the tooth or site level. Types of evidence required to establish risk factors in the causal pathway of a disease are discussed in Chapter 10.

Systemic risk factors and risk indicators for periodontal disease

- Systemic risk factors include smoking, diabetes mellitus, race, genetic factors, male gender, polymorphonuclear (PMN) functional abnormalities, low economic status, low educational level, acquired systemic infections such as human immunodeficiency virus (HIV), and severe malnutrition (Table 11.1).
- Systemic risk indicators or putative risk factors include low dietary calcium intake, postmenopausal osteoporosis and osteopenia, obesity, stress and inadequate coping, and decreased immunoglobulin 2 (IgG2) antibodies (Table 11.1).
- Regular dental visits, anaemia and anti-allergy medications protect against periodontal disease.
- Most of the risk factors for periodontal disease also affect risk for dental implant therapy.

Mechanisms by which systemic risk factors appear to be operating

Smoking

In the more than 4000 components of smoke, there are many that exaggerate the inflammatory responses to periodontal pathogens and others that suppress the immune response (Fig. 11.1). Local effects of smoking also include direct toxic effects to cells, thermal effects, increased stain and calculus, and effects on the flora. There are adverse effects of smoking on bone tissues resulting in reduced bone mineral density. Clinical features of smokers are illustrated in Chapter 36.

Diabetes

Both type 1 and type 2 diabetes are thought to lead to increased infections including periodontal disease by impairing protective immune responses, interfering with wound healing, and inducing a hyperinflammatory state associated with activated protein kinase C and advanced glycation of proteins. These adverse processes probably lead to increased tissue destruction and greater levels of infection in those with diabetes as compared to those without diabetes.

Obesity

The adverse effects of obesity appear to be associated with the production of adipokines and cytokines by adipose tissue and by macrophages in adipose tissues. These pro-inflammatory molecules lead to a hyperinflamed state, which probably increases tissue destruction triggered by periodontal and other infections. Some of the inflammatory mediators produced by adipose tissue such as tumour necrosis factor α (TNF-α) are thought to also bring about insulin resistance, which leads to diabetes and, in turn, leads to increased risk for periodontal disease.

Genetic factors

Twin studies show a significant contribution of genetic factors to risk for periodontal disease. There are over 40 associations between single nucleotide polymorphisms in candidate genes and periodontal disease. However, these are often not reproducible and differ among racial and ethnic groups. Genetic polymorphisms in the interleukin-1B (IL-1B) gene are the basis of the PST(R) test, which is marketed to assess periodontal risk.

Dietary calcium

Low dietary calcium is associated with increased periodontal disease in both men and women from cross-sectional studies. The mechanism may involve reduced bone mineral density which, in turn, renders the alveolar bone supporting the teeth more susceptible to periodontal infection.

Osteopenia and osteoporosis in post-menopausal women

A complex set of pathways, which affect bone mineral density, occur at menopause and it is likely that those brought about by reduced oestrogen levels lead to bone resorption outpacing bone deposition, which sets the stage for more advanced periodontal bone loss associated with periodontal infections. Calcium supplementation and bone-sparing agents have shown modest effects in reducing tooth loss in older adults, suggesting that the modification of osteopenia may have a beneficial effect on alveolar bone.

Stress and inadequate coping

Chronic stress and increased allostatic load appear to have many deleterious effects on the host including suppression of the immune response with increased susceptibility to infections.

Male gender

The mechanism for males being more susceptible to periodontal disease is unknown. However, it has been hypothesised that females, at least pre-menopausal females, are less susceptible to periodontal disease because of the protective effects of oestrogen on bone, thus resulting in an overall gender difference in periodontal disease.

Low socioeconomic status

For most chronic infections, low educational levels and low income levels are often associated with increased risk for disease. One possible mechanism may be increased stress with lack of locus of control in individuals of low socioeconomic status (SES). Another is reduced access to dental care in those of lower SES, since it is well known that lack of regular dental visits increases the risk for periodontal disease. Another possible explanation is lack of adequate oral hygiene, which may result from cultural differences or lack of adequate knowledge about healthy behaviours.

Clinical studies to assess the effects of risk factor modification on the initiation and progression of periodontal disease

It is clear that smokers are more difficult to treat, and many cases of refractory periodontitis and implant failures are found among smokers. It has been found that subgingival antimicrobial agents sometimes give an added periodontal treatment benefit in smokers over that achieved in non-smokers. Smokers are known to heal poorly and many clinicians will not perform major periodontal surgical, regenerative or implant procedures on heavy smokers until they demonstrate success in smoking cessation programmes.

Several studies show that patients with diabetes, especially if uncontrolled, heal more slowly and have more postoperative complications than non-diabetics after periodontal treatment. However, those patients with diabetes who have good glycaemic control most often heal at a similar rate and suffer no more complications than those who are non-diabetic after periodontal therapy. It is also clear that those with diabetes and periodontal disease have a tendency for the periodontal disease to recur more often after treatment, again especially in those who have uncontrolled diabetes. Hence, more frequent maintenance intervals and more intense attention to recurrent disease and its prevention are often necessary in patients with diabetes mellitus.

PMN abnormalities

Patients with PMN deficiencies, either congenital or acquired neutropenias, often have severe periodontal disease in childhood. Also, those with impaired PMN neutrophil function, including Chediak–Higashi syndrome, the lazy leukocyte syndrome and leukocyte adhesion deficiency, have severe periodontal disease, often before puberty. Patients with aggressive periodontitis (formerly called localised juvenile periodontitis) appear to have neutrophil abnormalities which, although not severe, probably increase susceptibility to early onset of periodontitis in the first molars and incisors. Patients with HIV infections also suffer from immune deficiencies and are more susceptible to periodontal disease.

Practice implications

It is clear that smoking cessation and diabetes control are an important part of the management of periodontal patients. Dentists can perform a great service to the patient by working with a physician in monitoring glycaemic control in diabetics and by instituting smoking cessation programmes in smokers. See Chapter 36 for details of smoking cessation programmes and Chapter 37 for management of patients with diabetes.

Key points

- Systemic risk factors for periodontal disease affect most, if not all, the tissues of the body. They may be modifiable (such as smoking) or non-modifiable (such as genetic factors)
- Modifiable systemic risk factors are important in managing periodontal disease
- Systemic risk factors may be associated with increased incidence, progression and recurrence of periodontal disease. They may also affect the prognosis of treatment
- Systemic risk factors are generally in the causal pathway and modify the expression of the disease by increasing susceptibility or decreasing resistance
- Present information supports the close monitoring of glycaemic control in patients with diabetes and instituting smoking cessation programmes as part of the management of periodontal disease

12 Periodontal diseases and general health

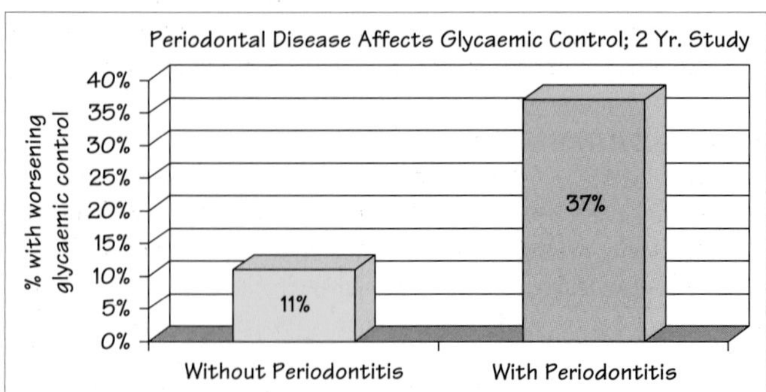

Figure 12.1 The effect of periodontal disease on glycaemic control: results from a 2-year study (Taylor *et al.*, 1996).

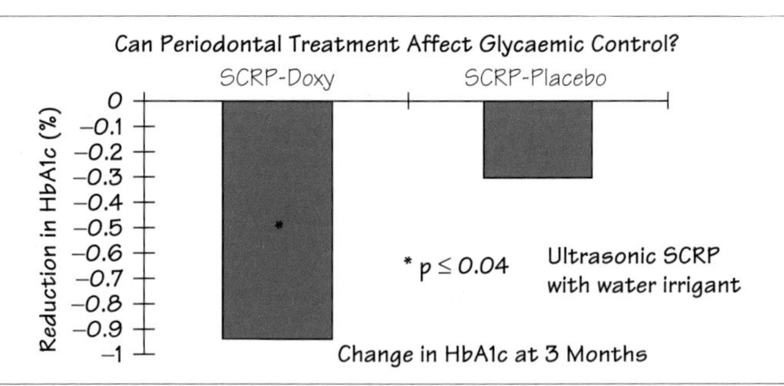

Figure 12.2 The effect of periodontal treatment on glycaemic control: results from a pilot randomised control study of 125 patients with type 2 diabetes mellitus showing the change in HbA1c at 3 months. SCRP, scaling and root planing.

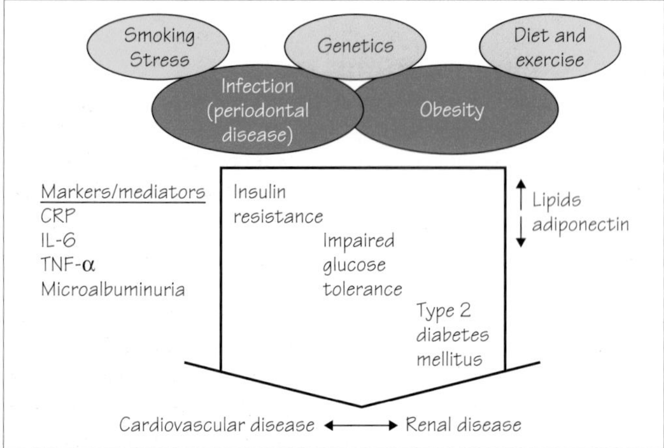

Figure 12.3 Periodontal infection and systemic disease – possible links.

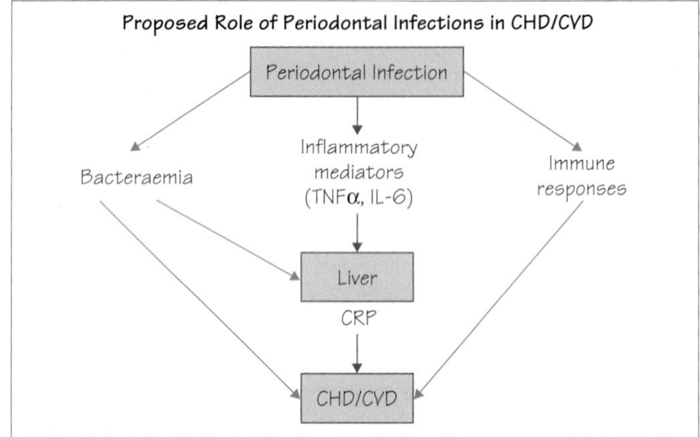

Figure 12.5 Proposed role of periodontal infections in chronic heart disease (CHD) and cardiovascular disease (CVD).

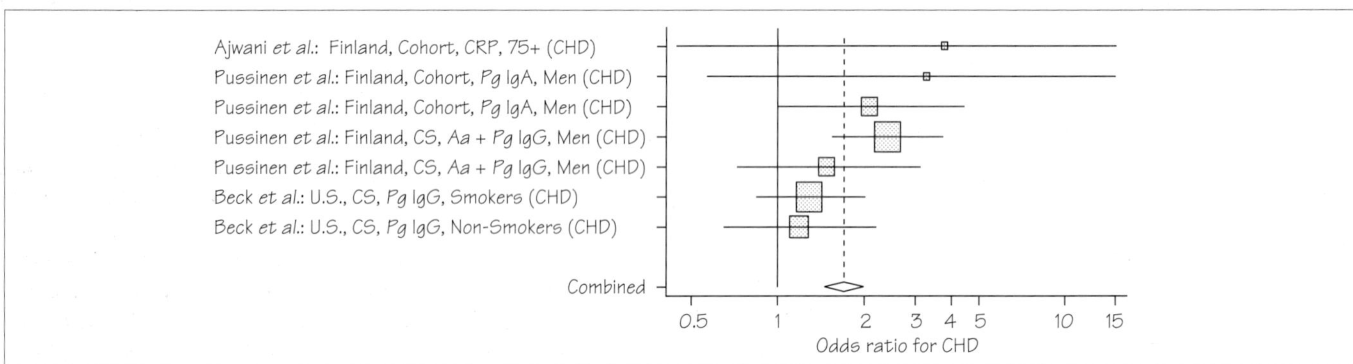

Figure 12.4 Markers of systemic periodontal bacterial exposure and chronic heart disease (CHD) risk. Details of the cited studies can be found in Mustapha *et al.* (2007).

Table 12.1 Systemic diseases or conditions where periodontal disease and other oral manifestations occur.

Diabetes mellitus types 1, 2 and gestational
Gingival changes in leukaemia
Immune dysfunction including neutrophil disorders
Chemotherapy
Head and neck irradiation
Medication therapy including phenytoin (dilantin), calcium channel blockers and bisphosphonates
Dermatological conditions including pemphigus and lichen planus
Severe neutrophil deficiencies

Table 12.2 Systemic conditions associated with periodontal disease.

Diabetes mellitus: diabetic complications including coronary artery disease and diabetic neuropathy
Atherosclerotic diseases including coronary artery diseases, ischaemic stroke and peripheral artery disease
Respiratory infections including nosocomial pneumonia and chronic obstructive pulmonary disease
Adverse pregnancy outcomes
Oral pharyngeal cancer

Periodontal diseases can be manifestations of systemic conditions and diseases. Periodontal diseases also may be closely associated with, and possibly independent risk factors for, some common, chronic systemic diseases and conditions.

Periodontal manifestations of diseases such as diabetes, gingivitis associated with leukaemia, gingival overgrowth as a complication of phenytoin (dilantin) therapy, and periodontitis associated with immune dysfunction (such as neutrophil disorders) are well documented. Other oral manifestations of systemic conditions include oral osteonecrosis seen in patients receiving head and neck radiation chemotherapies and intravenous bone-sparing agents. Gingival conditions are also associated with dermatological diseases such as pemphigus vulgaris, lichen planus and erythema multiforme (Table 12.1).

Clinical implications of periodontal and other oral manifestations of systemic conditions and diseases

The standard of care is to eliminate oral infection, including periodontal disease, before initiating radiation therapy for head and neck cancers and before initialising intravenous bisphosphonate therapy. It is becoming clear that treatment of oral infections including periodontal disease before instituting such therapies may reduce serious complications.

Gingival overgrowths associated with phenytoin (dilantin) medication of patients with epilepsy or calcium channel blockers are often treated by gingivectomy and gingivoplasty.

Periodontal diseases as risk factors for systemic conditions and diseases

The evidence for periodontal disease in the causal pathway of several major chronic systemic diseases is accumulating. These include diabetes mellitus, atherosclerotic diseases, nosocomial respiratory infections, adverse pregnancy outcomes and possibly oral pharyngeal and pancreatic cancers (Table 12.2).

Diabetes

Perhaps the strongest case for causation is in diabetes, where there is evidence that those patients suffering from diabetes types 1 and 2 who also have severe periodontal disease have poorer glycaemic control (Fig. 12.1). Furthermore, treatment of periodontal disease may contribute to glycaemic control by resolving the periodontal infection in these patients with diabetes (Fig. 12.2).

These effects on systemic diseases are thought to be mainly mediated by systemic inflammation as evidenced by elevated blood levels of C-reactive protein (CRP) and other acute phase proteins, and pro-inflammatory cytokines seen in patients with periodontal disease. For example, the elevation of tumour necrosis factor α (TNF-α) and interleukin-6 (IL-6) may well contribute to insulin resistance, a central pathology process in diabetes (Fig. 12.3). In the case of diabetes, there is also evidence that those patients with diabetes who suffer from periodontal disease also have increased risk of dying from cardiovascular disease or diabetic nephropathy.

Heart disease

There is strong association evidence, that periodontal disease is associated with and precedes cardiovascular disease (Fig. 12.4). There is similar evidence of the association of periodontal disease with ischaemic stroke and peripheral artery disease. There are *in vitro* and animal studies showing that periodontal infections could be in the causal pathway through induction of systemic inflammation and the effects of bacteraemia that occur in periodontal patients (Fig. 12.5). These, in turn, are thought to contribute to atheroma formation, a central pathology in heart disease, ischaemic stroke and peripheral artery disease. Randomised controlled trials are needed to determine if treating or preventing periodontal disease will have an effect on atherosclerotic conditions.

Respiratory infections

The association between poor oral hygiene and periodontal disease in institutionalised patients with respiratory infections such as pneumonia and bronchitis is well established. Furthermore, there are several small, randomised controlled trials that show that maintaining good oral hygiene in patients in intensive care units or nursing homes will reduce the incidence of respiratory infections, many of which are fatal. The mechanism is probably colonisation of the oral cavity of institutionalised patients with poor oral hygiene by respiratory pathogens, which are aspirated.

Clinical implications

It is reasonable to treat periodontal disease in patients with diabetes, not only to save the dentition, but also to help improve glycaemic control and thereby reduce other complications of diabetes. Furthermore, the institution of oral hygiene in patients who are institutionalised – in intensive care units or nursing homes – is justified to not only improve their oral condition, but it also may have beneficial effects in preventing or reducing respiratory infections.

The relationship of periodontal disease as either a complication of systemic diseases or as a risk factor for systemic diseases or conditions provides compelling reasons for urgent periodontal care in high risk patients. It also provides reason for dentists to expand their scope of activities and participate more fully as part of the health care team. Dentists may see patients more often than physicians and can be of great assistance in the initial screening for systemic conditions as well as in motivating patients to follow not only their dental regimes, but also their medical regimes.

Key points

- Periodontal disease may be a manifestation of diabetes, leukaemia, neutrophil disorders, dermatological diseases and medication therapies
- Periodontal disease may contribute to several major chronic diseases including diabetes and its complications, atherosclerotic disease, respiratory infections and the risk for adverse pregnancy outcomes
- There is strong evidence that periodontal infections induce a systemic inflammatory response as evidenced by elevated levels of acute phase proteins and pro-inflammatory cytokines. These may contribute to insulin resistance, atheroma formation and other adverse responses
- Pilot clinical trials show that treating periodontal disease can improve glycaemic control in diabetes. Other trials show a reduction in respiratory infections in institutionalised patients and in adverse pregnancy outcomes. Large randomised trials are needed to assess the extent to which periodontal intervention will affect these systemic conditions
- These associations between periodontal disease and several major chronic diseases, which are major causes of mortality and morbidity, call for an urgency in the diagnosis, prevention and treatment of periodontal diseases.

13 Diet and periodontal diseases

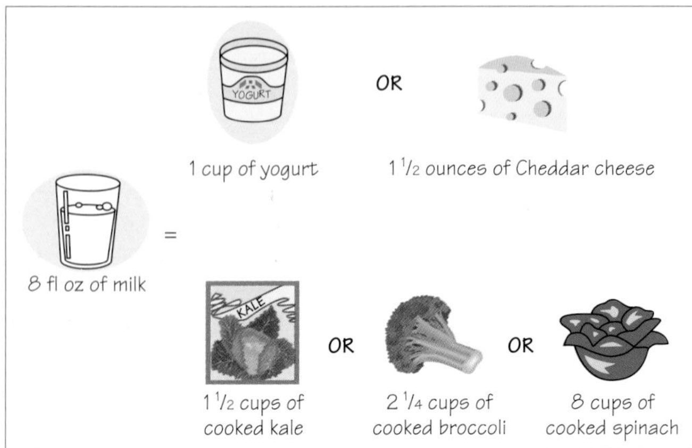

Figure 13.1 Amounts of milk and other food sources providing 300 mg of calcium (Weaver *et al.*, 1999).

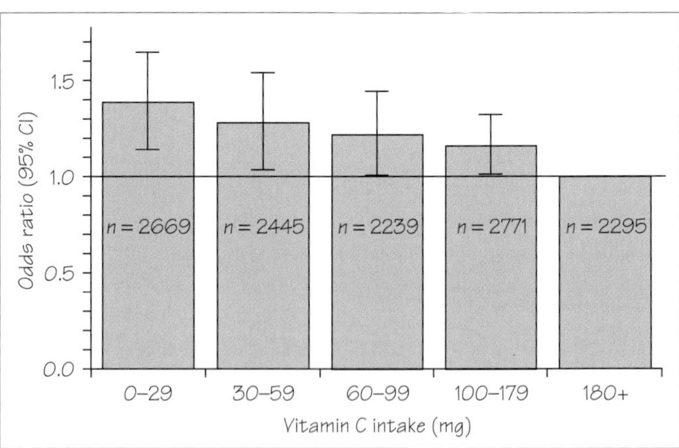

Figure 13.2 Odds ratio for periodontal disease (mean clinical attachment loss >1.5 mm) by level of dietary vitamin C intake after adjusting for age decade, gender, tobacco use, and gingival bleeding in the National Health and Nutrition Examination Survey (NHANES) III (Nishida *et al.*, 2000b). Weights provided in NHANES III data were used, and tobacco use, age decade, gender and gingival bleeding were adjusted for using multiple logistic regression. Dietary vitamin C intake was divided into five categories, and odds ratios are presented using the highest intake group as a reference. CI, confidence interval.

Tolerable upper limit = 2500 mg/day
Higher levels can result in:

- Hypercalcaemia
- Impaired kidney function
- Decreased absorption of iron, zinc, magnesium and phosphorus
- Interactions with other medications including digoxin, ciprofloxacin, tetracyclines, phenytoin and thiazide diruetics

Figure 13.3 Health risks of too much calcium.

- United Kingdom: 40 mg/day
- World Health Organisation: 45 mg/day
- Health Canada 2007: 60 mg/day
- **United States**
  - Adult male: 90 mg/day
  - Adult female: 75 mg/day
  - Smokers should take 35 mg/day more than above

Figure 13.4 Government recommended intake of vitamin C.

Table 13.1 Association of periodontal disease (mean clinical attachment loss of >1.5mm) with calcium intake in males and females of different ages after adjusting for tobacco use status and gingival bleeding in the National Health and Nutrition Examination Survey (NHANES) III (Nishida *et al.*, 2000a).

Age Range	Male	Female
20–30 years		
Odds ratio*	1.84	1.99
95% CI	1.36 – 2.48	1.34 – 2.97
P value	<0.001	<0.001
N	2727	3348
40–59 years		
Odds ratio*	1.90	1.31
95% CI	1.41 – 2.55	0.85 – 2.03
P value	<0.001	0.2401
N	1675	1863
60+ years		
Odds ratio*	1.11	1.13
95% CI	0.71 – 1.71	0.86 – 1.48
P value	0.6582	0.4037
N	1422	1384

CI, confidence interval.
* Computer software and weights provided in NHANES III data were used, and odds ratios were adjusted for tobacco use (categorized as 'never', 'former' and 'current') and gingival bleeding in multiple logistic regression.

Table 13.2 Recommended adequate intake for dietary calcium for males and females combined (Standing Committee on the Scientific Evaluation of Dietary Reference Intakes, 1997).

Age	Calcium (mg/day)	Pregnancy and lactation
0–6 months	210	N/A
7–12 months	270	N/A
1–3 years	500	N/A
4–8 years	1300	N/A
9–13 years	1300	N/A
14–18 years	1300	1300
19–50 years	1000	1000
51+ years	1200	N/A

In discussing the role of diet in periodontal disease, there are two main issues:
• The effect of diet on periodontal disease.
• The effect of tooth loss, which can impair chewing ability, leading to dietary intake changes.

The role of diet in periodontal disease

It is well known that nutritional status plays a major role in modulating the immune system, reducing inflammatory responses and maintaining tissue homeostasis. The studies of vitamin C deficiency and scurvy-associated gingivitis are well known, as are the devastating effects of severe malnutrition on the periodontium leading to diseases such as necrotising ulcerative periodontitis. In the developed world, such severe deficiencies are rare. However, inadequacies in the diet have been found to be risk factors for periodontal disease.
• One is the effect of low dietary calcium, which is common in the population today. Low dietary intake of calcium (Fig. 13.1) increases the risk for periodontal disease in women under the age of 30, and men under the age of 60 years (Table 13.1). Furthermore, calcium supplementation, especially in post-menopausal women who show osteopenia or osteoporosis, has been shown to prevent tooth loss related to periodontal disease. Direct evaluation of calcium supplementation to reduce periodontal disease, however, has not been carried out.
• There are large population studies showing that low levels of vitamin C in the diet increase the risk for periodontal disease slightly, but statistically significantly (Fig. 13.2). Large trials have not been carried out to determine if vitamin C supplementation will improve or modify periodontal disease.
• With respect to dietary protective factors, it has been shown in large epidemiological studies that increased fibre in the diet results in less periodontal disease. The mechanism is not entirely clear, but it may be that increased fibre in the diet leads to less dental plaque accumulation as well as having some nutritional effects on the periodontal tissues.
• It is proposed that hypovitaminosis D is linked to more periodontal disease as well as to other conditions as cancer, diabetes and cardiovascular disease. Again, intervention trials with vitamin D have not been carried out to determine the extent to which elevated dietary vitamin D in the diet would affect periodontal disease.

Dietary intervention in periodontal disease

Several studies have shown that dietary interventions including soya isoflavones and omega-3 fatty acids will improve periodontal status. Recent studies show that calorie restriction is associated with decreased periodontal disease, and it is not clear whether this effect is a nutritional effect or an effect on obesity which, in turn, is a risk factor for periodontal disease (Chapter 11). A recent study has shown that weight loss as well as exercise benefits the periodontal tissues.

Effects of adult tooth loss on diet

There are several studies that show that tooth loss in adults, especially if teeth are not adequately replaced, has effects on dietary intake. For example, tooth loss can lead to reduction of intake of hard to chew foods such as carrots, leaf salads, whole grains, fruits and vegetables. Large epidemiological studies have shown that an overall reduction in fibre intake as well as an increase in consumption of refined sugar and fats are associated with loss of teeth. The extent to which adequate dentures or implants improve mastication and moderate the diet is not clear. However, there are studies that show that denture wearers, if trained properly in dietary requirements, will consume a diet that is similar to those with a natural dentition.

The effects of high levels of refined sugar in the diet on dental caries are well known. Periodontal patients often suffer from gingival recession, exposing roots to the cariogenic microflora, and, in these patients, a diet rich in refined sugar has been shown to increase root surface caries. This is especially true in individuals who experience a dry mouth, or who have decreased salivary flow associated with medications or smoking.

The role of diet in healing after periodontal treatment

The importance of adequate diet in healing after periodontal or implant surgical procedures is often overlooked. Dietary intake may be transiently compromised by difficulty in chewing associated with post-operative pain and discomfort. Adequate nutrition should be dealt with by recommending soft foods that contain the macro- and micronutrients necessary for proper nutrition in the weeks after surgery.

Recommendations for dental patients

As part of the health care team, it is reasonable for dentists to advise patients on their diet, especially since there is clear evidence that refined sugars lead to increased coronal and root surface caries. There also is evidence that obesity, as well as calcium and vitamin C deficiency, contribute to the risk for periodontal disease. The well known benefits of adequate dietary calcium and weight control as part of the overall health of the patient are important also in the justification for dental professionals to assist their medical colleagues in counselling patients on adequate nutrition.

Therefore, the following recommendations are made for the management of diet in adult dental patients:
• Reduced intake of refined sugars, especially in those who have gingival recession and are prone to caries. This is also important in those who suffer from xerostomia associated with smoking or medications that reduce salivary flow.
• Proper intake of calcium. If dietary calcium is not at or near the recommended daily allowance (RDA) for the patient, calcium supplementation to bring them to the RDA should be recommended (Table 13.2; Figs 13.3, 13.4).
• Weight reduction for those who are overweight or obese, since obesity, especially visceral adiposity, is a risk factor for periodontal disease. Weight reduction may improve periodontal health, and it will clearly decrease the risk for several other chronic diseases such as diabetes and cardiovascular disease and hence will contribute to the overall health of the patient.
• Patients should include adequate fibre in the diet from fruits, vegetables and whole grains. The dentist should strive to provide an adequate dentition so that chewing these hard foods is possible.

Key points

• Diet may affect periodontal tissues, and tooth loss may affect diet
• There is evidence to suggest that inadequate dietary calcium and vitamin C levels leads to more periodontal disease
• Studies show that dietary calcium supplementation in post-menopausal women prevents tooth loss
• Tooth loss is associated with decreased dietary intake of fibre, and increased intake of refined sugars and fats. Tooth replacement reverses these effects
• It is recommended that dentists counsel their patients on dietary calcium, reduced intake of refined sugars and overall weight control

14 Local risk factors for periodontal diseases

VIII. Developmental or acquired deformities and conditions
A. Localised tooth-related factors that modify or predispose to plaque-induced gingival diseases/periodontitis
1. Tooth anatomical factors
2. Dental restorations/appliances
3. Root fractures
4. Cervical root resorption and cemental tears

The 1999 International Workshop for the Classification of Periodontal Diseases and Conditions (Armitage, 1999) is presented fully in Chapter 2. Above is section VIII.A from this classification on localised tooth-related factors that are associated with periodontal or gingival conditions. In addition to these there are a number of other factors that can be considered as local to sites or specific teeth which can result in a greater risk of periodontal diseases or that can modify the course of periodontal disease (discussed in this chapter).

Figure 14.1 Section VIII.A from the classification of periodontal diseases and conditions.

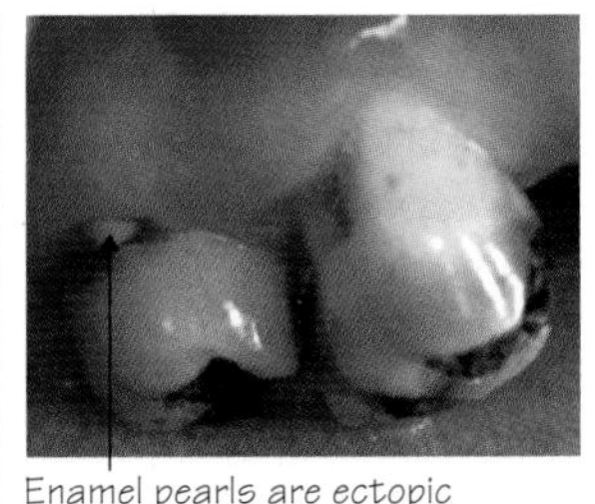

Enamel pearls are ectopic deposits of enamel that lie apical to the normal cement-enamel junction

Figure 14.2 An enamel pearl.

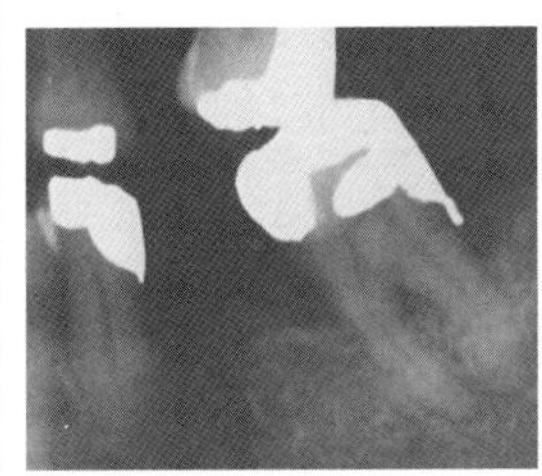

Overhanging restoration margins are seen on LL5 and particularly on the distal surface of LL7.

Figure 14.3 Overhanging restoration margins.

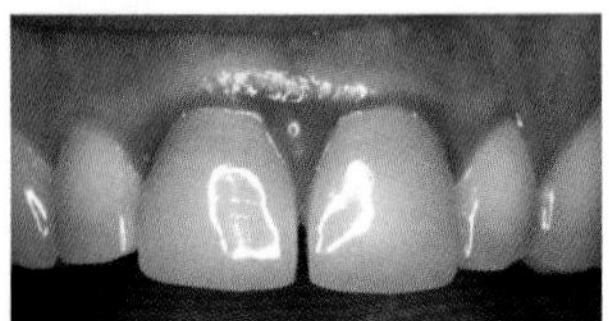

The subgingival crown margins on UR1 and UL1 are associated with gingival inflammation.

Figure 14.4 Subgingival crown margins.

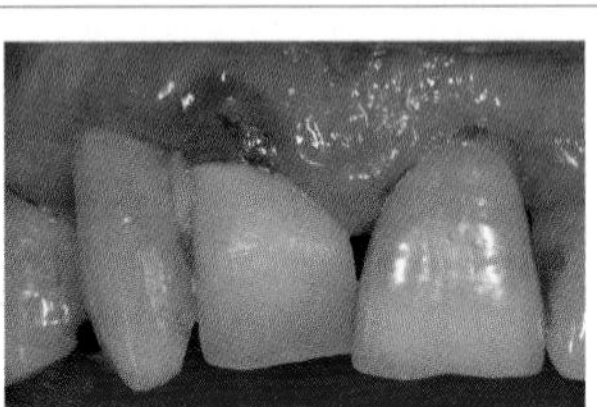

A crown on UR2 tries to mimic the appearance of a central incisor leading to an overbuilt mesial contour, plaque retention and gingival inflammation. Subgingival calculus can be seen for instance at the gingival margin of UL1, which acts as a plaque retention factor.

Figure 14.5 An overcontoured crown and subgingival calculus.

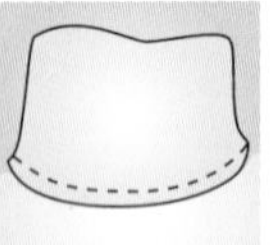

- Matrix bands and wedges should be used when placing plastic restorations
- Contact areas should allow for the normal gingival papilla
- Supragingival margins are to be preferred where possible
- Where aesthetics are of concern margins should be placed no more than 0.5 mm into the gingival crevice
- Sufficient tooth reduction is required to avoid overbuilt crowns
- A good impression technique with use of gingival retraction cord should be used for indirect restorations
  – soft tissue injury can occur from placement of gingival retraction cords but healing is generally rapid if the gingivae are initially healthy
- Excess cement should be removed on the placement of indirect restorations
- Extracoronal restorations (and bridge pontics) should be contoured to facilitate plaque control and allow for the normal dimensions of the gingival tissues

Figure 14.6 Minimising the periodontal consequences of restorative treatment.

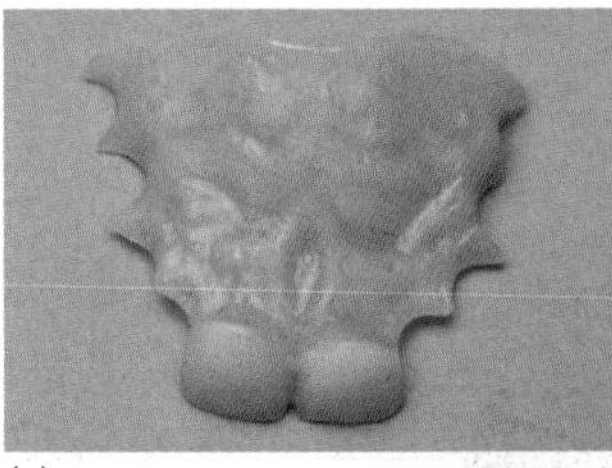

(a)

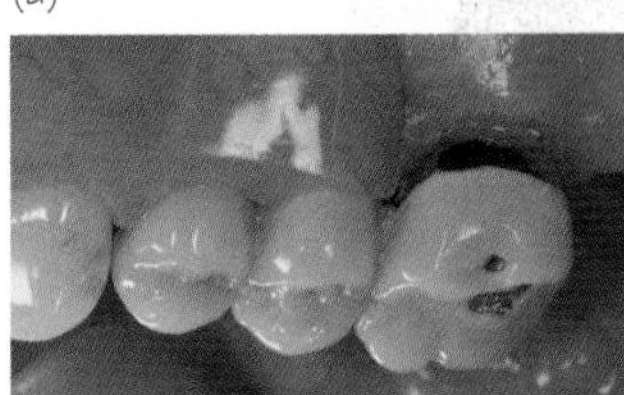

(b)

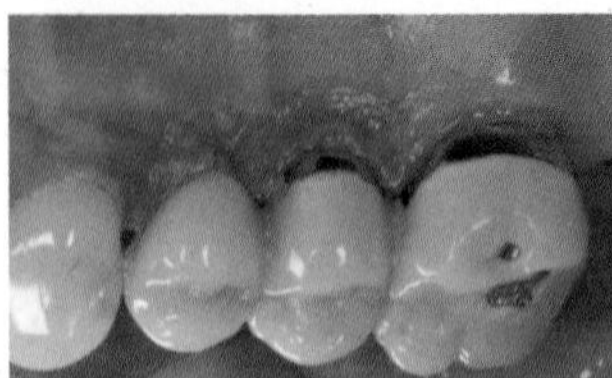

(c)

Figure 14.7 (a) Poorly designed acrylic partial denture with gingival coverage (shown out of the mouth). (b) Partial denture *in situ*; interproximal plaque is visible. (c) Following removal of the denture, the gingivae can be seen to be reddened and inflamed.

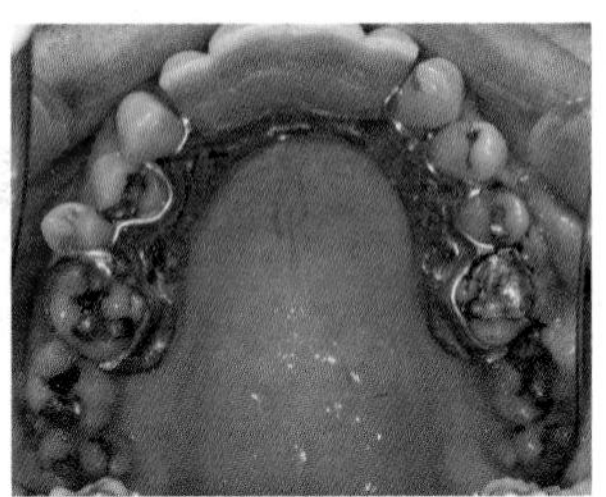

This upper cobalt chromium partial denture covers the palatal gingival margins which augments its role as a plaque retention factor.

Figure 14.8 Partial denture with extensive gingival coverage.

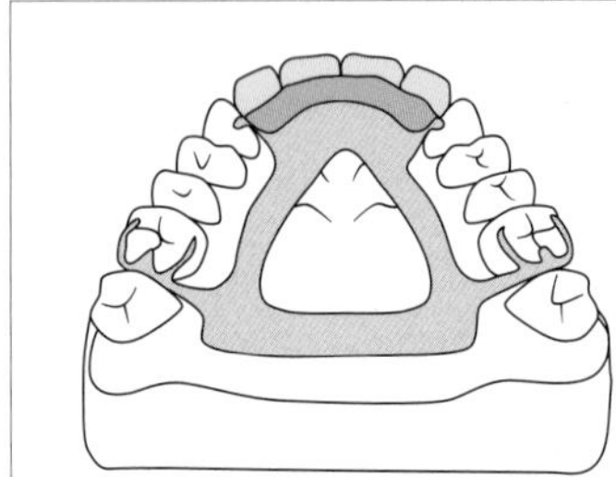

- Denture should be well supported with appropriate use of rest seats
- 3 mm clearance of the gingival margins should be provided where possible
- Denture design should be kept simple
- Partial dentures should be adequately maintained long term

Figure 14.9 Minimising the periodontal consequences of providing a partial denture.

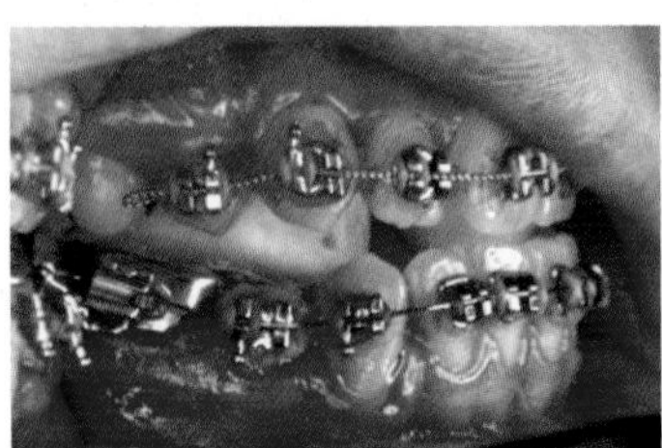

Figure 14.10 Orthodontic appliance acting as a plaque retention factor.

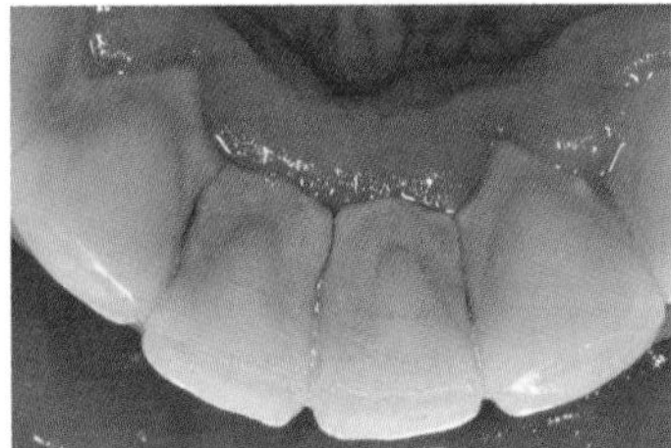

Figure 14.11 Supragingival calculus acting as a local plaque retention factor.

Local risk factors can increase the risk of development and progression of periodontal disease by acting as plaque retention factors. Local factors should be identified when carrying out a thorough dental examination of the patient and their removal or modification where possible should be included in the patient's management.

Figure 14.1 shows an extract from the 1999 International Workshop Classification of Periodontal Diseases and Conditions (Armitage, 1999) (Chapter 2). A number of additional factors that can be considered as local to sites or specific teeth are also discussed in this chapter.

Local risk factors for periodontal diseases include the following:

- Anatomical factors.
- Restorations.
- Removable partial dentures.
- Orthodontic appliances.
- Root fractures and cervical root resorption.
- Calculus.
- Local trauma.
- Frenal attachments.
- Mouth breathing and lack of lip seal.

Anatomical factors

A number of anatomical variations may be associated with localised gingivitis and attachment loss:

- Enamel pearls or projections (Fig. 14.2).
- Cemental tears occur either within the cementum layer or as full thickness separation of the cementum from the dentine.
- Root grooves are most commonly seen palatally on the upper lateral incisors.
- Furcation lesions can act to retain plaque, making sites harder to maintain.
- Untreated periodontal pockets and post-treatment residual pockets harbour subgingival plaque.

Tooth position

- Oral hygiene measures can be harder to implement where teeth are crowded with imbrication, rotations or marked angulation.
- Some malocclusions can cause direct soft tissue trauma (e.g. occlusion of the upper incisors on the lower labial gingivae in a marked class II division 2 malocclusion).
- Some studies have shown an association between tooth malalignment and loss of periodontal support.
- Open contacts are associated with increased pocketing and loss of attachment.

Restorations

- Restoration margins can be associated with gingivitis and attachment loss related to:
  - roughness of the restorative material and at the tooth–restoration interface due to increased plaque retention;
  - overhanging restorative material (Fig. 14.3);
  - marginal discrepancies;
  - exposed cement margins.
- Subgingival margins are potentially more damaging than supragingival ones and are often associated with gingival inflammation (Fig. 14.4).
- Overcontoured crowns are often associated with increased gingival inflammation (Fig. 14.5).

Restorations must be placed with great care to avoid the creation of local risk factors for periodontal disease (Fig. 14.6).

Removable partial dentures

Removable partial dentures (RPDs) can enhance plaque accumulation and increase the risk of periodontal diseases (Figs 14.7, 14.8). Proximal surfaces are most at risk. Factors to be considered to minimise the periodontal consequences of providing RPDs are shown in Fig. 14.9.

Orthodontic appliances

Fixed and removable orthodontic appliances may be worn for several years and can potentially have reversible or irreversible effects on the periodontal tissues (see Chapter 29). Aspects to be aware of with the wearing of orthodontic appliances are:

- Access to interdental cleaning is usually compromised leading to plaque accumulation.
- Components of the orthodontic appliances, especially bands, can lie close to the gingival margin leading to plaque accumulation (Fig. 14.10).
- Good oral hygiene will minimise the effect on periodontal tissues.
- Coronal attachment loss can occur during orthodontic treatment (0.05–0.3 mm annually).

Root fractures and cervical root resorption

Vertical root fractures can be associated with periodontal lesions. Periodontal breakdown can occur at the site of cervical external root resorption where there is a communication with the oral environment.

Calculus

Supragingival and subgingival calculus act as local plaque retention factors (Figs 14.5, 14.11). The surfaces of the calculus offer large irregular areas harbouring plaque close to the gingival margins. These sites are also relatively sheltered from host defences. Much of periodontal therapy is directed at calculus detection and removal.

Local trauma

This can be associated with overzealous tooth brushing or habits such as direct picking of the gingivae with a fingernail. The results may be gingival recession, attachment loss and bone loss.

Frenal attachments

A prominent frenum can act as a local plaque retention factor reducing access for the patient's oral hygiene measures. Frenal pull acting directly on the gingival margin has been described as a factor in the development of gingival recession but the associated increased plaque retention may be of greater aetiological significance.

Mouth breathing and lack of lip seal

Mouth breathing and a lack of lip seal at rest can lead to dehydration of the oral tissues and higher levels of dental plaque. This results in greater gingivitis in the associated anterior region.

Key points

- Local factors that can act as risk factors for periodontal diseases are:
  - anatomical factors
  - restorations
  - removable partial dentures
  - orthodontic appliances
  - root fractures and cervical root resorption
  - calculus
  - local trauma
  - frenal attachments
  - mouth breathing and lack of lip seal
- Local factors act by increasing plaque retention
- Local factors may need to be prevented, modified or eliminated where possible

15 Occlusion and periodontal diseases

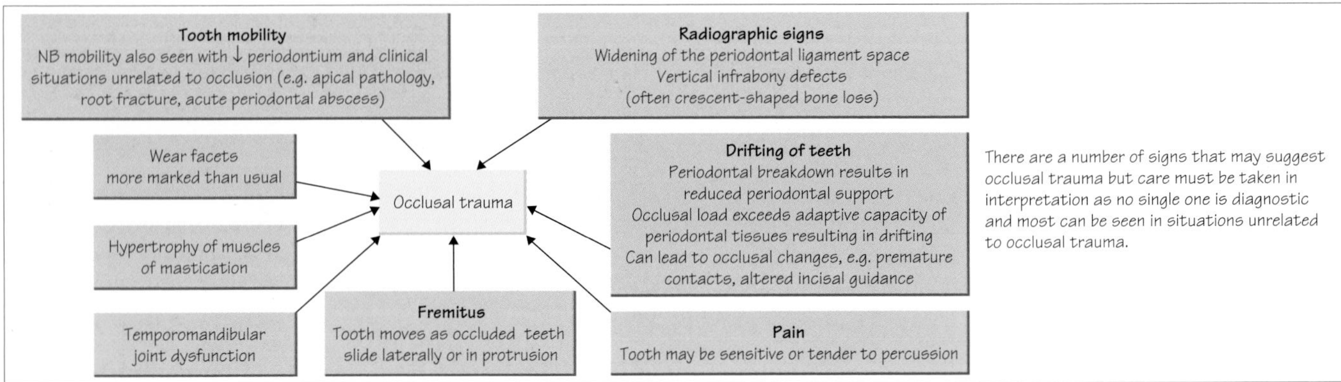

Figure 15.1 Diagnosis of occlusal trauma.

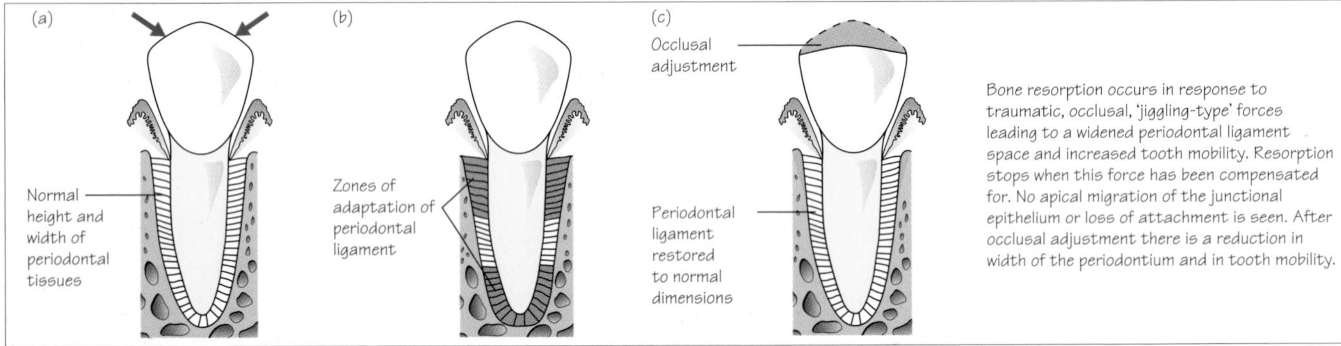

Figure 15.2 Tooth with healthy periodontal tissues: (a) prior to application of traumatic alternate mesial and distal occlusal forces, (b) following application of traumatic occlusal forces, and (c) following occlusal adjustment. From Lindhe *et al.* (2008).

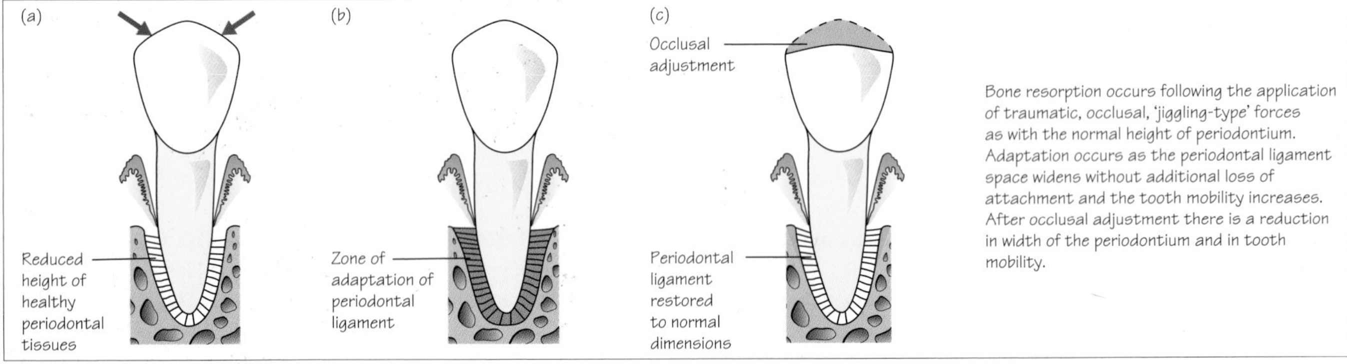

Figure 15.3 Tooth with reduced height of healthy periodontal tissues: (a) prior to application of traumatic occlusal forces, (b) following application of traumatic occlusal forces, and (c) following occlusal adjustment. From Lindhe *et al.* (2008).

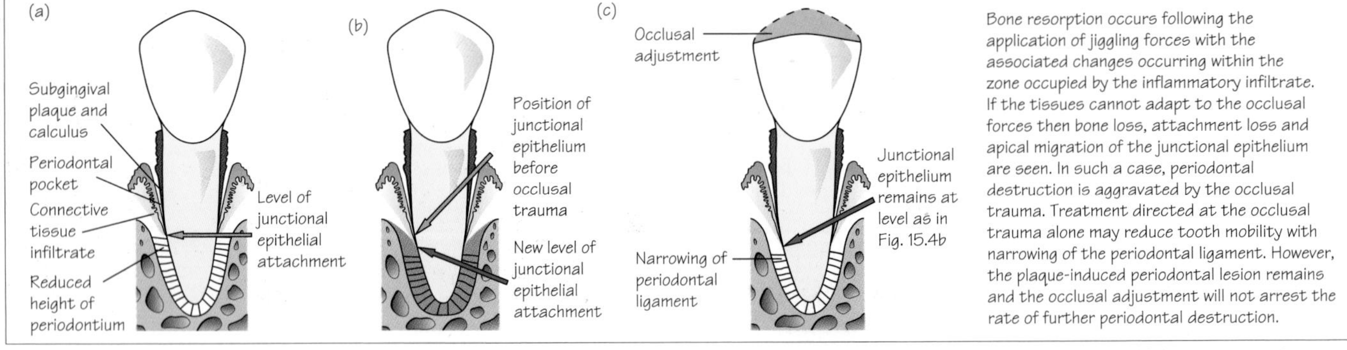

Figure 15.4 Tooth with periodontal disease: (a) prior to application of traumatic occlusal forces, (b) following application of traumatic occlusal forces, and (c) following occlusal adjustment. From Lindhe *et al.* (2008).

The periodontium attaches the tooth to the alveolar bone and dissipates the forces of occlusion to the surrounding tissues. If the occlusal load is abnormally high or the periodontium is reduced in height due to periodontal disease, tissue changes may be seen (Fig. 15.1) (Lindhe *et al.* 2008).

Tissue changes in response to occlusal load

Experiments in beagle dogs designed to mimic prolonged traumatic occlusion by applying alternate mesial and distal 'jiggling-type' trauma to a tooth (Lindhe & Ericsson, 1982) have shown the following:

- A healthy periodontium remodels in response to the occlusal forces.
- The periodontal ligament space widens if:
  - the periodontium is of normal height (Fig. 15.2a, b);
  - the periodontium is of reduced height due to past periodontal disease (Fig. 15.3a, b).
- The tooth shows non-progressive increased mobility.
- The periodontal ligament returns to its normal width following occlusal adjustment (Figs 15.2c, 15.3c).

It can be concluded from this that occlusal trauma does not initiate periodontal destruction.

When jiggling-type trauma is applied to a tooth with plaque-associated periodontal disease (Fig. 15.4a):

- There is remodelling of the periodontium.

And either:

- Remodelling stops if the periodontium can adapt to the forces.
- The tooth shows non-progressive increased mobility but no further loss of attachment.

Or:

- Remodelling may continue if the periodontium cannot adapt to the forces (Fig. 15.4b).
- The tooth may show progressive mobility and attachment loss with trauma from occlusion acting as a co-factor in periodontal destruction.
- Removal of the occlusal trauma alone may reduce tooth mobility but it will not stop the rate of further periodontal breakdown (Fig. 15.4c).

Similar work by another research group in monkeys found that there was no difference in the connective tissue attachment loss between animals with periodontitis alone and those with periodontitis and excessive occlusal forces; so occlusal trauma was not a co-factor in periodontal destruction (Polson & Zander, 1983). These conflicting results highlight the difficulties in using animal models and applying results to humans.

Nonetheless, both research groups found that the control of plaque in a lesion with periodontitis and occlusal trauma led to gains in attachment and bone levels but removal of the occlusal trauma had little effect.

The conclusion was that the successful treatment of periodontal disease will arrest periodontal destruction even if occlusal trauma persists.

Occlusal analysis

Having identified potential occlusal interferences and trauma, occlusal analysis is carried out to assess the occlusion clinically and on study models. The models should be mounted on a semi-adjustable articulator, usually in the retruded contact position as this position is reproducible. The intercuspal position is the position of maximum interdigitation and end point of functional movement but it may have been reached by deviated mandibular closure compensating for occlusal disharmonies. The teeth should be examined for wear facets and tooth surface loss, tooth loss, rotations, drifting and tilting. The lateral and incisal guidance should be reviewed. Clinically the muscles of mastication and temporamandibular joints should be assessed.

Occlusal adjustment

The occlusion may be altered by selective grinding, restorative treatment or orthodontics. Detailed assessment of the occlusion is required and premature contacts identified. Any occlusal modifications that are considered should be carried out on a duplicate set of articulated models to fully investigate the consequences. Larger changes can be achieved by restorative or orthodontic means.

Management of tooth mobility

Treatment of periodontal disease

One of the signs of periodontal disease is tooth mobility in association with loss of the supporting tissues. Periodontal therapy should be instituted and following treatment mobile teeth may respond with a reduction in mobility due largely to the reduction in inflammation of the supporting tissues. However, where significant support has been lost the tooth is still likely to exhibit some mobility. Where mobility is not progressive or does not interfere with function this mobility is generally acceptable to the patient.

Splinting

If function is compromised or the mobility is progressive, splinting can be considered. A mobile tooth can be splinted to adjacent teeth using composite resin alone or with an orthodontic wire. Such a splint is likely to be temporary, with debonding common. The composite also acts as a plaque retention factor, particularly across the interdental spaces, and needs excellent plaque control to avoid worsening the periodontal condition.

Permanent splinting can be achieved by the construction of a removable splint or by linked crowns as described by Lindhe and Nyman (1979). Such restorations require significant tooth preparation and are technically demanding.

For a very mobile tooth, consideration should be given to elective replacement. A conservative replacement by the provision of a cantilevered adhesive bridge or immediate partial denture may be preferable to attempting to retain a compromised tooth.

Key points

- The periodontal tissues respond and adapt to occlusal loading even when there is reduced periodontal support following periodontal disease
- Occlusal forces cannot initiate periodontal breakdown
- The successful treatment of periodontal disease will arrest destruction even if occlusal trauma persists
- Where forces are too great for adaptation, teeth may become mobile or drift
- Occlusal analysis has a role in identifying occlusal interferences
- Occlusal adjustments can be made by selective grinding, restorative treatment or orthodontics
- Tooth mobility is seen in teeth with reduced periodontal support resulting from periodontal disease
- Splinting can be used when tooth mobility is progressive or compromising function but has limitations

16 Periodontal history, examination and diagnosis

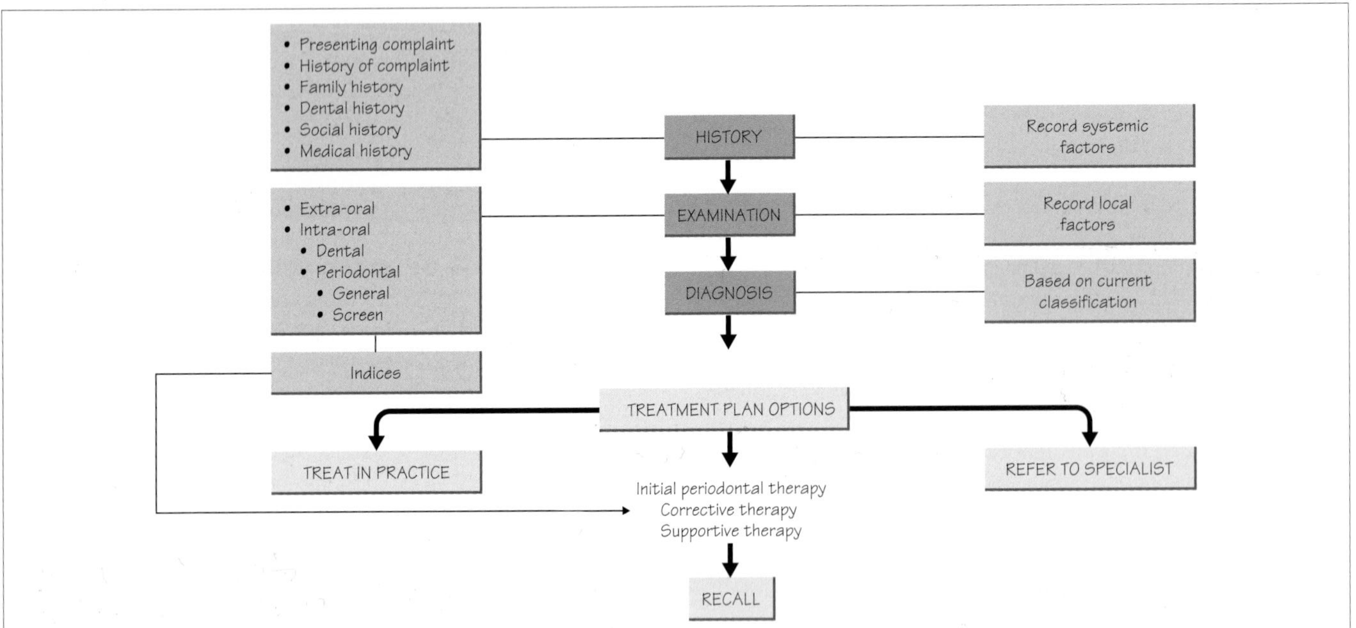

Figure 16.1 Steps in taking a periodontal history, examination and diagnosis.

- Qualitative assessment of oral hygiene and presence of supragingival calculus deposits
- Presence of obvious
  - gingival inflammation, swelling, loss of contour
  - gingival recession
  - suppuration
- Occlusal problems, drifting / tooth migration and related aesthetic problems
- Identification of local periodontal risk factors

Figure 16.2 Points a general description of a periodontal condition should cover.

- Probing pocket depths in millimetres
  - from gingival margin to base of pocket
- Clinical attachment loss in millimetres
  - from cement–enamel junction to base of pocket
- Bleeding on probing within 10–15 seconds of probing
- Suppuration on gentle palpation of tissues or following probing
- Furcation using codes 1, 2, 3
- Recession in millimetres
  - from cement–enamel junction to gingival margin
- Mobility using codes I, II, III

Figure 16.3 A detailed examination of periodontal tissues and recording of periodontal indices.

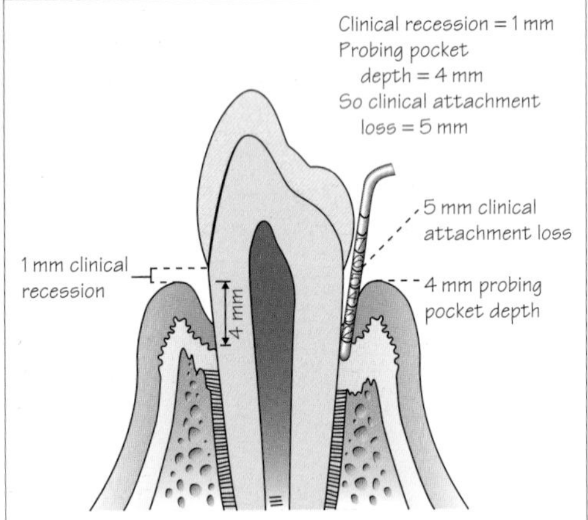

Figure 16.4 Diagram of probing pocket depth, recession and clinical attachment loss.

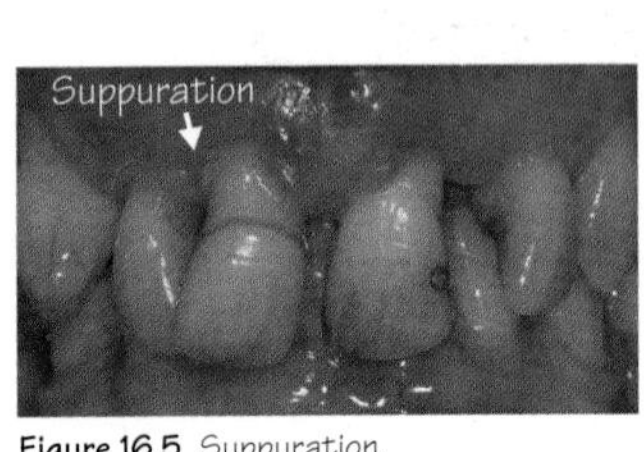

Figure 16.5 Suppuration.

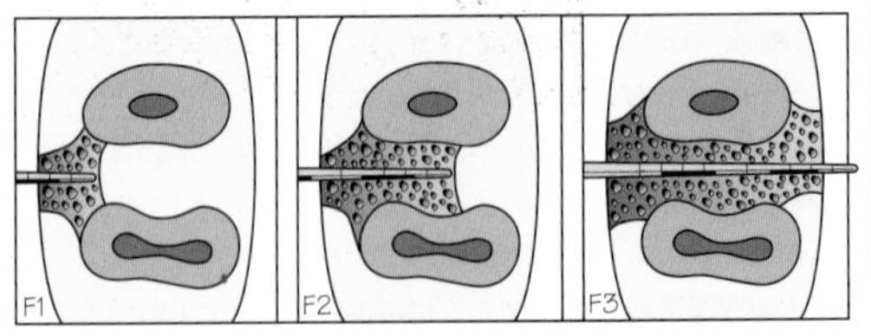

The probe is inserted between the roots of a multi-rooted tooth. A class 1 involvement (F1) is where a probe can be inserted less than 3 mm between the roots. A class 2 involvement (F2) penetrates more than 3 mm but not fully through the furcation, and a class 3 (F3) involvement extends completely between the roots.

Figure 16.6 Classification of furcation involvement.

Handles of two instruments placed on tooth and mobility graded according to movement in horizontal (buccolingual) and vertical direction:

- Grade I = 0.2–1 mm movement in horizontal direction
- Grade II = more than 1 mm movement in horizontal direction
- Grade III = more than 1 mm movement in horizontal direction + vertical movement

Figure 16.7 Mobility.

Features of periodontal significance to note:

- Degree and pattern of bone loss (horizontal or vertical)
- Progression of bone loss (serial radiographs)
- Subgingival calculus
- Overhanging restoration margins or deficiencies
- Furcation defects
- Periodontal–endodontic lesions
- Widened periodontal ligament space
- Root morphology

Features of dental significance to note:

- Teeth present
- Caries, recurrent caries, root caries
- Periapical radiolucencies
- Root fractures
- Root resorption
- Retained roots
- Impacted or unerupted teeth
- Cysts
- Other pathology affecting bone, temporomandibular joint or sinuses

Figure 16.8 Radiographic assessment.

The history and examination should provide relevant information to enable the clinician to formulate a clinical diagnosis and treatment plan (Fig. 16.1).

Periodontal history

Eliciting a good history requires a structured approach, good communication skills and building up a rapport with the patient. The history for a patient presenting for a periodontal assessment should include details of:

1 *Presenting complaint*:
• If there is not a complaint, the reason for attendance should be noted.
• If there are other dental complaints these should also be noted.

2 *History of complaint/reason for attendance*: the onset, duration, severity and any triggers of the presenting complaint should be noted.

3 *Family history* of periodontal problems or early tooth loss.

4 *Previous dental history*:
• Past experience and the nature of dental work including restorative, prosthodontic and orthodontic treatment should be noted and the reason for any extractions should be sought.
• A record should be made of any previous periodontal treatment, whether plaque control advice has been given and what type.
• The patient should be asked about any adverse reaction or difficulties accepting local analgesia.
• The pattern of attendance for dental treatment (regular or irregular) should be noted, which may indicate compliance.

5 *Social history*: the social history should include a summary of any personal circumstances that may influence dental management or provision of treatment:
• Availability for treatment.
• How, and how often, tooth brushing is carried out and whether interdental aids are used.
• Tobacco smoking history (how many cigarettes smoked, for how many years, if tried to stop/interested in stopping); also smokeless tobacco habits.
• Alcohol consumption and number of units.
• Dietary factors relevant to caries risk, e.g. frequency of consuming sucrose-containing snacks or carbonated sucrose-containing drinks.

6 *Medical history*:
• A full medical history should be taken systematically, noting any relevant points. This permits the identification of patients who may:
  • be at risk from receiving a periodontal examination/treatment (e.g. on anticoagulants and needing INR (international normalised ratio) prior to treatment to avoid excessive bleeding);
  • pose an infection risk to the dental professional/other patients (e.g. carrier of blood-borne viruses human immunodeficiency virus, hepatitis B or C); universal cross-infection control is implicit;
  • have systemic risk factors for periodontal diseases (e.g. poorly controlled diabetes).
• If there is uncertainty about any drugs in the UK, the *British National Formulary* (http://www.bnf.org/bnf/) can be consulted.
• The medical history should be checked and updated every visit.

7 *Informed consent* needs to be obtained from the patient before proceeding with the subsequent periodontal management.

Periodontal examination

The dental examination begins with an extra-oral examination followed by an intra-oral examination of the soft and hard tissues, occlusion and any fixed or removable prostheses. The periodontal examination should be an integral component of the dental examination and can be considered in three parts:

1 General description of the periodontal condition (Fig. 16.2).
2 Periodontal screening using the Basic Periodontal Examination (UK, Europe) or Periodontal Screening and Recording (USA) (Chapter 17).
3 Detailed examination of the periodontal tissues and recording of periodontal indices (Fig. 16.3):
• Probing pocket depths, clinical attachment loss and recession (Fig. 16.4).
• Bleeding on probing.
• Suppuration (Fig. 16.5).
• Furcation (Fig. 16.6).
• Mobility (Fig. 16.7).

These indices are usually measured on six sites per tooth (mesiobuccal, buccal, distobuccal, mesiolingual, mid-lingual, distolingual) and recorded on a periodontal chart. There is no universally accepted periodontal chart, indeed many versions of charts exist.

Time may not permit the detailed periodontal indices to be examined at the same visit as the history and examination, so they are often recorded at the start of the initial therapy.

Special tests

In order to reach a diagnosis, additional information may be needed:
• Radiographs.
• Vitality tests.
• Other special tests.

Radiographs

Periapical radiographs, horizontal bitewings, vertical bitewings, panoramic views or combinations of these may be suitable for periodontal assessment but should only be taken when they are clinically justified and would change the management or prognosis of the patient (Chapter 18). The key findings of the radiographic examination must be concisely recorded in the notes (Fig. 16.8).

Vitality tests

Pulpal vitality can be tested by thermal (primarily cold) stimuli or electric pulp testers, and together with radiographic assessment may be useful in determining management options such as root canal therapy.

Other special tests

Other tests may include blood tests, e.g. full haematological screen, blood glucose levels, INR or microbiological plaque sampling.

Diagnosis

The diagnosis is dependent on the findings from the history and examination and should include the periodontal diagnosis based on the current classification and also any dental condition that needs management (Chapter 2).

Following the diagnosis, the treatment plan can be drawn up and agreed with the patient's consent.

Key points

• History taking requires a structured approach and good communication skills
• Periodontal examination is an integral part of the dental examination and comprises: general assessment of the periodontium, periodontal screening and detailed periodontal indices
• Periodontal diagnosis is based on classification and may need special tests; other dental diagnoses should also be made

17 Periodontal screening

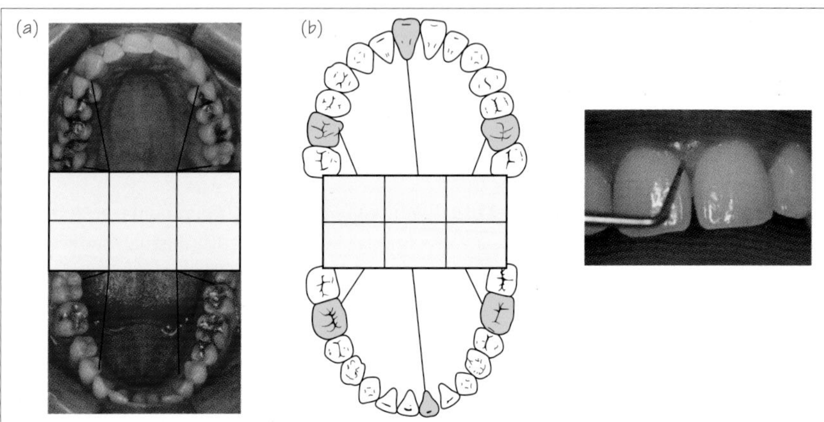

Figure 17.1 (a) Sextants and grid for recording BPE in adults. (b) Index teeth highlighted in yellow on UR6, UR1, UL6, LL6, LL1 and LR6 for recording BPE in teenagers and children.

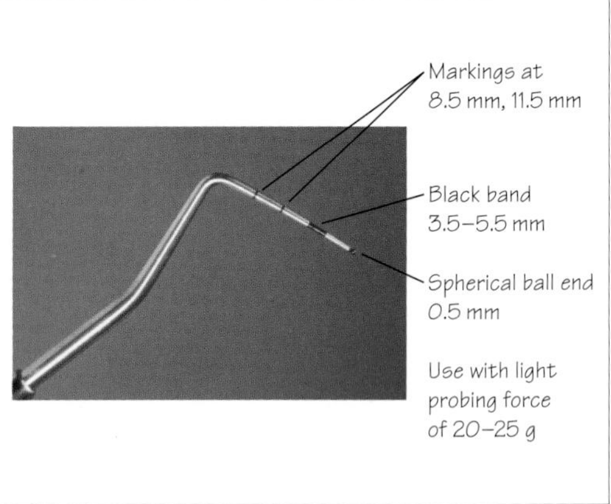

Figure 17.2 Features of the probe used for periodontal screening using BPE.

BPE code	Criteria
0	Healthy periodontal tissues No bleeding after gentle probing
1	Bleeding after gentle probing Black band remains completely visible above gingival margin No calculus or defective margins detected
2	Supragingival and/or subgingival calculus and/or other plaque retention factor Black band remains completely visible above gingival margin
3	Shallow pocket (4 or 5 mm) Black band partially visible in the deepest pocket in the sextant
4	Deep pocket (6 mm or more) Black band disappears in the pocket
*	Furcation involvement Recession + probing depth = 7 mm or more

Figure 17.3 BPE codes and criteria.

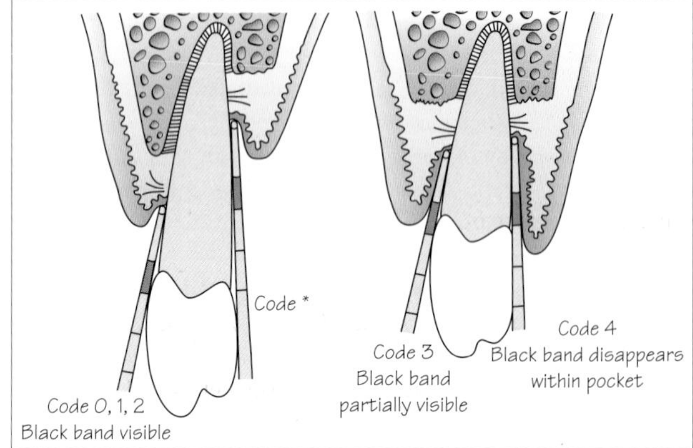

Figure 17.4 Use of probe and codes for BPE.
Code * Recession and probing depth = 7 mm or more.

Healthy

0	0	0
0	0	0

Gingivitis

1	1	1
1	2	1

Periodontitis – early to moderate

3	3	3
3	2	3

Periodontitis – severe

4	4	4
4	4	4

Figure 17.5 Examples of BPE codes for various periodontal diagnoses.

BPE code	Management options
0	Appropriate preventive care
1	Chart gingival bleeding. Disclose and chart plaque. Oral hygiene instruction. Prophylaxis
2	Chart gingival bleeding. Disclose and chart plaque. Oral hygiene instruction. Remove defective margins, plaque retention factors. Scale and prophylaxis
3	Manage as for code 2 plus record probing depths and bleeding on probing in code 3 sextant(s). Treatment will take longer
4	Full periodontal charts. Oral hygiene instruction. Remove defective margins, plaque retention factors. Scale, prophylaxis and root surface instrumentation as appropriate. Consider referral to specialist
* With 0, 1, 2	As for code 0, 1, 2 above, plus periodontal charts of furcation and/or recession and treat as appropriate. Consider referral
* With 3, 4	Full periodontal charts. Scale, prophylaxis and root surface instrumentation as appropriate. Consider referral to specialist

Figure 17.6 Management options for BPE codes.

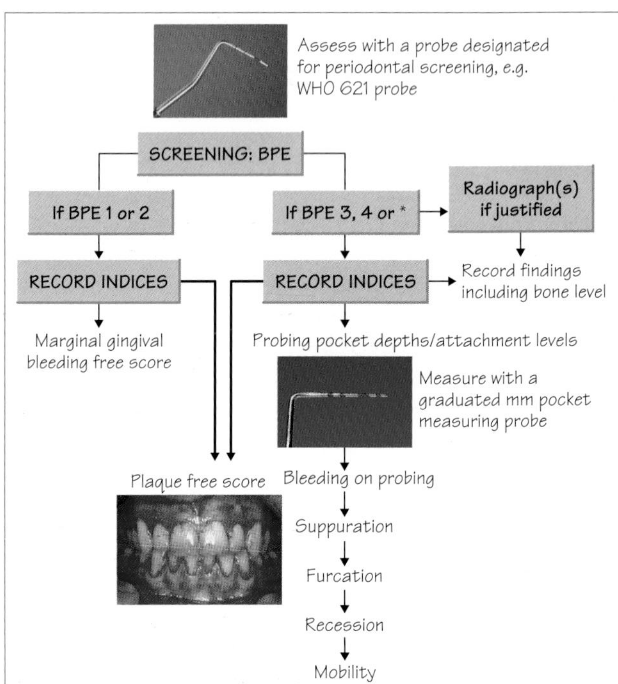

Figure 17.7 Suggested periodontal indices to use for BPE codes.

Periodontal screening provides a quick and easy method of detecting periodontal disease so that appropriate treatment and patient education can be started at the earliest opportunity. In the United Kingdom, periodontal screening has been recommended for use in general dental practice by the British Society of Periodontology since 1986. The system initially employed was the Community Periodontal Index of Treatment Needs (CPITN) but this has since been reconfigured for use in individual patients as the Basic Periodontal Examination (BPE). It is also used in Europe. The equivalent system in the United States of America is Periodontal Screening and Recording (PSR), which was introduced by the American Dental Association and the American Academy of Periodontology into general dental practice in 1992.

Why use periodontal screening

- It is a simple, rapid and cost-effective method of assessing patients for periodontal diseases.
- It is comfortably tolerated.
- Periodontal screening summarises the necessary information with minimal documentation.
- It helps determine patients who would benefit from a more detailed periodontal examination and who may require more complex periodontal therapy.
- It helps avoid dento-legal problems when used as recommended for screening, recording and further evaluations.
- In children and adolescents its use takes less time and is better accepted than full probing with a graduated probe and research has shown no differences in diagnosis and clinical management.

Limitations of periodontal screening

- It is not intended as a replacement for the full periodontal examination/periodontal indices.
- It is not able to signify the extent of periodontal involvement.
- Periodontal screening does not record plaque levels or details of attachment loss/recession.
- It is not suitable to monitor the periodontal status or response to treatment.

Who to screen

- All new patients.
- All recall patients as an integral part of a routine dental examination.

How to screen using the BPE

Sextants/index teeth

In adults, the mouth is divided into sextants (Fig. 17.1a). At least two teeth (or implants) must be present in a sextant for it to be scored, otherwise the single tooth/implant should be included in the score for the neighbouring sextant (www.bsperio.org.uk).

In teenagers and children, following full eruption of the teeth, screening can be undertaken on the index teeth: all four first permanent molars plus the maxillary right central incisor and mandibular left central incisor (Fig. 17.1b) (Clerehugh, 2008).

Probe

To be suitable for periodontal screening, a number of features should be present, based on the original WHO 621 probe devised for the CPITN (Fig. 17.2):

- A 0.5 mm spherical ball tip to aid detection of subgingival calculus deposits and limit penetration at the base of the pocket.
- A black band at 3.5–5.5 mm to delineate the normal sulci (<3.5 mm) and periodontal pockets (>3.5 mm).
- Sometimes additional marks at 8.5 and 11.5 mm are present on the 'C-type' probe version for clinical use.
- Lightweight.
- Recommended probing force of 20–25 g (0.20–0.25 N).

Recording BPE

The probe should be gently walked around all the teeth in each sextant in adults, or around the index teeth in children/teenagers, covering six sites per tooth: distobuccal; mid-buccal; mesiobuccal; distolingual/palatal; mid-lingual/palatal; mesiolingual/palatal.

This should take no more than 2–3 minutes in adults, and even less time in children and teenagers.

What to record for the BPE

The screening procedure assigns codes 0, 1, 2, 3, 4 or * according to the presence or absence of bleeding after gentle probing; supragingival or subgingival calculus, defective restoration margins or other plaque retention factors; shallow pockets (4 or 5 mm); deep pockets (6 mm or more); and furcation involvement or extensive recession (Figs 17.3, 17.4).

Adults

The worst finding in each sextant is recorded in a six box grid (Fig. 17.1a).

Teenagers and children

The worst finding around each index tooth is recorded in a six box grid (Fig. 17.1b). Only codes 0, 1 or 2 should be determined up to the age of 11 years because of the likelihood of false pockets associated with newly erupting teeth. However, if the black band disappears into any unusually deep pockets, then further periodontal investigation is required, irrespective of age. In adolescents aged 12 years or over, the full range of codes can be used on the index teeth to facilitate early detection of periodontal pockets.

How to use the screening information

- To assist in reaching a basic periodontal diagnosis such as gingivitis or periodontitis (Fig. 17.5), along with other information from the history and examination.
- To assist in formulating a treatment plan or decision to refer to a periodontal specialist (Fig. 17.6).
- To determine whether further periodontal indices are indicated (Fig. 17.7), also if special tests such as radiographs may be required.

Key points

- Screening provides a simple, rapid method of assessing a patient's periodontal condition using:
  - Basic Periodontal Examination (BPE) in UK and Europe
  - Periodontal Screening and Recording (PSR) in the USA
- The mouth is divided into sextants in adults or index teeth in children/teenagers
- A probe based on the WHO 621 probe with a spherical ball tip and black band is gently walked around six sites per tooth
- The worst score is recorded for each sextant/index tooth in a six box grid
- BPE and PSR do not replace the need for a full periodontal examination
- Information gathered helps the clinician reach a diagnosis and form a treatment plan

18 Role of radiographs in periodontal diagnosis

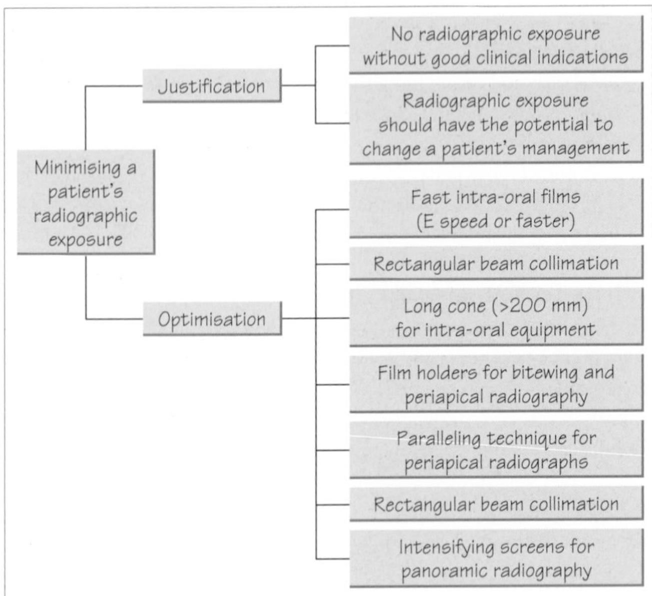

Figure 18.1 Ways of minimising radiation exposure when using radiographs.

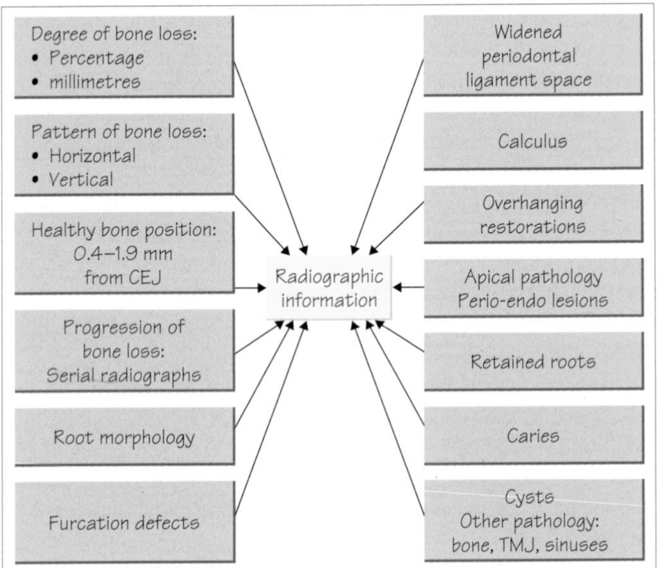

Figure 18.2 Key aspects of a radiographic periodontal assessment. CEJ, cement–enamel junction; TMJ, temporomandibular joint.

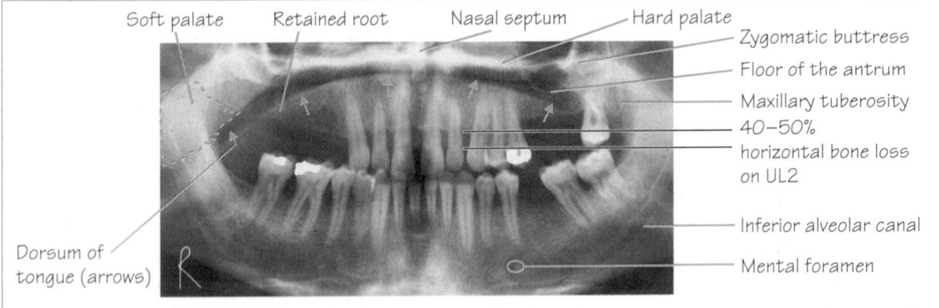

Panoramic radiograph showing some of the normal anatomical structures. A generalised horizontal pattern of bone loss is seen around the teeth. Percentage bone loss is estimated from an assessment of total root length relative to the degree of bone remaining, so for instance an estimate of 40–50% bone loss is seen around UL2.

Figure 18.3 Panoramic radiograph showing bone loss.

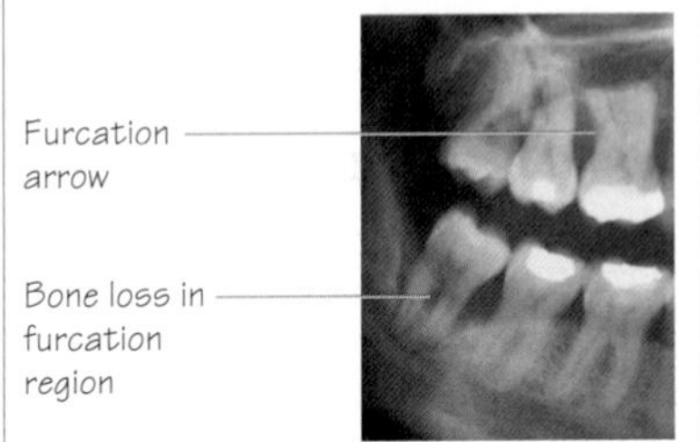

Part of a panoramic radiograph showing furcation defects with bone loss clearly evident between the roots of LR8. The furcation arrow indicates early furcation involvement in a three-rooted molar (UR6).

Figure 18.4 Furcation defects.

Figure 18.5 Calculus and deficient crown margin.

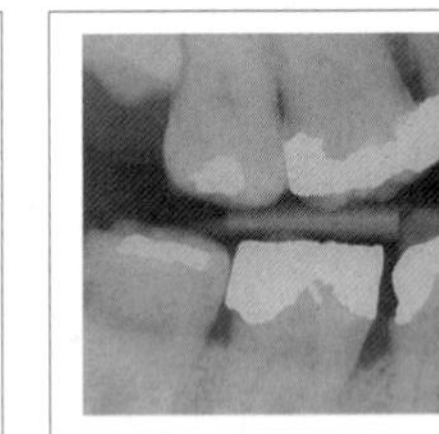

Horizontal bitewing radiograph showing multiple, heavily restored teeth, including poorly restored LR6 with distal open contact and deficient distal margin LR7.

Figure 18.6 Plaque retention factors. Courtesy of Ms V. Yorke.

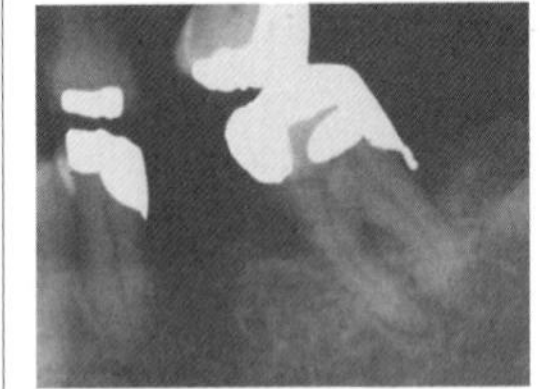

Part of a panoramic radiograph showing overhanging restorations distally on LL5 and particularly on LL7.

Figure 18.7 Overhanging restoration margins.

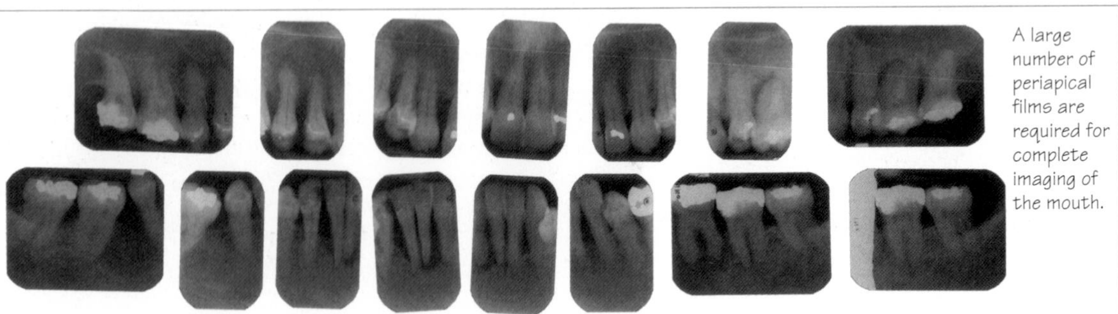

A large number of periapical films are required for complete imaging of the mouth.

Figure 18.8 Full mouth periapical radiographs for a patient with advanced bone loss.

Radiographs are used as an adjunct to a thorough clinical examination in order to make a diagnosis and draw up a treatment plan. The details of national regulations governing the use of radiographs vary in different countries, but in principle they all seek to protect the workforce and general public and to limit the radiation dose to patients.

Patients are protected by application of the principles of justification and optimisation (Fig.18.1):

- *Justification* of a medical exposure is based on the practitioner's understanding of the hazards associated with taking a radiograph and the clinical information. Radiographs are justified when they can be demonstrated to have the potential to change the patient's management.
- *Optimisation* is applied by employing a range of measures to minimise the radiation dose once it has been established that the radiograph should be taken.

Radiographic information

Radiographs can provide considerable information that may assist in the diagnosis and management of a patient's periodontal condition (Figs 18.2–18.7). The degree of bone loss can be expressed either as a percentage of the root length if the apex of the tooth can be visualised or in millimetres on a bitewing radiograph. The pattern of bone loss is not diagnostic but irregular bone loss can be suggestive of more rapid destruction than a horizontal pattern of loss. Angular or infrabony defects have been considered to be associated with occlusal trauma but this is not inevitable. The exact pattern of bone loss is often more dependent on the amount of separation between the roots.

Sequential radiographs can give information on disease progression; for instance serial bitewing radiographs primarily taken for caries detection can provide information about bone levels over time. It is important that any radiographs taken solely for periodontal follow up are justified.

Radiographic views

The selection of views should be based on the diagnostic information required. Radiographs can be used alone or in combination as appropriate.

- Horizontal bitewing.
- Vertical bitewing.
- Periapical.
- Panoramic.

Horizontal bitewing

Horizontal bitewing radiographs are frequently prescribed primarily for caries detection. The alveolar crest can be visualised even if there have been several millimetres of bone loss. These radiographs provide a good image with consistent positioning and they may allow monitoring of bone changes if a series of these radiographs is available.

Vertical bitewing

Vertical bitewing radiographs are taken by rotating the conventional bitewing film through 90° so that more extensive bone loss can be seen while still imaging several teeth on one film.

Periapical

Periapical radiographs can be taken at selective sites or throughout the mouth to produce a full series (Fig. 18.8). The long cone paralleling technique enables a consistent image to be taken. Good clarity of the image is obtained by this technique although it can take time to obtain several films.

Panoramic

Panoramic radiographs enable all teeth to be seen on one film (Fig. 18.3). Newer machines generate films of good quality although detail is less fine compared to intra-oral techniques. There is a tendency for overlap of teeth and reduced image quality in the anterior regions. Having reviewed the panoramic radiograph, selected periapical films can be taken to supplement the information obtained if necessary.

Digital radiography

The use of digital radiography is becoming more widespread. There are two main types of digital receptors. The first uses a charge coupled device (CCD). A wire connects it to a computer. The receptor tends to be smaller than a normal film and bulkier. The second sensor is wireless and uses a storage phosphor plate. Receptors are thinner than film and come in different sizes, comparable to conventional film. Digital radiography generally has dose advantages and the capability for image enhancement. Thin bone that may escape detection can be rendered visible by adjusting contrast and brightness. Serial radiographs can be manipulated and used to detect changes in bone which may be valuable in monitoring bone loss.

Selection of radiographs

Radiographic selection or referral criteria have been available for some years in the UK, Europe and the USA. The objectives for their use are to limit unnecessary radiation to the patient and increase the diagnostic value of the radiographs taken. They are used following completion of a thorough clinical assessment of the patient. The results of this examination are then used to determine whether radiographs should be taken and to aid selection of views.

In compiling guidelines, the convened bodies in the UK, Europe and the USA found limited evidence on which to base their recommendations and so the referral criteria available are derived largely from expert opinion and differ in specific detail. Having undertaken the radiographic examination all films must be examined and the diagnostic findings should be reported in a written form in the patient's notes, producing what is termed a radiographic report. This ensures that all valuable diagnostic information is extracted regardless of the primary reason for taking the radiographs.

Key points

- Radiographs are used with a thorough clinical examination to make a diagnosis and draw up a treatment plan
- Radiographs must be taken in accordance with principles of justification and optimisation
- Radiographs can provide information on bone levels, local plaque retention factors and other features that can assist diagnosis and treatment planning of periodontal conditions
- Different radiographic views can provide different information, radiation exposure and image quality
- Referral criteria may help in deciding when to take radiographs and which views to use

19 Principles of periodontal diagnosis and treatment planning

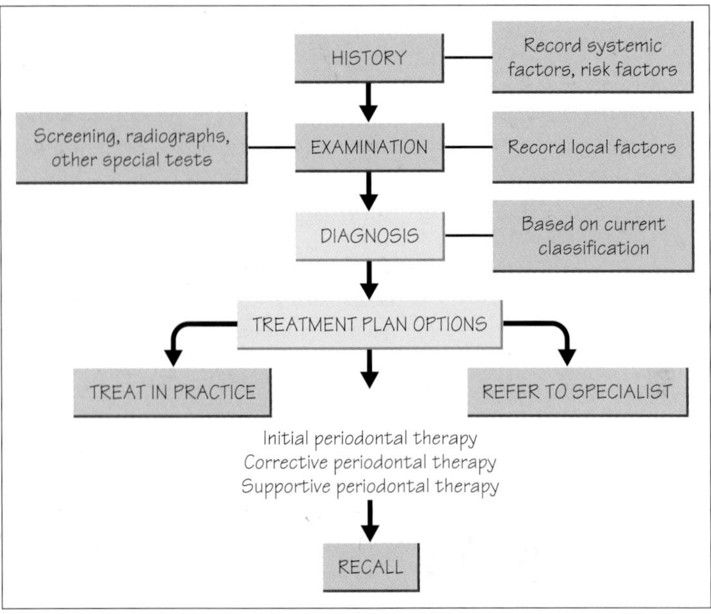

Figure 19.1 Flow diagram showing diagnosis and treatment plan options.

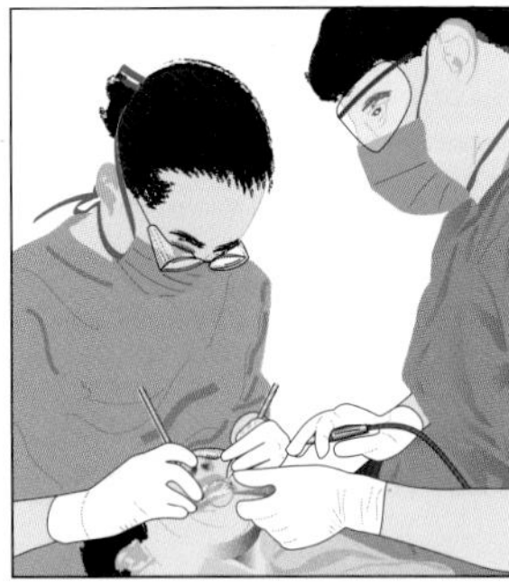

Figure 19.2 Dental examination of a patient.

- Gingival diseases
- Chronic periodontitis
- Aggressive periodontitis
- Periodontitis as a manifestation of systemic diseases
- Necrotising periodontal diseases
- Abscesses of the periodontium
- Periodontitis associated with endodontic lesions
- Developmental or acquired deformities and conditions

Figure 19.3 Classification of periodontal diseases based on the 1999 International Workshop for the Classification of Periodontal Diseases and Conditions (Armitage,1999).

First decide which disease or condition is present (may be more than one disease or condition present)
- Use main classification categories (Fig. 19.3) and sub-classifications (Chapter 2)
- If any uncertainty, list differential diagnoses i.e. other possible diagnoses, ranked from the most to the least likely
  - Provides other options if initial diagnosis proves to be incorrect

Then describe severity
- Designate as slight (or initial or mild), moderate or severe (or advanced)
  - e.g. for chronic periodontitis, slight = 1–2 mm CAL, moderate = 3–4 mm CAL, severe ≥ 5 mm CAL
  - e.g. for gingivitis, comment on degree of gingival redness, swelling, bleeding

Then state whether disease is localised or generalised
  - e.g. for chronic periodontitis, localised is where ≤30% sites involved, generalised > 30% sites
  - Can specify precise location and sites
  - e.g. for aggressive periodontitis, there are specific features for localised and generalised forms

Note if disease is associated with any local, systemic or other periodontal risk factors
  - e.g. overhanging restoration margin, diabetes mellitus, cigarette smoking, stress

Figure 19.4 Periodontal diagnosis and descriptors. CAL, clinical attachment loss.

- Control or elimination of plaque infections
  - Baseline indices of periodontal status
  - Instruction in oral hygiene techniques
  - Smoking cessation counselling (if needed)
  - Scaling and root surface debridement and elimination of plaque retention factors
  - Monitor response to treatment
  - Review prognosis
- Provisional treatment plan may include:
  - Extractions +/– immediate dentures
  - Endodontics
  - Occlusal adjustments
  - Treat dentine hypersensitivity

Figure 19.5 Initial periodontal therapy.

- Periodontal therapy may include:
  - Further non-surgical therapy
  - Periodontal surgery
  - Adjunctive local antimicrobials (chronic periodontitis)
  - Adjunctive systemic antibiotics (aggressive periodontitis)
- Review outcome and prognosis
- Definitive treatment plan may include:
  - Occlusal adjustments
  - Endodontics
  - Extractions
  - Definitive restorative work, fixed and/or removable prosthodontics
  - Implants
  - Orthodontics
- Arrange periodontal supportive therapy

Figure 19.6 Corrective periodontal therapy.

Supportive therapy
- Recall at time interval appropriate to diagnosis (e.g. more frequent for aggressive periodontitis than chronic periodontitis)
- Monitor periodontal status
- Re-motivate and re-educate patient
- Repeat plaque control instruction
- Re-treat disease
- Arrange next recall

Figure 19.7 Supportive periodontal therapy.

The periodontal diagnosis follows a thorough history and examination (Figs 19.1, 19.2; Chapter 16) and should be based on the current classification derived from the 1999 International Workshop for the Classification of Periodontal Diseases and Conditions (Fig. 19.3; Chapter 2). If more than one disease is present, more than one diagnosis should be made. If there is any uncertainty, a differential diagnosis can be made. For each condition diagnosed additional descriptors can be used (Fig. 19.4), such as the severity, extent and location of disease or description of associated risk factors.

It is also important for other non-periodontal diagnoses to be made based on the extra-oral and intra-oral examination of soft and hard oral tissues, e.g. temporomandibular joint disorders, oral mucosal diseases, caries/root caries, deficient, fractured or overhanging restorations, apical pathology, retained roots, unerupted or impacted teeth, oral pathology such as cysts or tumours, and problems relating to fixed or removable prosthodontics.

The treatment plan is based on the periodontal and dental conditions diagnosed.

Periodontal treatment plan

The periodontal treatment plan is usually in three phases:
- Initial therapy (Fig. 19.5).
- Corrective therapy (Fig. 19.6).
- Supportive therapy (Fig. 19.7).

Initial therapy

The remit of the initial therapy is to control the microbial plaque and to identify and deal with any modifiable risk factors (Chapters 11, 14). At the start of the treatment, baseline indices of periodontal status are recorded (Chapter16) and the patient is given personal instruction in oral hygiene techniques, including the type of toothbrush and the use of interdental aids, dentifrice or mouthwash (Chapter 20). This is a crucial aspect of the treatment and without compliance and motivation from the patient to control their plaque levels, the outcome of the initial and subsequent phases of the therapy will be jeopardised. The ultimate goal is to achieve 85–90% of surfaces free from plaque, with a concomitant reduction in marginal inflammation.

Smoking cessation counselling is provided if needed (Chapter 36) and the patient informed of the risks to their oral and general health from smoking and the detrimental effects to the success of periodontal treatment. If a periodontal risk factor such as diabetes mellitus is identified, then the patient should be advised of the link between diabetes control and their periodontal health. Liaison with the patient's diabetes consultant, specialist nurse or general medical practitioner can be helpful and prudent (Chapter 37).

Scaling and root surface debridement are undertaken using local analgesia as required in conjunction with elimination of plaque retention factors (Chapter 20). The response to therapy is monitored 8–12 weeks after treatment; 6 weeks is the minimum period to allow for initial healing to occur before re-probing the tissues (Chapter 22). The prognosis of individual teeth can be reviewed and decisions made about management. At this stage, the decision is made to undertake corrective therapy if there is residual disease and further therapeutic measures are indicated. If initial therapy has been successful, then the patient can move to the supportive phase of therapy.

The provisional treatment plan needs tailoring to the individual, e.g. extraction(s) with or without immediate denture(s), endodontics, occlusal adjustments where teeth have drifted due to periodontitis, and the management of dentine hypersensitivity following recession resulting from periodontitis or root surface debridement.

Corrective therapy

Various therapeutic measures can be applied during the corrective phase of therapy. Further non-surgical therapy may be needed to treat residual active pockets. In some cases, periodontal surgery may be indicated.
- Reparative surgery such as the modified Widman flap technique involves a flap being raised to allow better access and direct vision to the root surface for thorough debridement (Chapters 24, 25).
- Resective surgery such as gingivectomy involves surgical removal and reshaping of tissue.
- Regenerative surgery techniques aim to regenerate the periodontium, for example using guided tissue regeneration or enamel matrix derivatives (Chapter 26).

Adjunctive local antimicrobials may be indicated in some selected sites in cases of chronic periodontitis, although clinical gain in attachment is usually small (Chapter 23). Adjunctive systemic antibiotics have very limited application, aggressive periodontitis being one such possibility (Chapter 23).

Following review of the outcome of this phase of periodontal therapy, and consideration of the prognosis, the definitive treatment plan can be constructed. This may involve a range of options such as:
- Occlusal adjustment(s).
- Endodontics.
- Extractions.
- Final restorative work, and fixed and/or removable prosthodontics.
- Implants (Chapter 28).
- Orthodontics (Chapter 29).

Supportive therapy

This is directed at the prevention of recurrence of disease and maintenance of periodontal health and is arranged at a time interval appropriate to the periodontal diagnosis (e.g. more frequent for aggressive periodontitis than chronic periodontitis). It is important to re-motivate/re-educate the patient, repeat plaque control instruction, re-treat any recurrent or new disease and then arrange a further recall to review the patient and monitor their periodontal status.

Key points

- Periodontal diagnosis:
  - follows a thorough history and examination
  - is based on current classification
- Initial periodontal therapy:
  - relates to cause of disease, control of infection and management of aetiological factors
  - involves provisional treatment plan
- Corrective periodontal therapy:
  - comprises therapeutic measures, option for periodontal surgery and option for adjunctive treatments
  - involves definitive treatment plan
- Supportive periodontal therapy:
  - prevents recurrence of disease
  - stabilises periodontal condition
  - maintains optimum periodontal health
- Non-periodontal diagnoses should also be made and treatment arranged

Plaque control and non-surgical periodontal therapy

- *Scaling*: aims to remove plaque and calculus from the tooth surfaces and can be supragingival or subgingival depending on the location of the deposits
- *Root planing*: a technique that aims to remove deposits but also softened cementum leaving a smooth and hard root surface. The need for cementum removal has been questioned and rendering the root surface clean is now the primary aim
- *Root surface debridement*: a term used to describe removal of deposits from the root surface to leave the surface clean but without a specific aim of cementum removal.

Figure 20.1 Terms in use relating to plaque and calculus removal.

(a)

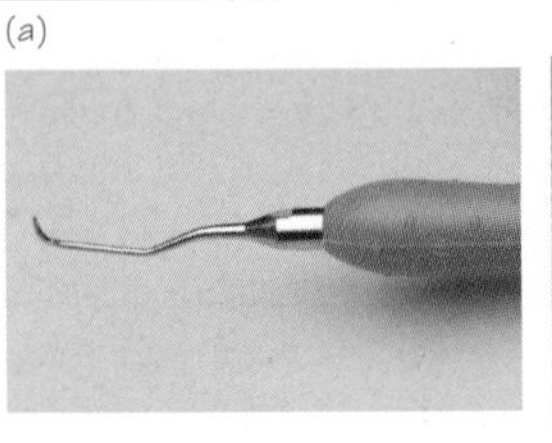

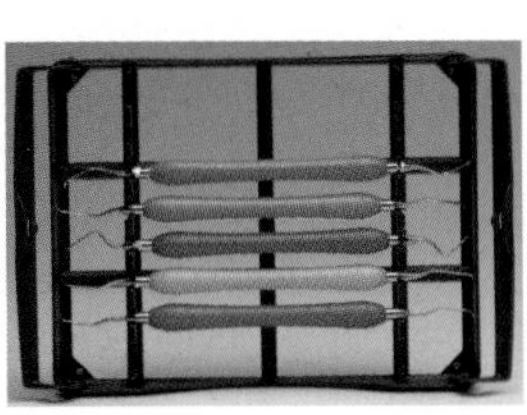

- Hand instrumentation allows the operator tactile sensitivity which is lost with ultrasonic instruments
- Hand instruments are cheaper to buy and maintain than ultrasonics
- Hand instruments are less likely to cause discomfort in sensitive teeth
- No aerosol is generated

(b)

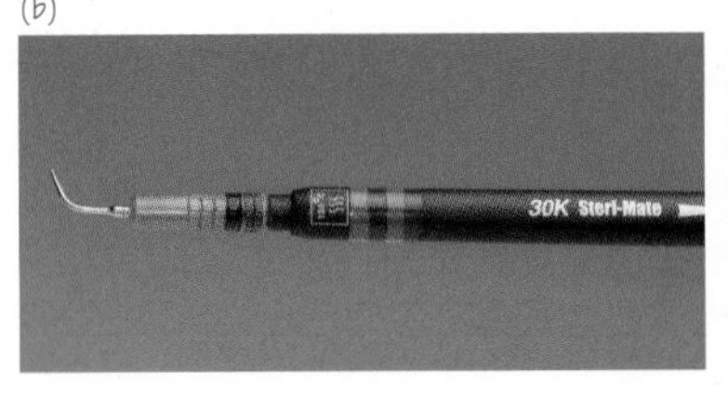

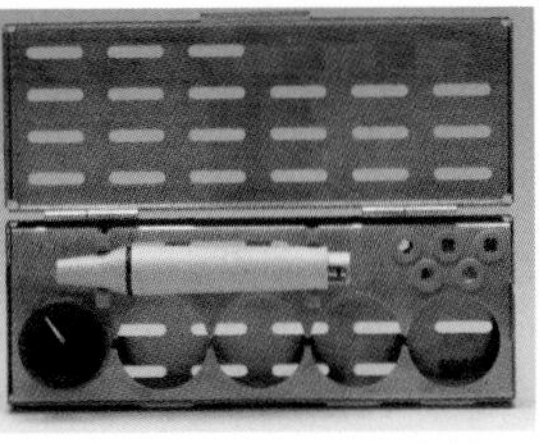

- Irrigation with water (or another coolant) in ultrasonic instruments clears the field of debris and blood but can in itself obscure vision
- Magnetostrictive ultrasonics are contraindicated in patients with some cardiac pacemakers
- Piezoelectric and sonic instruments can be used in patients with cardiac pacemakers
- Ultrasonic instruments can generate contaminated aerosols
- Ultrasonics can be useful to bring about quick removal of gross deposits (especially supragingivally)
- Ultrasonics can be less tiring for the operator
- Ultrasonics can be used to remove overhanging margins on amalgam restorations

Clinical studies show similar improvements in pocket depth and bleeding on probing achievable with both hand and ultrasonic instruments.

Figure 20.2 (a) Hand instruments. (b) Ultrasonic instruments.

Lovdal *et al.* (1961)
- 1500 subjects in Norway
- Oral hygiene instruction and scaling and root planing repeated 2–4 times a year, over 5 years
- Reduced gingivitis and tooth loss even in patients whose home care was not substantially improved

Badersten *et al.* (1984)
- 16 subjects with moderate–advanced periodontitis
- Oral hygiene instruction and root surface debridement of single rooted teeth
- After 2 years, elimination of gingivitis and pocket reduction even at very deep sites (> 9 mm)

Figure 20.3 Two classic studies demonstrating the effectiveness of plaque control (Lovdal et al., 1961; Badersten et al., 1984).

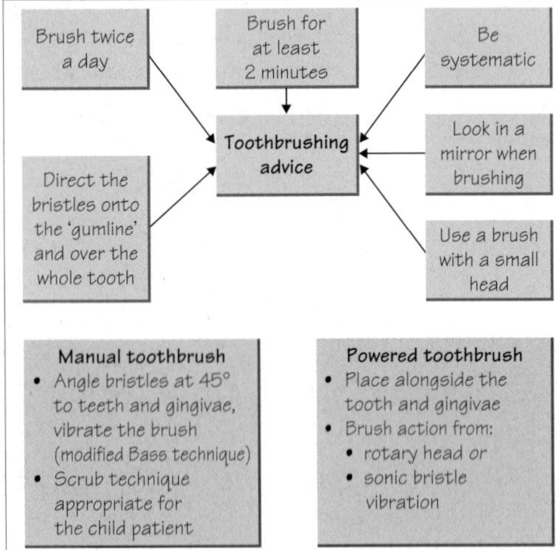

Figure 20.5 Toothbrushing advice to patient.

(a)

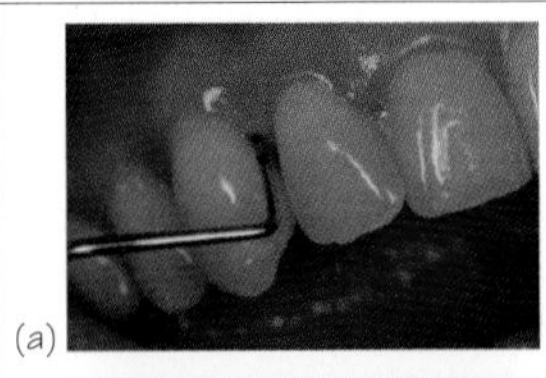

(b)

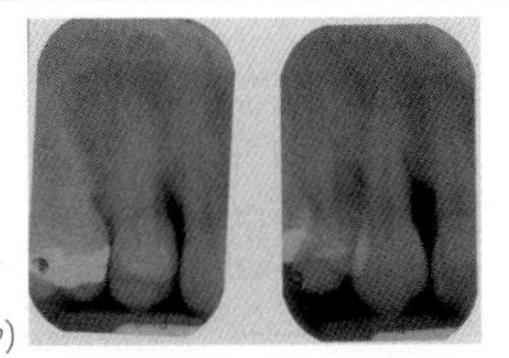

(c)

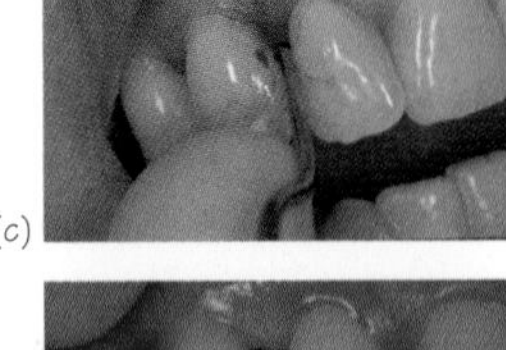

(d)

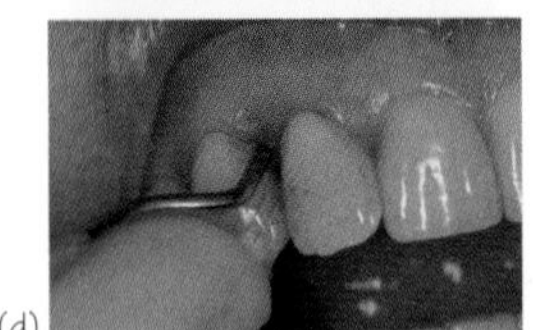

(e)

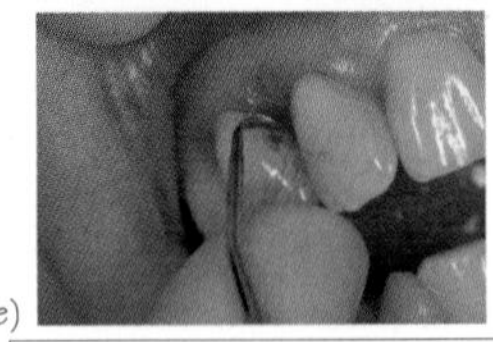

(f)

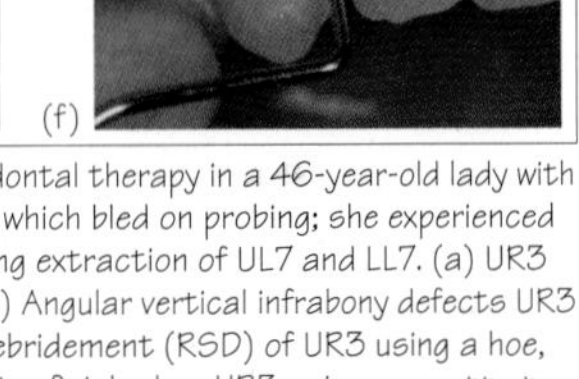

(g) (h)

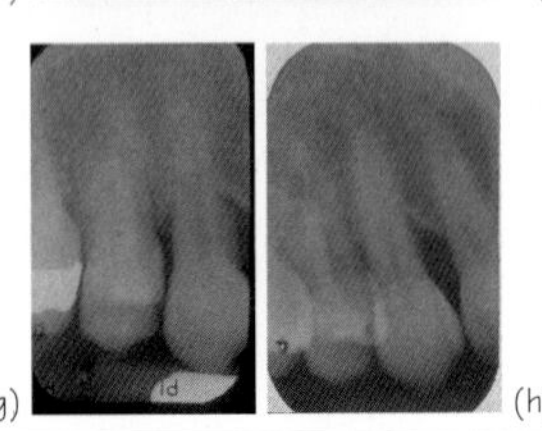

Figure 20.4 Non-surgical periodontal therapy in a 46-year-old lady with deep pockets on UR3 and UR4, which bled on probing; she experienced occlusal trauma on UR4 following extraction of UL7 and LL7. (a) UR3 probing depth (PD) of >7 mm. (b) Angular vertical infrabony defects UR3 and UR4. (c, d) Root surface debridement (RSD) of UR3 using a hoe, following ultrasonic. (e) RSD being finished on UR3 using a curette to create a clean smooth root surface; occlusal adjustment was undertaken on UR4 as part of the initial therapy. (f) PD at 2 years follow up is less than 4 mm on UR3 (shown) and UR4. (g, h) Bone level stability and corticated crest on UR3 at 2 years (g) and 5 years (h) follow up.

Enzymes:	Protease, dextranase
Bisbiguanides:	Chlorhexidine gluconate
Quaternary ammonium compounds:	Cetyl pyridinium chloride
Phenols:	Triclosan
Essential oils:	Thymol, eucalyptol
Metal ions:	Zinc, stannous fluoride
Oxygenating agents:	Peroxide

Figure 20.7 Pharmacological plaque control agents.

Corsodyl® mouthwash
Rinse with 10 ml of 0.2% for 1 minute twice daily
Peridex® mouthwash, PerioGard® mouthwash
Rinse with 15 ml of 0.12% for 30 seconds twice daily

- When brushing is not possible for limited periods
- To help with acutely inflamed gingivae
- To relieve pain from ulcers or minor oral problems
- Specific cases of the medically compromised, physically or mentally handicapped patient
- Prior to ultrasonic scaling to reduce microbial load of aerosol spray
- Post-periodontal/oral surgery

Figure 20.8 Use of chlorhexidine mouthwash.

- Patients with adequate oral hygiene skills should be instructed in the method they use rather than changed unnecessarily
- Patients who seem unable to improve their cleaning with a manual brush may benefit from making a change and investing in a powered brush. Timer helps patient to brush for sufficient time
- Powered toothbrushes can improve long-term compliance
- Patients with reduced manual dexterity such as sufferers of arthritis may benefit from a powered toothbrush
- Some mentally handicapped patients or a carer may find a powered brush easier to use
- Some patients, especially children, like using gadgets so may be more motivated to brush with a powered brush though the novelty may wear off

Figure 20.6 Potential use of powered toothbrushes: points to consider.

Plaque is the primary aetiological factor in the periodontal diseases. Periodontal therapy is then directed at cleaning the root surfaces and removing plaque retention factors. Patient homecare – including toothbrushing, interdental cleaning and adjunctive pharmacological agents delivered as toothpastes and mouthwashes – is necessary after periodontal therapy to maintain the health of the periodontium. Good communication with the patient is essential to establish good hygiene practices (Chapter 21).

Non-surgical periodontal therapy

Non-surgical periodontal therapy is directed at the removal of supragingival and subgingival plaque and calculus deposits, plus local plaque retention factors, and forms the mainstay of periodontal management in general dental practice (Greenstein, 2000). Terms relating to this are shown in Fig. 20.1. It was previously thought that endotoxin was firmly bound to cementum and that extensive cementum removal by scaling and root planing was required. However, studies have shown that endotoxin is weakly bound to the root surface and can readily be removed by powered or manual scalers and even by washing or polishing. Therefore, complete cementum removal is no longer a goal of periodontal therapy (Drisko, 2000).

The removal of deposits is technically demanding. Effectiveness is dependent on the depth of pocket, skill of the operator, root anatomy, time spent and instrument sharpness (for hand instruments). Scaling and root surface debridement are routinely carried out using hand instruments (Fig. 20.2a) (sickle scalers, curettes and hoes) and ultrasonic or sonic instruments (Fig. 20.2b) (Drisko, 2000). The latter operate by tip vibration and a spraying/cavitation effect of the fluid coolant. The vibrations of ultrasonic tips are generated by an electromagnetic field (magnetostrictive) or crystal transducer (piezoelectric); sonic tips are air driven with the vibrations generated mechanically.

Overhanging restoration margins are associated with greater bone loss (Chapter 14) and may be removed with burs and ultrasonic/sonic scalers, though sometimes a properly contoured replacement restoration is required.

Effectiveness of plaque control and root surface instrumentation

Many studies have shown the effectiveness of plaque control and instrumentation in the treatment of periodontal diseases. Two classic papers are summarised in Fig. 20.3 (Lovdal *et al.*, 1961; Badersten *et al.*, 1984). Traditional therapy is delivered over a series of appointments and a successful outcome results in reduced probing depth, elimination of bleeding on probing, gain in attachment and stability of bone levels, even infill in some infrabony defects (Fig. 20.4). Some more recent studies have used full mouth disinfection strategies to minimise reinfection of treated pockets from areas with pathogens by completing treatment within 24 hours (Mongardini *et al.*, 1999); this approach has its advocates. The success of non-surgical periodontal therapy may be limited by technical, local or systemic factors, in which case adjunctive antimicrobials (Chapter 23) or surgical approaches (Chapters 24–26) may be indicated.

Toothbrushing

Manual and powered toothbrushes are available. Both can be effective in plaque removal although a systematic review concluded that oscillating, rotating, powered toothbrushes have shown improved efficacy (Robinson *et al.*, 2005). Any recommendation should be based on assessment of the individual patient (Figs 20.5, 20.6).

Interdental cleaning

An effective toothbrushing technique can only clean about 65% of the tooth surface and cannot remove interproximal plaque so interdental cleaning is also necessary. Interdental brushes, dental floss, tape and powered flossing devices are all available for interproximal use. Wood sticks have a triangular cross-section and although they can be used in open interdental embrasures, they can be damaging or break if used too aggressively and therefore have limited value.

Dental floss and tape are advised when the interdental papillae completely fill the embrasures. Where there is space for brushes these are recommended; compliance is better than floss and improved periodontal clinical outcomes were found in a randomised controlled clinical trial of patients with chronic periodontitis using customised pre-curved interdental brushes of different sizes even prior to root surface debridement (Jackson *et al.*, 2006). Structural equation modelling analysis showed that the reductions in probing depths and bleeding on probing were mainly due to the greater efficiency of the interdental brushes in removing interdental plaque rather than compression of the interdental papillae (Tu *et al.*, 2008).

Adjunctive pharmacological agents

Many agents have been incorporated into mouthwashes and toothpastes and key groups are shown in Fig. 20.7. Most are used to supplement brushing and interdental cleaning but some (e.g. chlorhexidine gluconate) can be used when toothbrushing is not possible, for instance after oral or periodontal surgery.

Chlorhexidine gluconate is generally considered the gold standard anti-plaque/anti-gingivitis agent. It is most usually used as a mouthwash but is also available in some toothpastes or gels. It exhibits substantivity, i.e. the ability to adsorb to hard and soft tissues and subsequently desorb in a biologically active form, and this prolongs the antibacterial activity following rinsing. Side effects that limit its use include altered taste sensation, staining of teeth or tooth-coloured restorations, increased supragingival calculus formation, and, rarely, mucositis. Prolonged usage is not generally recommended but the mouthwash is useful in specific clinical situations (Fig. 20.8).

A meta-analysis (Gunsolley, 2006) reported that other adjunctive agents with proven anti-plaque and anti-gingivitis efficacy include: (i) essential oils; (ii) triclosan 0.3% with a co-polymer (2.0% polyvinyl methyl ether and maleic acid) in a dentifrice formulation; this also has anti-inflammatory effects and has been shown to have subgingival benefits which can help retard or prevent periodontitis (Rosling *et al.*, 1997; Ellwood *et al.*, 1998; Cullinan *et al.*, 2003).

Key points

- Non-surgical periodontal therapy is the mainstay of periodontal practice, but adjunctive antimicrobial or surgical treatment may be indicated
- Hand, ultrasonic and sonic instruments can be equally effective for scaling and root surface debridement
- Both toothbrushing and interdental cleaning are necessary for optimal plaque control; advice should be specific to each patient
- Pharmacological plaque control agents may be useful adjuncts

21 Patient communication in dental care

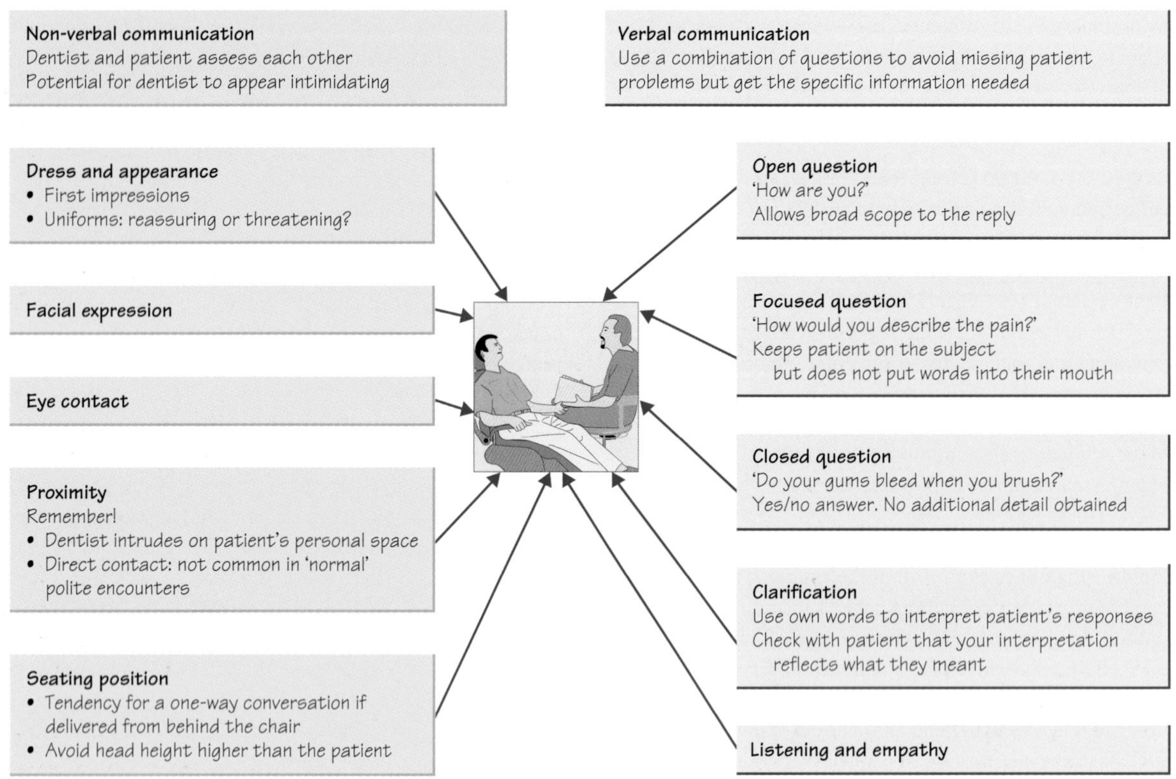

Figure 21.1 Communication with the patient

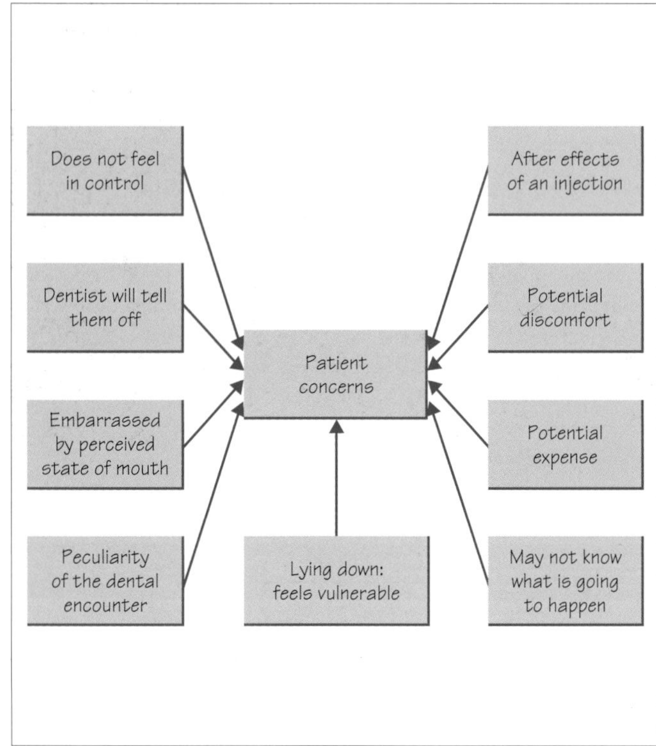

Figure 21.2 A patient's potential concerns about a visit to the dentist.

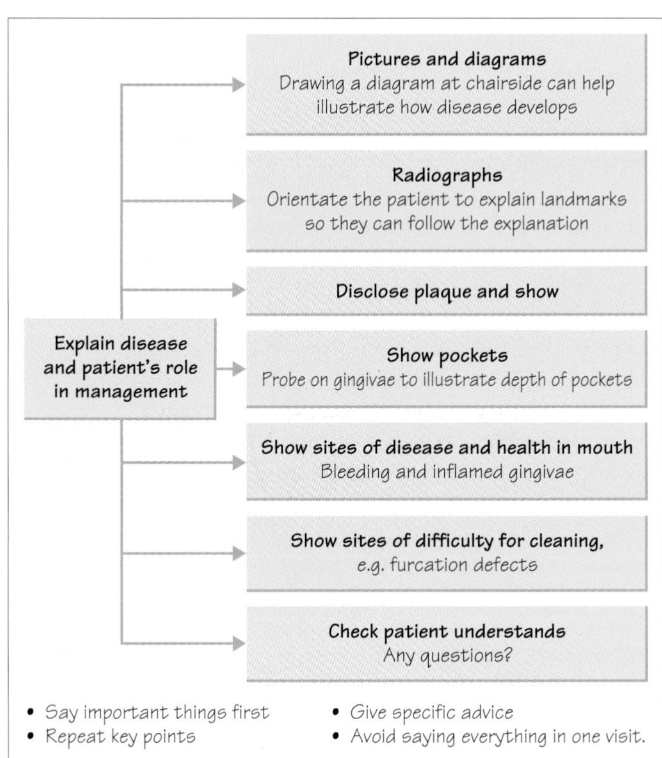

Figure 21.3 Tailor-made patient information.

As dentists we wish to establish a good rapport with our patients. Doing so makes both the patient and dental team's experience more positive and also more productive. The dental team is discussed further in Chapter 42. Oral hygiene advice for patients is discussed in Chapter 20. It is important to be aware of the importance of non-verbal communication in achieving a reassuring and welcoming environment for the patient. Verbal communication must seek to identify and explore the patient's dental complaint while empathising with their concerns and building up a trusting relationship (Fig. 21.1).

Patient concerns

There are plenty of reasons why a patient may have some negative thoughts about an impending dental visit, as shown in Fig. 21.2. Organising the practice or hospital set-up and structure of the dental visit with these in mind can help to improve the patient's experience:

- Prior information: directions to the practice or hospital, parking situation, where to report and what the visit may involve if appropriate.
- Avoid 'telling the patient off'.
- The patient needs to understand their role in disease and management but avoid blaming the patient: putting their condition into the context of the population at large or the dentist's own experience can help the patient see that they are not the only one with this problem and the dentist has seen it all before.
- Inform the patient during the visit of what is going on.
- Avoid jargon.
- Warn the patient of any after effects so that there are no nasty surprises.
- Ensure that the patient feels that they do have some control. This could be done by telling the patient that they can determine what is done in the visit, or can stop the dentist by a prearranged signal.
- Give the patient time to consider treatment options and come back with any questions.

Patient's involvement in dental care

Active patient involvement is fundamental to successful periodontal care. This means that the patient must have an understanding of the nature of their disease, the treatment and their role in its outcome. Figure 21.3 shows how the information provided should be made relevant to an individual patient. Verbal advice can be supported by providing more general resources such as leaflets or details of appropriate web resources on periodontal disease or oral hygiene methods. The dentist should try not to overload the patient with information on any one visit and should follow up advice at subsequent appointments.

Communication with the young patient

Although periodontal diseases are most common in adults they are also found in young patients (Chapter 40). When communicating with a child patient it is important to address the child and not solely the accompanying adult. The nature of the visit and treatment planned should be explained as simply as is appropriate to the child's understanding and development. Long-term health goals will seem remote to the young patient and other motivating factors should be used. The child patient may respond to praise and encouragement from parents or teachers, simple rewards such as stickers and can be encouraged to brush by using a brushing chart to mark off each time they brush. Adolescents value peer group acceptance, and are becoming very conscious of appearance and attractiveness and these concepts can be linked to the health messages that are given.

Changing behaviour

Most of us know how hard it is to comply with, for instance, a sensible diet or exercise regime even if we know the benefits. Information and explanation are fundamental but not always enough to change a person's behaviour. This is sometimes disappointing to the dental team who, having provided oral heath advice, can take a patient's failure to change as a personal insult and brand them as non-compliant.

Positive encouragement from the dental team, other health care workers, family and peers can help to support a change in behaviour. Additional support, for example for smoking cessation, may be found from telephone helplines or other organisations.

Positive consequences to a change in behaviour help to promote the change. However, the dentist's perception of the main benefits may differ from the patient's. Wanting an attractive smile and not having bad breath may be more influential drivers to a patient for making a change in life style.

The dentist can help the patient to set realistic goals so that a change in behaviour may be staged. This can be by agreeing targets for plaque scores or introducing interdental cleaning in a specific area of the mouth first.

The dental team also needs to appreciate that relapse is part of the process of changing behaviour. It is at this point that the patient may feel they have failed and will need support rather than a reprimand.

Key points

- Communication occurs by non-verbal and verbal means
- Careful planning of a practice and dental visit can address many patient concerns about attending a dental appointment
- Patients need tailor-made information and advice on their periodontal condition and their role in its management
- Communication with young patients should reflect their development and understanding and those factors that motivate them
- Identify benefits that the patient considers positive and set realistic goals when attempting to change established behaviour patterns

22 Periodontal tissue response, healing and monitoring

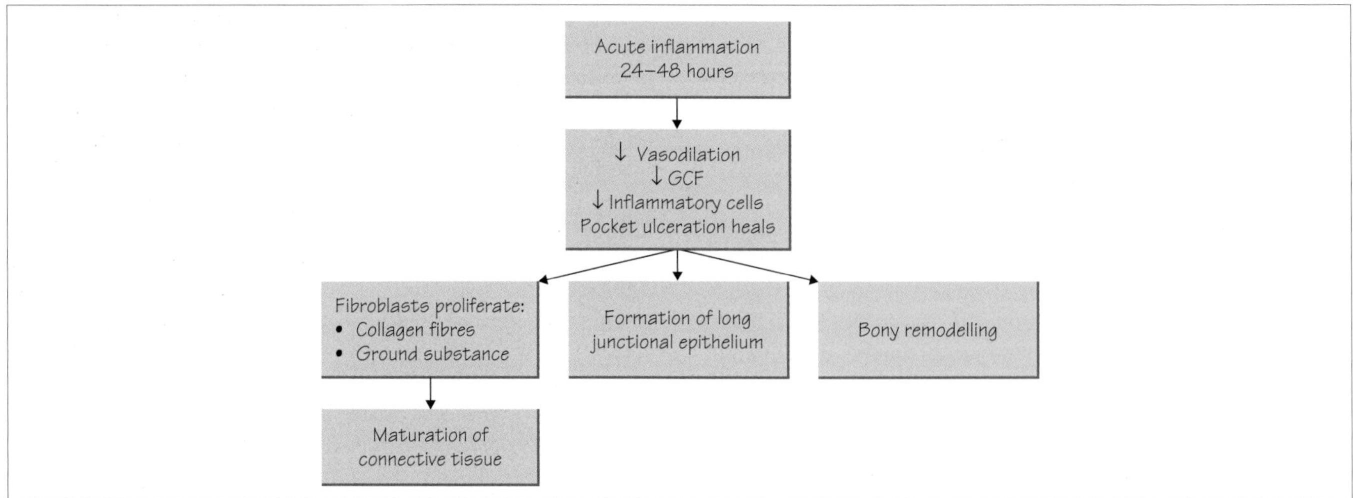

Figure 22.1 Healing of the periodontal tissues. GCF, gingival crevicular fluid.

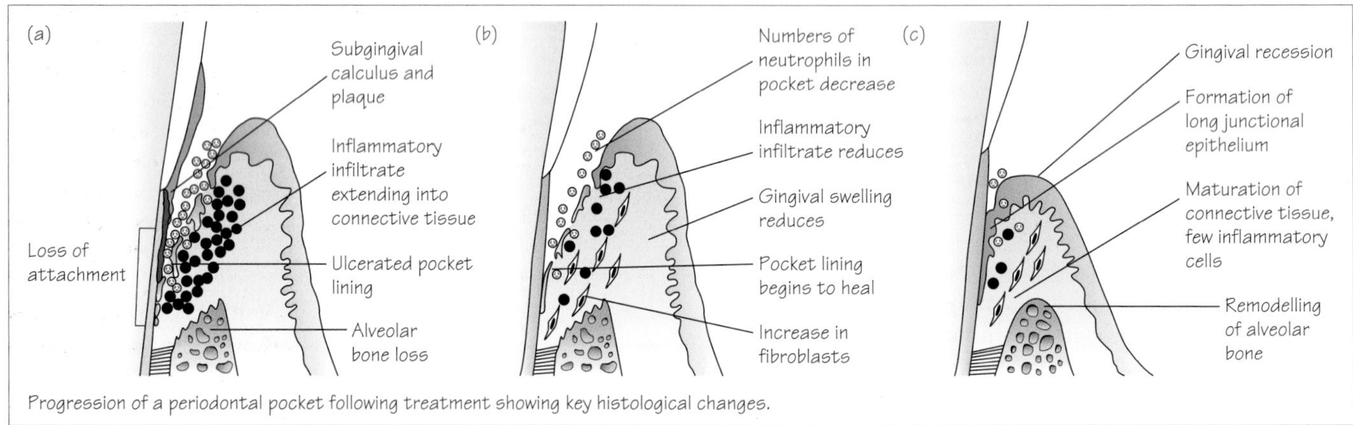

Progression of a periodontal pocket following treatment showing key histological changes.

Figure 22.2 (a) A periodontal lesion before treatment. (b) Early healing of a periodontal pocket. (c) Further healing of a periodontal pocket.

Response to oral hygiene instruction
- Plaque free score
- Gingival bleeding free score

Response to root surface debridement
- Probing pocket depths
- Attachment levels
- Bleeding on probing
- Suppuration
- Furcation lesions
- Mobility
- Recession

Figure 22.3 Indices for monitoring the response to periodontal therapy.

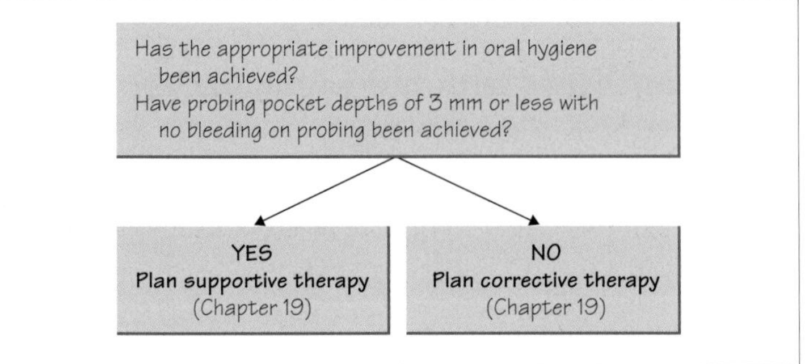

Figure 22.4 Decision making following monitoring the response to periodontal therapy.

Following oral hygiene measures and root surface debridement there are two potential outcomes:

1 The tissue may respond by healing.

2 The tissue may fail to heal.

Response to treatment

Following thorough root surface debridement and implementation of good oral hygiene, changes will occur in the bacterial flora and periodontal tissues.

Bacterial flora

There is a reduction in the total numbers of microorganisms in the periodontal pockets. The residual bacterial flora shifts from predominantly Gram-negative anaerobic to one that is largely Gram-positive aerobic and associated with periodontal health, partly because of the reduction in plaque bulk allowing in higher oxygen concentrations within the plaque.

Tissue response and healing

The response to root surface debridement is summarised in Figs 22.1 and 22.2. As the periodontal tissue heals there is a reduction in redness and swelling and the tissue becomes pink and firm. Clinically it feels more fibrous and the gingival cuff tightens. Bleeding on probing and suppuration subsides.

A reduction in pocket depths results from a combination of events:

- Shrinkage of tissue following resolution of the inflammation with the development of gingival recession.
- Formation of a long junctional epithelium which attaches the gingiva to the cleaned root surface.
- Tightening of the gingival cuff as the gingival collagen fibre bundles reform.
- A small amount of gain in attachment may occur at the base of the pocket.

Healing can result in resolution of inflammation in the pocket without much shrinkage, leaving a persistent pocket without bleeding. Such a site will be healthy but plaque may enter the deep residual pocket leading to recurrence of inflammation. Scrupulous patient home care and a good supportive programme are required to ensure stability of such a site.

Healing following conventional periodontal surgery is essentially the same and is discussed in Chapter 25. Healing following regenerative periodontal surgery is discussed in Chapter 26.

Studies have shown that:

- Initially deeper sites show more recession than shallow sites.
- Initially deeper sites achieve more gain in clinical attachment.

Failure of treatment

Failure to heal will result in persistence of inflammation with the following signs:

- Bleeding on probing.
- Redness.
- Swelling.
- Persistent deep pockets or increasing depths.
- Suppuration.
- Increasing mobility.

The most common reasons for failure to respond are:

- Inadequate patient plaque control:
  - lack of compliance;
  - lack of dexterity.
- Residual subgingival calculus deposits harbouring subgingival plaque:
  - deep pockets;
  - furcation lesions, concavities and root grooves;
  - inexperienced operator.

It can be hard to tell by probing if a root surface has been cleaned of subgingival calculus. Studies examining extracted teeth following debridement show that achieving a completely calculus-free root surface is very difficult. Only 20–30% of sites that bleed on probing will go on to demonstrate further attachment loss. Nonetheless, bleeding on probing from the base of the pocket suggests a site which is not responding, particularly if the bleeding persists at the same site with sequential monitoring.

Systemic risk factors (e.g. continued smoking, uncontrolled diabetes) may also contribute to treatment failure. In aggressive conditions failure to eradicate key pathogens such as *Aggregatibacter actinomycetemcomitans* may impact on healing and the patient's individual host response will also determine treatment outcome.

Monitoring

To assess a patient's response to the therapy that has been carried out the periodontal condition needs to be monitored. This is achieved by repeating the indices taken at baseline (Fig. 22.3). The findings are then compared.

Healing will be indicated by a reduction in pocketing and bleeding indices. Pocketing may persist but if bleeding at the site has resolved this is a sign of healing, though such a site is harder to maintain than one where the pocketing has reduced. The patient's ability to implement plaque removal at home is assessed by repeating the plaque score.

Furcation and mobility indices are also repeated. Although these may improve following treatment, successful healing may in many cases not be associated with a significant change in these indicators. Mobility can be present in the presence of a healthy but reduced periodontal support (Chapter 15). Recession may well increase with healing.

Probing should be avoided in the first few weeks following treatment to allow early healing and tissue maturation. The indices can be repeated 8–12 weeks (minimum of 6 weeks) after treatment to assess response. Bony changes will take significantly longer to become apparent and radiographs will not detect early changes and healing. Any decision to take radiographs to monitor bone levels must be based on the principles discussed in Chapter 18, and radiographs should not be taken unless they can be clinically justified.

When the response to treatment has been monitored the clinician will have the answers to the questions posed in Fig. 22.4 and can make further treatment decisions.

Key points

- Following successful treatment:
  - the bacterial flora shifts from one that is principally Gram negative and anaerobic to Gram positive and aerobic
  - pocket depths and bleeding are reduced
  - the gingivae become more pink and fibrous
- Treatment failure may result from poor plaque control, residual calculus or other local and systemic factors
- Monitoring 8–12 weeks after treatment identifies responsive and non-responsive sites and enables subsequent treatment decisions to be made

23 Role of antimicrobial therapy in periodontal diseases

a) Systemic Antimicrobials

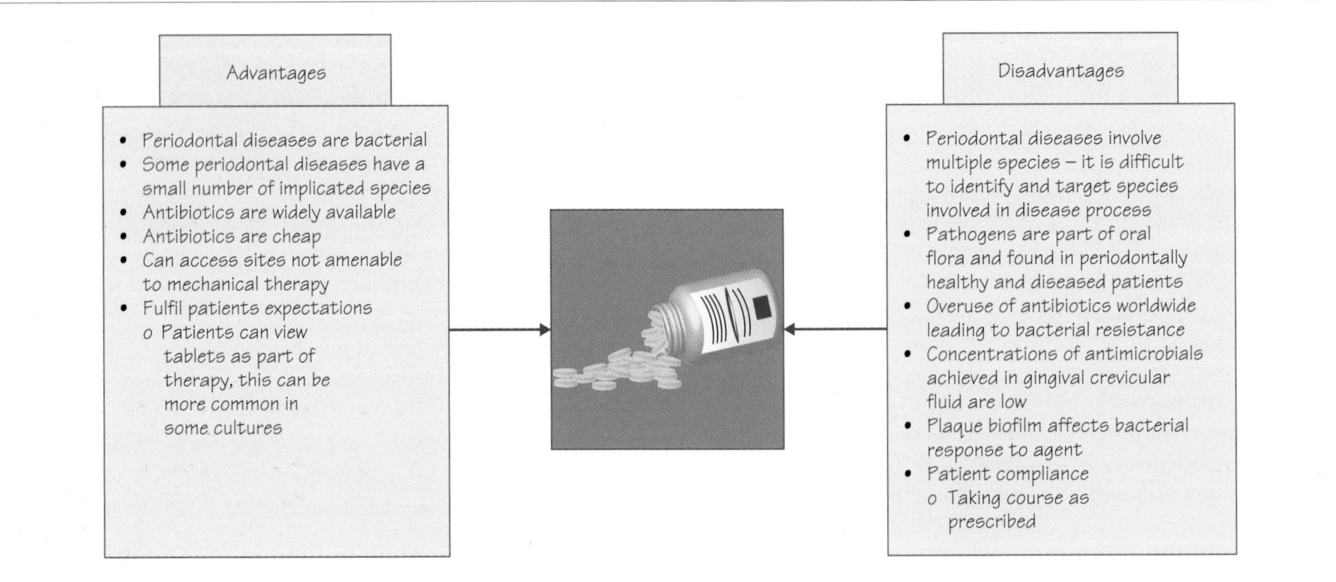

b) Local Antimicrobials

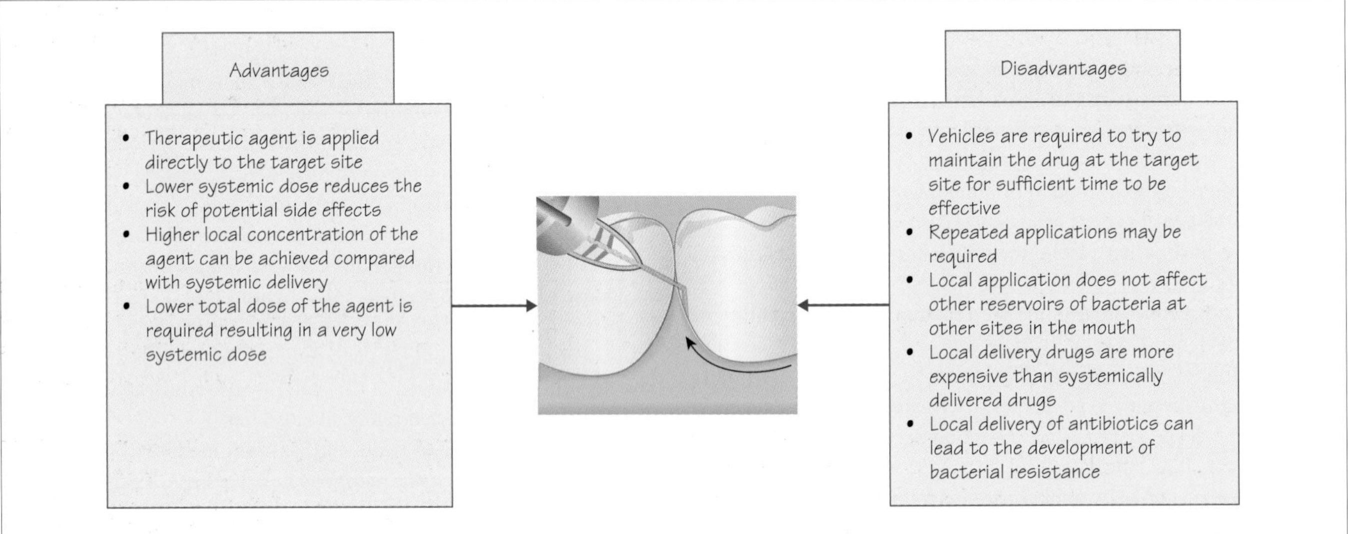

Figure 23.1 Advantages and disadvantages of using antimicrobials for periodontal diseases.

Periodontal disease has a bacterial aetiology and therefore much work has been done to investigate the potential role of antimicrobial drugs in the management of periodontal diseases. Mechanical therapy can not always access all subgingival deposits or reach bacteria that may have invaded soft tissue or dentinal tubules. Also, treated sites can be recolonised by pathogens from non-dental sites. Antimicrobial agents can be delivered by systemic or local routes.

Systemic antimicrobial therapy

Systemic antimicrobial agents have a role in periodontal therapy in a few specific clinical situations:

- Aggressive periodontitis.
- Necrotising ulcerative gingivitis and periodontitis.
- Acute periodontal abscess.

They are not indicated for the treatment of chronic periodontitis.

Aggressive periodontitis

Systemic antimicrobials can be used as an adjunct to root surface debridement. It is important to remove the plaque biofilm in order for antimicrobials to be most effective. Although root surface debridement in these cases can improve the clinical condition, a number of studies have shown that this alone can fail to significantly reduce the number of *Aggregatibacter actinomycetemcomitans* in the subgingival flora. The use of systemic antimicrobials can be effective in reducing *A. actinomycetemcomitans*. The effectiveness of treatment may be enhanced if debridement can be completed in a short time period while the drug is being taken.

Antibiotic regimes that are supported by the literature include:

- Tetracycline 250 mg four times daily for 14 days.
- Doxycycline (in the tetracycline family) 200 mg loading; 100 mg daily for 13 days – this is more convenient but there is less evidence of benefit.
- Metronidazole 250 mg (200 mg in UK) + amoxicillin 375 mg (250 or 500 mg in UK) three times daily for 7 days.

Antibiotics can also be used in combination with surgery in aggressive periodontitis.

Necrotising ulcerative gingivitis and periodontitis

- Necrotising ulcerative gingivitis (NUG) is an endogenous infection by mainly anaerobic bacteria (Chapter 38). Where there is lymph node involvement, it is effectively treated with metronidazole in conjunction with non-surgical debridement (e.g. 200 mg three times daily for 3 days). A mouthrinse such as chlorhexidine should also be used to control the plaque until the painful infection subsides.
- Necrotising ulcerative periodontitis (NUP) is a more destructive condition and antimicrobials are indicated as part of the overall management.

Acute periodontal abscess

Antibiotics may be used in the treatment of an acute periodontal abscess where adequate drainage cannot be achieved and there are signs of a spreading infection such as lymph node enlargement (see Chapter 39).

Other uses of systemic antimicrobials

Systemic antibiotics have been prescribed by some clinicians following periodontal surgery such as post guided tissue regenerative surgery. There is limited evidence to indicate the efficacy of use in these situations.

Low dose systemic antimicrobial therapy

Tetracyclines have a number of non-antibiotic properties that can have therapeutic benefit. Tetracyclines can:

- Inhibit host collagenases and metalloproteinases.
- Inhibit collagenases from other sources such as neutrophils, macrophages, osteoblasts and osteoclasts.
- Inhibit bone resorption.

A product called Periostat® (Collagenex International/Alliance Pharmaceuticals, Chippenham, UK) (20 mg doxcycline hyclate) seeks to utilise these non-antimicrobial properties at a dose lower than would affect the microbial flora. This drug is advocated for use as an adjunct in chronic periodontitis. Some work has indicated that even with a low dose there is a shift in flora, though other studies have shown no effect on bacterial resistance. The clinical benefits and long-term effect on the bacterial flora of such a regime needs further investigation.

Local antimicrobial therapy

These agents have been developed for the treatment of chronic periodontitis in adults. Clinical trials have used local delivery agents either as the sole treatment or in conjunction with root surface debridement. The reported levels of additional gain in clinical attachment and pocket depth reduction are modest, ranging from studies showing no additional benefit to an additional mean gain of attachment in the order of 1 mm.

Several commercial local delivery antimicrobial agents have been developed. These have included the following (though not all these systems have been continuously available in the marketplace since their original launch):

- Metronidazole gel (25%): Elyzol® (Colgate-Palmolive, Guildford, UK).
- Minocycline gel (2%): Dentomycin® (Blackwell Supplies, UK).
- Minocycline HCl (1 mg) encapsulated spheres: Arestin® (OraPharma Inc., Warminster, PA, USA).
- Tetracycline (25%) in ethylene vinyl acetate fibres: Actisite® (Alza Corporation, Palo Alto, USA).
- Doxycycline hyclate (8.8%) gel: Atridox® (Atrix Laboratories Inc.).
- Chlorhexidine (2.5 mg) in biodegradable polymer: Perio Chip® ((Dexcel Pharma).

The first five systems use antibiotics, and the last uses the antimicrobial agent chlorhexidine, which is available in mouthwashes. Chlorhexidine products have not shown the development of bacterial resistance.

Local delivery agents might be indicated in patients with chronic periodontitis who have isolated active pockets that are unresponsive to non-surgical therapy. Other indications might be in cases where surgery is not considered appropriate, for example in a smoker, where there are other systemic contraindications to surgery or where patient tolerance of a surgical procedure is in doubt.

Although the average potential clinical improvement anticipated from the use of local delivery agents may be small, in an individual site or patient this may be enough to change a progressive situation into a manageable one.

A possible disadvantage of antimicrobial use is that periodontal diseases are chronic and therefore antimicrobial therapy may have to be administered long-term, however, the long-term effects of antimicrobial usage are not yet known.

New developments

Photodynamic disinfection systems combine a non-thermal laser light with a photosensitising solution to target periodontal pathogens that remain after conventional instrumentation. (Periowave, Ondine Biopharma Corporation. Ondine Biopharma Corp. Vancouver, Canada).

Key points

- Despite the bacterial aetiology of periodontal disease, the involvement of indigenous species restricts the use of antibiotics in their management
- Systemic antimicrobials may have an adjunctive role in the management of:
  - aggressive periodontitis
  - necrotising ulcerative gingivitis and periodontitis
  - acute periodontal abscess
- Local antimicrobials can be applied directly to the target site
- Local antimicrobials have shown modest gains in clinical attachment

24 Periodontal surgery

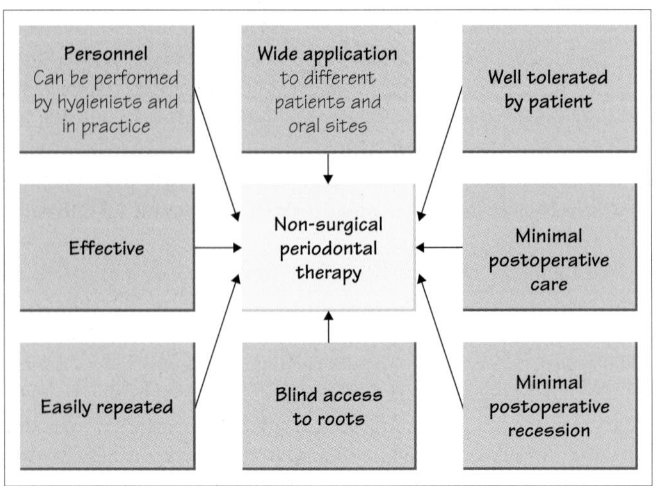

Figure 24.1 Advantages and disadvantages of non-surgical periodontal therapy.

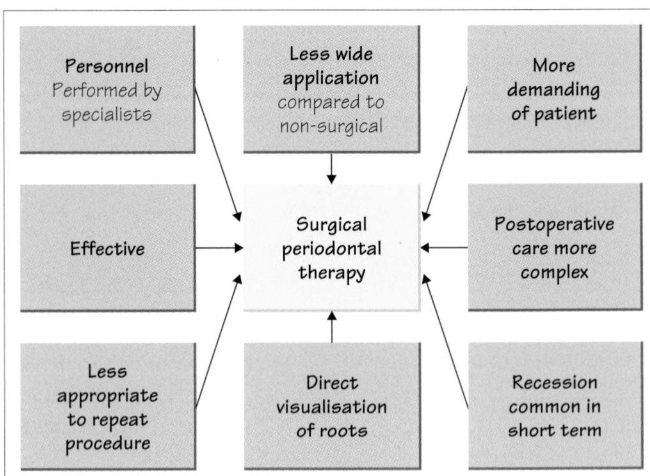

Figure 24.2 Advantages and disadvantages of surgical periodontal therapy.

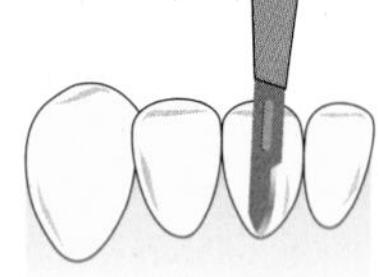

- Postoperative oral hygiene is decisive for outcome of surgical therapy
- Surgical procedures result in a decrease in probing pocket depths
  - Greater reduction occurs at initially deeper sites
  - Greater short-term reduction than non-surgical therapy
  - Long term, some studies show greater reduction compared with non-surgical therapy, others show no differences
- Surgical procedures may show superior outcomes to non-surgical for molar teeth but benefits become less apparent over time
- The deliberate excision of a soft tissue lesion does not improve the healing
- Bony infill can occur in two- and three-walled intrabony defects following surgical therapy

Figure 24.3 Clinical outcomes of surgical therapy.

In the first 24 hours:

- Take care until local analgesia wears off
- Avoid vigorous rinsing of the mouth
- Avoid vigorous exercise
- Avoid alcohol
- Pain relief can be gained by paracetomol 500 mg to 1 g or ibuprofen 400–600 mg and repeated 6 hours later if required. Do not exceed doses as recommended on the packet. Avoid aspirin
- Some oozing of the surgical site is not unusual
- Bleeding can be controlled by application of pressure with a clean handkerchief or pack placed on the site for 20 minutes. Seek help if bleeding continues

After 24 hours

- Rinse around site with chlorhexidine mouthwash twice daily (for 1–2 weeks as advised) (Chapter 20)
- Clean other teeth as normal as close to the surgical site as is reasonable but avoid the site itself (for 1–2 weeks as advised)
- Seek advice if there any concerns

Figure 24.4 Postoperative instructions to patients.

As described in Chapter 22, non-surgical root surface instrumentation is effective in controlling periodontal disease in many situations. Nonetheless there are limitations as to what can be achieved and in specific circumstances surgical techniques have a role to play in disease management (Figs 24.1, 24.2). Non-surgical techniques are generally most effective in shallow and moderate pockets and less so in deep pockets (greater than 6 mm). However, there is no absolute cut-off depth of pocket at which non-surgical debridement is ineffective. Non-surgical therapy may be unable to achieve thorough root debridement if there is reduced access to a pocket or if furcation defects or root grooves are present.

Thorough non-surgical therapy should be used in the first instance and the outcome assessed. If a site fails to respond to non-surgical debridement (indicated by suppuration, bleeding, loss of attachment, or persistent or increasing pocketing) it may be amenable to surgical intervention (Fig. 24.3).

Uses of periodontal surgery

Periodontal surgery can be used to:

- Provide access to a site for debridement by the operator.
- Make a site accessible to the patient for cleaning.
- Correct gross gingival morphology.
- Gain regeneration of tissues.
- Improve aesthetics.

Access to a site for debridement

Non-surgical debridement is a blind procedure and direct visualisation of the root surfaces and residual deposits can improve the effectiveness of deposit removal. Direct access may be useful where there is a furcation defect or suspected root groove.

Access to a site for cleaning

Following periodontal destruction the patient may be left with tissue contours that are hard to maintain, e.g. thickened flaps after recurrent episodes of necrotising gingivitis or partial access to a furcation area. Periodontal surgery can re-contour the tissues for optimal plaque removal by the patient.

Correction of gross gingival morphology

Excess tissue removal may be required subsequent to gingival overgrowth (Chapter 33).

Regeneration of tissues

Regenerative techniques can enable new supporting structures to develop, though the techniques are only appropriate in specific instances (Chapter 26).

Improve aesthetics

Aesthetics may be improved by root coverage following gingival recession using a variety of mucogingival surgical techniques (Chapter 32).

Contraindications for periodontal surgery

- If patient plaque control is not of a high standard.
- In patients with systemic diseases such as severe cardiovascular disease, malignancy, kidney and liver disease, bleeding disorders and uncontrolled diabetes. Consultation with the general medical practitioner and specialists is essential.
- Pregnancy: surgery is best delayed until after the birth.
- Smoking is known to adversely effect healing. Smokers have shown a poorer short- and long-term response to surgical treatment than non-smokers. Many clinicians do not perform periodontal surgery on smokers.
- Where the long-term prognosis and value of the tooth to the dentition is questionable.

Surgical flaps

Many of the surgical procedures require the raising of tissue flaps. Flaps allow access to the underlying root and bony defects. The soft tissue can then be manipulated in such a way that the flap is either replaced approximately back to the original position or moved to an adjacent site.

Flaps should be raised with the following factors in mind:

- The flap should be large enough to provide good access to the roots and bony defects.
- A flap that is too small will not enable adequate vision and may be liable to tearing.
- A wide flap base will enable sufficient blood supply to maintain the flap during healing.
- The flap must be raised avoiding other key nerves and blood vessels.
- The flap must be moveable without tension.

A full thickness flap is one comprising all the soft tissue, which is lifted from the underlying bone using a periosteal elevator. This flap is used commonly. A split thickness flap is one that is dissected so that the gingiva is separated from the mucoperiosteum which remains on the bone. This flap is used in some of the surgical procedures described in Chapter 32.

Periodontal dressings

A periodontal dressing may be used after many periodontal surgical procedures. The dressing material performs the following functions:

- Protects the wound.
- Keeps the wound clean.
- Controls bleeding.
- Helps to maintain the close approximation of flaps or grafts to the underlying tissue.

The dressing material needs to have a slow setting time to allow placement and be adapted to the surrounding tissues. Previously, many dressing materials were zinc oxide eugenol based, but most widely available materials are now eugenol free.

Postoperative care

Information regarding the surgical procedure will be given to the patient prior to undertaking surgery and as part of gaining the patient's consent. Following periodontal surgery patients require postoperative care. The patient should be given verbal and written instructions on how to care for the mouth in the postoperative period (Fig. 24.4) and arrangements should be made for a follow-up visit. The patient should be provided with contact details should they have any concerns following the treatment.

Key points

- Periodontal surgery can be used to:
  - provide access to a site for debridement by the operator
  - make a site accessible to the patient for cleaning
  - correct gross gingival morphology
  - gain regeneration of tissues
  - improve aesthetics
- Postoperative oral hygiene is decisive for the outcome of surgical therapy
- Clear postoperative instructions should be provided to the patient

25 Types of periodontal surgery

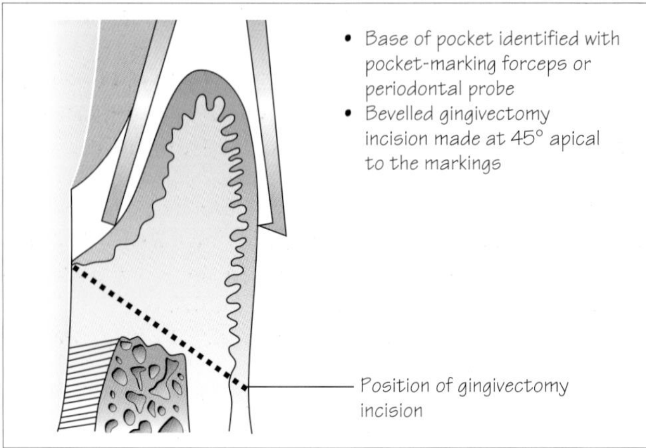

Figure 25.1 Gingivectomy.

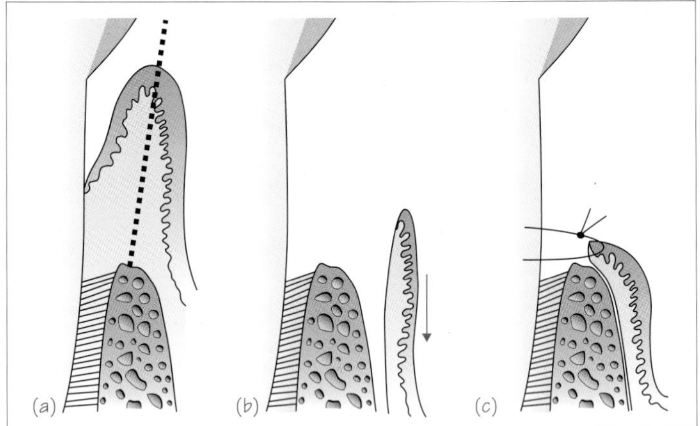

Figure 25.2 (a–c) Apically repositioned flap. (a) inverse bevel incision to alveolar crest (dashed line), (b) flap moved apically (arrow), (c) flap sutured just above the alveolar crest.

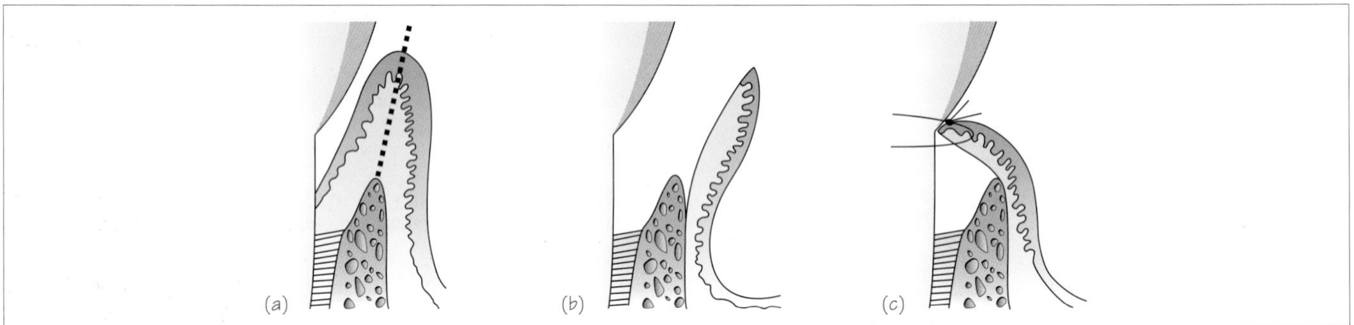

Figure 25.3 (a–c) Modified Widman flap. (a) inverse bevel incision to alveolar crest (dashed line), (b) following removal of inner lining of pocket the root surface can be accessed for cleaning, (c) flap is replaced at or close to its presurgical position.

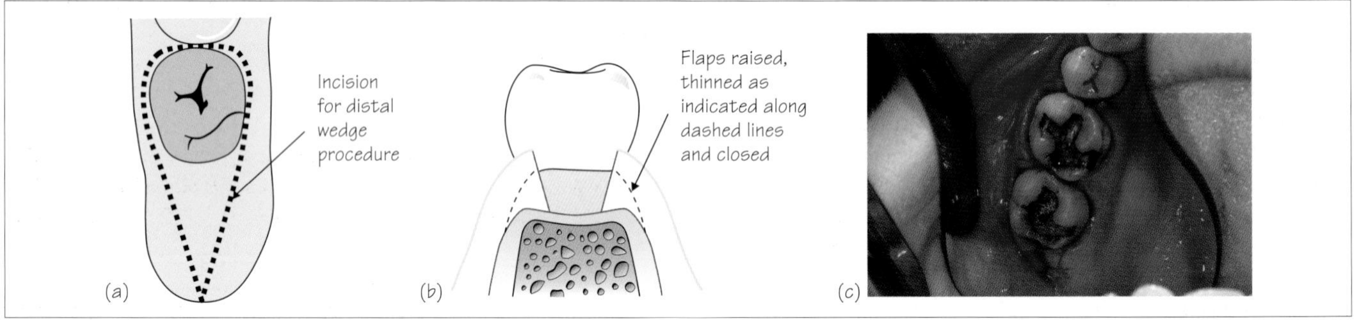

Figure 25.4 Distal wedge procedure: (a) occlusal view. The incision is made around the last standing molar and the wedge of tissue is removed. (b) vertical section. The tissue wedge is removed and the flaps thinned and approximated over the underlying bone. (c) clinical image. Incisions for distal wedge procedure. Photograph courtesy of Mr P J Nixon.

The techniques used can be divided as follows:

1 *Surgery to eliminate disease and produce conditions to minimise its recurrence* (outlined in this chapter):

- Pocket elimination or reduction:
  - gingivectomy (Fig. 25.1);
  - apically repositioned flap (Fig. 25.2).
- Accessing root for cleaning:
  - replaced flap (modified Widman flap) (Fig. 25.3).
- Distal wedge excision and tuberosity reduction (Fig. 25.4).

2 *Surgery to eliminate disease and regenerate lost periodontal structures* (Chapter 26):

- Guided tissue regeneration.
- Enamel matrix derivative (Emdogain®, Biora).
- Bone grafting.

3 *Surgery for root coverage* (mucogingival surgery) (Chapter 32):

- Pedicle grafts:
  - rotational flaps: laterally repositioned flap or double papilla flap;
  - advanced flaps: coronally advanced flap or coronally advanced flap plus enamel matrix derivative.
- Free epithelialised gingival grafts.
- Guided tissue regeneration.
- Subepithelial connective tissue graft.

Gingivectomy

This can be used for:

• Persistent gingival enlargement such as drug-induced gingival overgrowth.

• Exposing a furcation involvement with a wide zone of attached gingiva for access to oral hygiene measures.

• Persistent active sites with suprabony pockets of >5 mm, where adequate attached gingiva would be left following surgery.

This technique reduces the width of the attached gingiva so should not be used where this zone is limited. Gingivectomy for pocket elimination not associated with gingival deformity or overgrowth has largely been replaced by flap surgery.

Procedure

• The base of the pocket is identified with pocket marking forceps or a periodontal probe (Fig. 25.1).

• A bevelled gingivectomy incision is made at 45° apical to the markings both buccally and lingually/palatally. It is made as a continuous not scalloped incision.

• Tissue is removed with curettes.

• The exposed root surfaces are debrided.

• The dressing is placed.

Healing

The connective tissue becomes covered with blood clot. There is transient acute inflammation with reorganisation of the blood clot. The open wound epithelialises, covering the site in 7–14 days and keratinising in 2–3 weeks.

Apically repositioned flap

This procedure eliminates pockets by displacing the flap apically and the flap is sutured just coronal to the alveolar crest. This technique preserves the zone of attached gingiva. The roots are left exposed so aesthetics and postoperative sensitivity are poorer than with the more widely used modified Widman flap.

Procedure

• Two vertical, parallel, relieving incisions are made to the bone at either end of the flap. These are carried out buccally and lingually. Care is required lingually with the distal relieving incision to prevent damage to the lingual nerve.

• An inverse bevel incision is made along the gingival margin, and scalloped around the necks of the teeth to separate the pocket lining and inflamed connective tissue from the flap (Fig. 25.2).

• The flaps are raised leaving the separated pocket lining *in situ*.

• The separated pocket lining and connective tissue are removed from the roots with curettes.

• The roots are debrided.

• The buccal and lingual flaps are displaced apically and sutured. The palatal flap cannot be displaced so it is treated by inverse bevel incision alone.

• A dressing is placed to help maintain apical displacement.

Healing

There is transient acute inflammation with reorganisation of the blood clot between the tooth and flap into granulation tissue (1 week).

There is replacement of granulation tissue by connective tissue (2–5 weeks).

The epithelial migration commences from the margin of the flap and gives rise to new junctional epithelium (approximately 4 weeks).

There is some resorption of the alveolar bone margin resulting from raising a flap. This is minimised by a careful surgical technique.

Long term the gingival margin may shift coronally by about 1 mm.

Replaced flap (modified Widman flap or modified flap)

This technique is widely used as it allows access to the roots for cleaning and, since it conserves tissue, it can be used when aesthetics are important. It is indicated when there is persistent deep active pocketing.

Procedure

• An inverse bevel incision is made up to 1 mm from the gingival margin buccally and palatally/lingually to separate the pocket epithelium and inflamed connective tissue from the flap (Fig. 25.3).

• The separated tissue can be removed either directly by a curette or after two further incisions:

  • an incision from the base of the pocket to the bone crest;

  • a horizontal incision after the flap is reflected from the crest of the bone to the tooth surface.

• Reflection of the flap (note there are no relieving incisions in this technique).

• Debridement of the root surfaces.

• The flap is replaced at the original level and is sutured. Try to gain complete interdental coverage avoiding root exposure.

• A dressing is placed if it is considered necessary.

Healing

There is transient acute inflammation with reorganisation of the blood clot between the tooth and flap into granulation tissue (1 week) which is replaced by connective tissue (2–5 weeks).

The epithelial migration commences from the margin of the flap and gives rise to new long junctional epithelium. This occurs over several weeks and is easily disrupted by premature probing. Pocket reduction is achieved by long junctional epithelial attachment to the cleaned root surface. Long term the gingival margin may shift coronally by about 1 mm.

Distal wedge excision and tuberosity reduction

Excess flabby tissue distal to the last standing tooth can be excised to reduce a pocket and enable root surface debridement of the site. Flaps are raised and a wedge of tissue is removed (Fig. 25.4). The flaps are thinned and approximated to the underlying bone.

Key points

• The categories of periodontal surgery are:

  • surgery to eliminate disease and to produce conditions to minimise its recurrence

  • surgery to eliminate disease and regenerate lost periodontal structures

  • surgery for root coverage

• Gingivectomy is used to excise excess tissue and reduce pockets

• An apically repositioned flap is used to eliminate pockets

• A replaced flap is used to gain access to roots without achieving immediate postoperative pocket reduction

  • pocket reduction occurs following healing with the formation of long junctional epithelium

26 Regenerative periodontal therapy

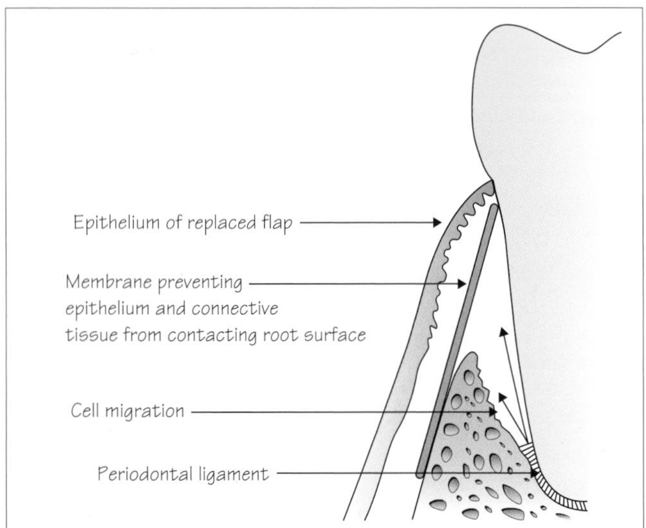

Figure 26.1 Guided tissue regeneration.

Non-resorbable	**Resorbable**
• Flexible Teflon® (ePTFE): Gore-Tex®	• Lactide/gylycolide co-polymer: Resolut® • Polylactic acid + citric acid ester: Guidor® • Polylactic acid (made at chairside for custom fit): Atrisorb® • Collagen: Bio-Gide®

Figure 26.2 Types of membrane for guided tissue regeneration.

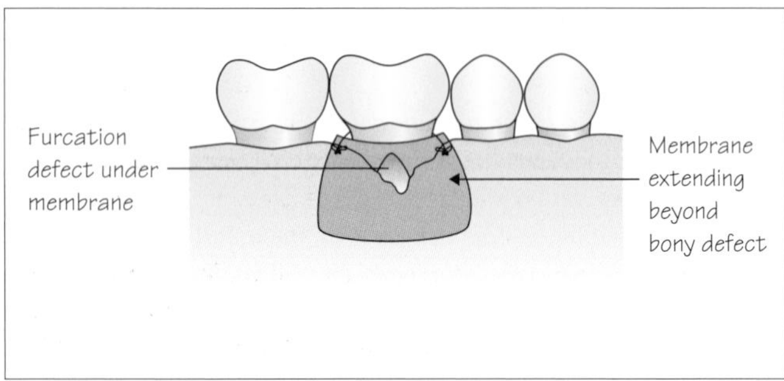

Figure 26.3 Guided tissue regeneration: membrane placement.

- After gaining surgical access to the site the cleaned root surfaces are conditioned with an EDTA (ethylene diamine tetra acetate) gel to remove the smear layer
- The Emdogain® gel is syringed directly onto the washed roots and the flap replaced

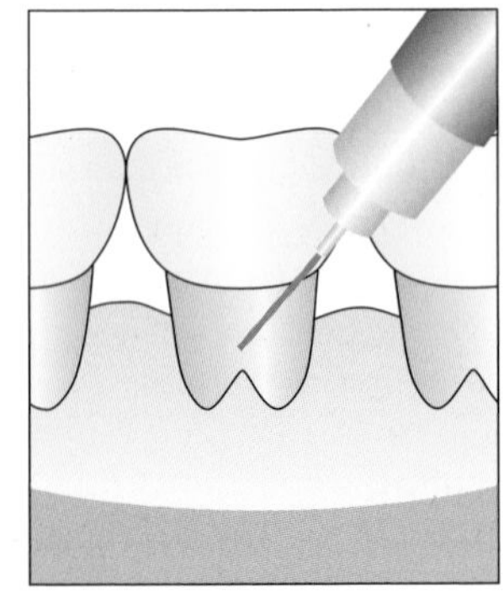

Figure 26.4 Procedure for use of Emdogain®.

- Platelet-derived growth factor (PDGF)
- Insulin-like growth factor (IGF)
- Fibroblast growth factors (FGFs)
- Transforming growth factor-β (TGF-β) – including bone morphogenetic proteins

Figure 26.6 Potential growth factors for periodontal regeneration. Growth factors are known to affect osteogenic cells and are being actively investigated for a potential role in periodontal regeneration.

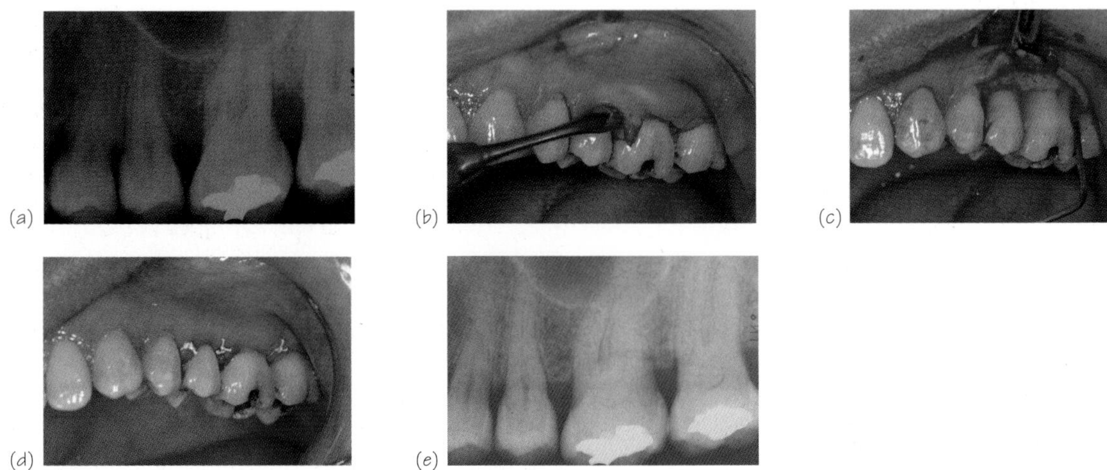

Figure 26.5 A case treated by the use of Emdogain® and PerioGlas®. (a) Preoperative radiograph of the surgical site. (b) Reflection of the buccal flap. (c) Application of Emdogain® following the use of ethylene diamine tetra acetate (EDTA) conditioner. (d) Flaps replaced and secured with sutures. (e) Radiograph taken 18 months' postoperatively. Courtesy of Mr P. J. Nixon.

Regenerative periodontal therapy encompasses a number of surgical procedures that aim specifically at gaining healing of periodontal destruction by developing new periodontium rather than by repair with a long junctional epithelial attachment. These techniques include:

- Guided tissue regeneration.
- Enamel matrix derivative (Straumann®, Emdogain).
- Bone grafts (Chapter 27).
- Growth factors.

Guided tissue regeneration

Following conventional flap surgery, cells from the overlying epithelium rapidly migrate apically. A long junctional epithelium results and this attaches onto the cleaned root surface resulting in healing by repair which does not mimic the original periodontal attachment.

Guided tissue regeneration (GTR) attempts to reorder the migration of cells so that cells from the periodontal ligament are able to proliferate and migrate into the healing site, resulting in a reformed periodontium rather than a repaired periodontium (Fig. 26.1).

The technique consists of the placement of a membrane which excludes the migrating epithelium and connective tissue, creating a space around the cleaned root surface. This is repopulated by cells that can then mature to form new periodontal ligament fibres, which insert into bone.

Types of membrane

There are two types of membrane (Fig. 26.2):

- Non-resorbable.
- Resorbable.

Non-resorbable membranes

The first membranes to be developed were non-resorbable. Titanium reinforcement was added to create and maintain the space between the flap and root more effectively. A disadvantage of this type of membrane is that a second surgical procedure is required to remove it.

Resorbable membranes

These were devised to avoid the second surgical procedure for removal of the membrane. Polylactic membranes are degraded by enzymes in the Krebs cycle. Collagen membranes are broken down by collagenases and subsequently by other proteinases. Collagen membranes are made from animal collagen and have to be produced in a way that ensures they are antigen free.

Use of GTR

- Treatment of two- or three-walled intrabony defects (Chapter 27).
- Treatment of furcation defects (Chapter 27): most predictable in class II lesions).
- Treatment of recession defects (Chapter 32).
- For alveolar ridge defects and limited generation of new bone for implant placement.

Procedure

- Intracrevicular incisions are used and the flaps are raised at the site of the defect. This is in order to achieve the following:
  - to preserve as much of the keratinised attached gingiva as possible;
  - to separate the pocket epithelium.
- The root surfaces are cleaned.
- The membrane is cut to fit the area so that it covers the defect and extends slightly beyond it (Fig. 26.3).
- Most membranes are then sutured into place (Atrisorb® (Tolmar Inc.) does not need sutures).
- Flaps are replaced so that none of the membrane is exposed to the oral cavity.
- Non-resorbable membranes are removed 4–6 weeks after placement. The healing tissue appears as a red gelatinous material, which needs to be carefully separated from the membrane to allow the membrane to be removed.
- The resorbable membranes break down over time.

GTR can be used alone or with enamel matrix derivatives or bone grafts.

Outcomes

Although studies have shown significant gains in bone levels and clinical attachment with GTR, there is a great variability in the gains reported. Complete resolution of intrabony defects is only rarely found. GTR has shown attachment gains in class II furcation defects, particularly at lower molar sites, but results are unpredictable in class III defects (Chapter 27). Factors that may influence the outcome include plaque levels, the morphology of the site and factors relating to the surgical technique. Membrane stability is very important in achieving success, and exposure of the membrane with subsequent bacterial contamination is associated with reduced attachment gains.

Recent studies have shown similar results from non-resorbable and resorbable membranes.

Enamel matrix derivative (Emdogain®)

Enamel matrix proteins have been found to induce cementum formation and periodontal regeneration. This has been used to formulate the commercial product Straumann®, Emdogain. Similar clinical results to GTR have been reported but the surgical technique is much simpler (Fig. 26.4).

Straumann®, Emdogain can also be used in conjunction with bone graft materials (Chapter 27) such as Bio-Oss® (Geistlich Pharma AG), PerioGlas® (Nova Bone) or Straumann BoneCeramic 400–700® (Straumann, Crawley, UK) that act as scaffolds for bone deposition (Fig. 26.5). Emdogain® can also be used with the technique of GTR.

Growth factors

Growth factors and cells mediators regulate cellular activities such as migration and proliferation (Fig. 26.6). They function in low concentrations and act locally. They bind to high affinity cell membrane receptors and activate cellular mechanisms.

Bone morphogenetic proteins are a group of the proteins belonging to the transforming growth factor β (TGF-β) group. These factors are able to stimulate bone and cartilage and cementogenesis. In the periodontal site they may be able to stimulate cells not only from the remaining periodontal ligament but also from other tissue such as the flaps. Research is very active in this area and commercial products may be developed in the future.

Key points

- Guided tissue regeneration involves the placement of a membrane to create a space for the migration of cells from the periodontal ligament
- Enamel matrix derivative is available as Emdogain®, which induces cementum and periodontal regeneration
- Growth factors may have the future potential to regenerate the periodontium

27 Bone defects and furcation lesions

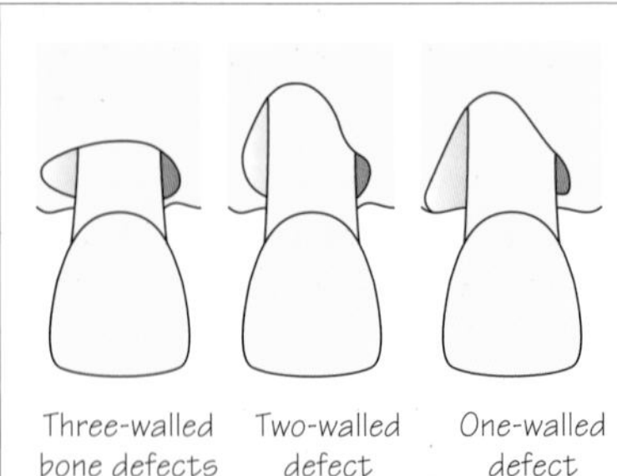

Bony defects are often described according to the number of supporting bone walls that surround the tooth: one-, two- or three-walled defects. A three-walled defect is bounded by one tooth surface and three osseous surfaces. Clinical and radiographic investigations can aid the diagnosis of a bone defect but the actual anatomy can only fully be assessed if a surgical flap is raised.

Figure 27.1 Anatomy of bone defects.

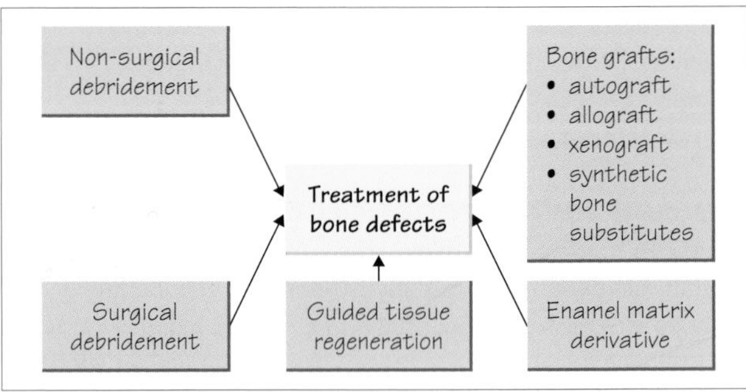

Figure 27.2 Treatment of bone defects.

(a)

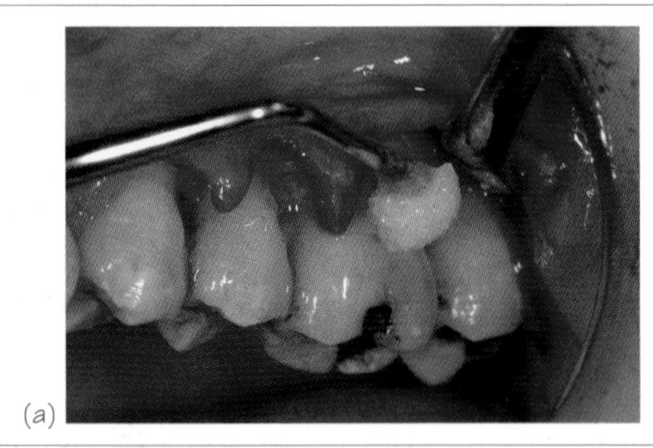

(b)

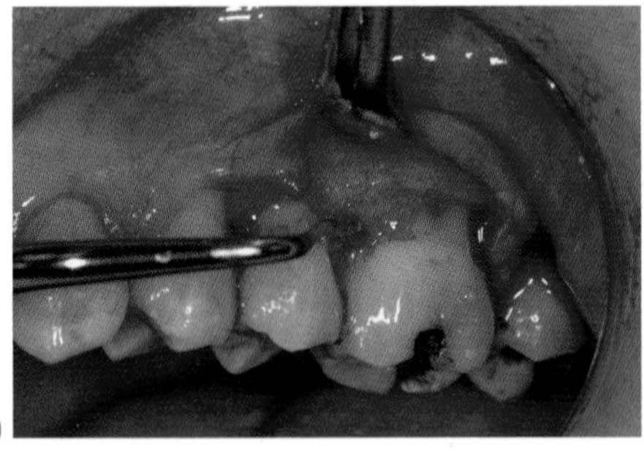

This case was treated using Emdogain® and PerioGlas®. The placement of Emdogain® and the subsequent healing following the use of both materials is shown in Fig. 26.5.

Figure 27.3 Use of synthetic bone graft (PerioGlas®). (a) Synthetic bone graft material on an instrument prior to placement. (b) Placement of the synthetic bone graft material. Courtesy of Mr P. J. Nixon.

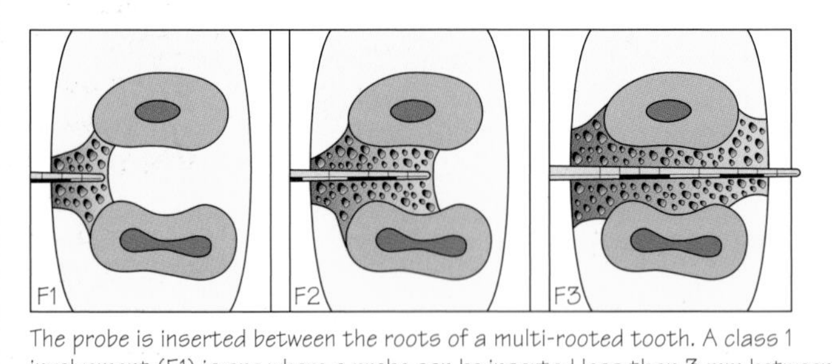

The probe is inserted between the roots of a multi-rooted tooth. A class 1 involvement (F1) is one where a probe can be inserted less than 3 mm between the roots. A class 2 involvement (F2) penetrates more than 3 mm but not fully through the furcation, and a class 3 (F3) involvement extends completely between the roots.

Figure 27.4 Classification of furcation involvement.

- Non-surgical debridement
- Surgical debridement
- Surgical exposure of furcation ± soft tissue modification
- **Treatment of furcation lesions**
- Regeneration
  - Guided tissue
  - Enamel matrix proteins
- Tunnel preparation
- Root resection, tooth division and hemisection
- Extraction

Figure 27.5 Treatment of furcation lesions.

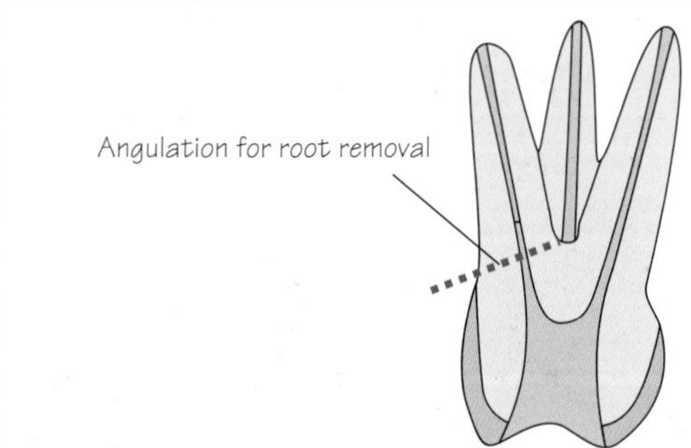

Endodontic treatment is required. Flaps are raised and the root to be removed is sectioned along the line indicated. The root is elevated. The remaining tooth is contoured to give access to cleaning and the flaps are replaced leaving the tooth supported on the two remaining roots. A permanent restoration is placed to seal the cut root canal. Careful oral hygiene measures are needed to clean under the crown at the amputation site.

Figure 27.6 Root resection.

Bone defects

Alveolar bone resorption leads to the creation of bony defects (infrabony or intrabony), which differ in anatomy from one tooth site to another (Fig. 27.1).

Treatment of bone defects

The different methods of treatment are depicted in Fig. 27.2.

Non-surgical debridement

• Bone defects can be treated as at any other site by non-surgical debridement.
• Healing is with a long junctional epithelium and potentially some bony infill, particularly where there are several walls to the defect.

Surgical access for debridement

• Raising a surgical flap can improve access to the site and enable thorough removal of the inflammatory tissue.
• Healing is as for non-surgical debridement.
• The bony defect can be reshaped during the procedure.
  – May result in further bone loss so use with caution to create an architecture that allows better flap adaptation.
• Bone fill may be obtained in two- and three-walled defects but great variability in the degree of fill has been found.

Simple debridement of the defect (either indirectly or directly) is most successful if the defect is not too large and there are several bone walls.

Bone grafts

Bone grafts can be used with a surgical technique to access the bony defect. The graft may be derived from a number of sources:

• *Autografts* (from same individual) taken from other oral sites or the iliac crest (an invasive procedure). Fresh marrow often leads to ankylosis and tooth resorption so it is frozen before use. Bony infill can be gained but the site generally heals with a long junctional epithelial attachment.
• *Allografts* (from same species) have included freeze-dried bone allograft (FDBA) and freeze-dried demineralised bone allograft (FDDBA). Studies have shown bony infill and some regeneration of new bone, periodontal ligament and cementum. The possibility of disease transfer is a potential problem though probably a very low risk. The graft is likely to act as a scaffold which is replaced by new tissue.
• *Xenografts* (from different species) have been commercially produced from the mineral component of bovine bone (Bio-Oss®, Geistlich Pharma AG). There is potentially a risk of transmission of infective agents. However, this material has been used widely and appears to have osteogenic potential in periodontal infrabony defects.
• *Synthetic bone substitutes* include hydroxyapatite, ceramics and bioactive glasses (e.g. PerioGlas®, NovaBone) (Fig. 27.3). The bioactive materials show formation of new cementum and bone and periodontal ligament, while hydroxyapatite tends to result in bony infill with a long junctional epithelial attachment.

Enamel matrix derivative and guided tissue regeneration

See Chapter 26.

Furcation lesions

Bone loss around multi-rooted teeth can expose part or the entire furcation region where the roots divide. This complicates the anatomy of the bony defect, creating a site that is potentially hard for the patient and operator to clean. Furcation lesions can be diagnosed by probing or radiographically. They are usually classified according to the degree of horizontal involvement (Fig. 27.4).

Treatment of furcation lesions

The different methods of treatment are depicted in Fig. 27.5.

Non-surgical and surgical access for debridement

• Class 1 and 2 defects can be managed by scaling and supportive therapy.
• Access to a furcation defect may be improved by raising a flap for thorough scaling of the site.

Surgical exposure (± soft tissue modification)

A gingivectomy or apically repositioned flap can be used to uncover a furcation defect to produce a site accessible to plaque control by the patient.

Regeneration

• Guided tissue regeneration (GTR) can be used to treat class 2 furcation involvement and with other graft materials (Chapter 26).
• GTR has been used to treat class 3 defects but with less predictable results.
• Enamel matrix proteins have been used to treat class 2 defects.

Tunnel preparation

Can be used in the lower molars to produce a furcation accessible from buccal to lingual for cleaning.

• The buccal and lingual flaps are raised and displaced apically.
• The furcation defect may be recontoured for a brush to pass through easily.
• A periodontal pack in the furcation maintains the site during healing.

Root resection, tooth division and hemisection

These are used where there is advanced bone loss around one of the roots and the remaining roots will have enough support to allow the tooth to function. The value of the tooth to the patient should be assessed. Endodontic treatment is undertaken so unfavourable canal morphology can be a contraindication.

• *Root resection* is used generally for the three-rooted upper molars with a loss of the mesiobuccal or distobuccal root (Fig. 27.6).
• *Tooth division* is used infrequently in lower molars where bone loss is severe in the furcation region but roots individually have reasonable bone support. The tooth is divided and each part is subsequently prepared for a single tooth crown.
• *Hemisection* is used in lower molars with advanced bone loss around one root. Following division of the tooth, one root is retained and the other elevated. The remaining root can then be used as a bridge retainer to support a pontic replacing the missing portion or as a premolar-sized crown.

Extraction

Extraction may be the appropriate management of a tooth with advanced furcation involvement where the tooth is compromised.

Key points

• Bone defects can be managed by non-surgical and surgical therapy aimed at debridement of the defect
• Regeneration in bony defects may be achieved by the use of:
  • bone grafts
  • guided tissue regeneration
  • enamel matrix derivative
• Furcation defects can be managed by non-surgical and surgical therapy aimed at debridement of the defect
• Regeneration in furcation lesions may be achieved using guided tissue regeneration and enamel matrix derivative
• Advanced furcation defects may be managed by tunnel preparation, resection of part of the tooth or extraction

28 Dental implants and peri-implantology

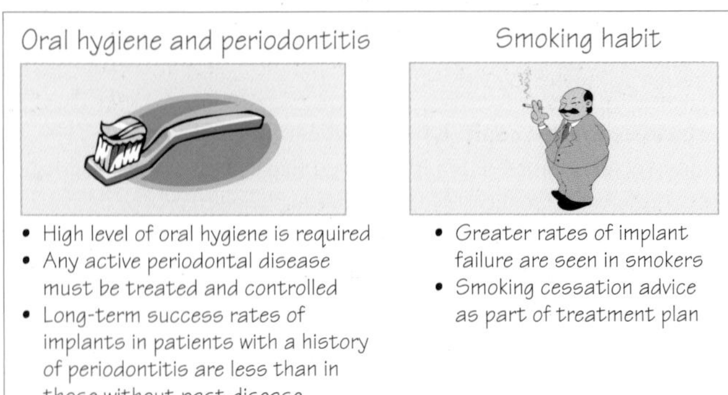

Figure 28.1 Factors to consider prior to implants.

(a)

(b)

(c)

Figure 28.3 Implant replacing an upper left lateral incisor. (a) Implant at UL2 with impression coping *in situ*. (b) Final restoration of UL2. (c) Radiograph showing the healthy implant with final restoration at 1 year post placement. Courtesy of Mr P. J. Nixon.

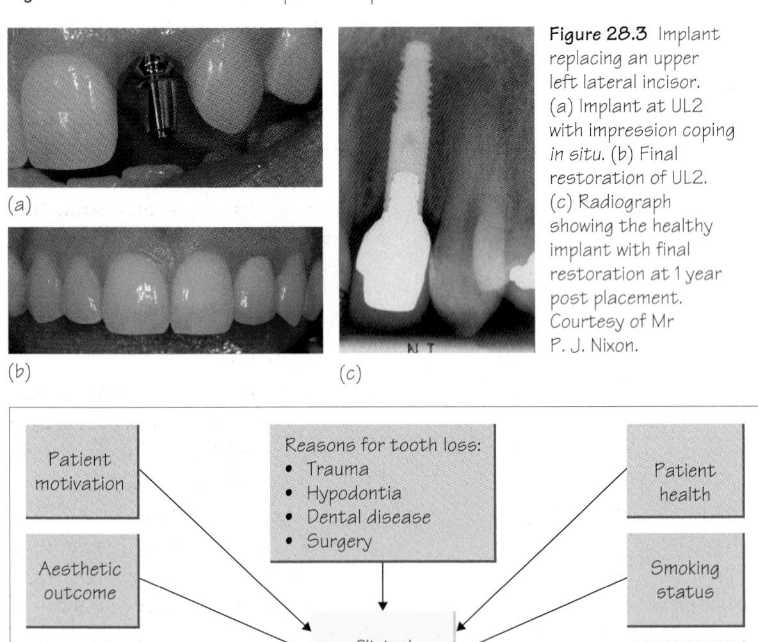

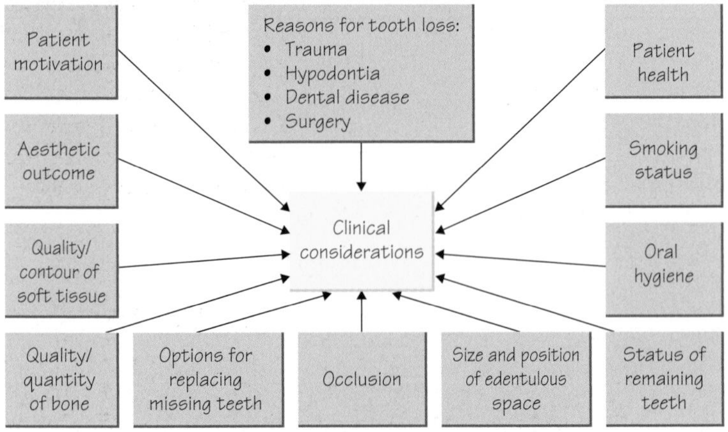

Figure 28.4 Clinical considerations for implant therapy.

The barrier epithelium is about 2 mm long with an underlying zone of connective tissue of about 1.5 mm. The epithelium is attached to the implant via hemidesmosomes. The fibres in the connective tissue run parallel to the implant surface with no attachment to its surface.

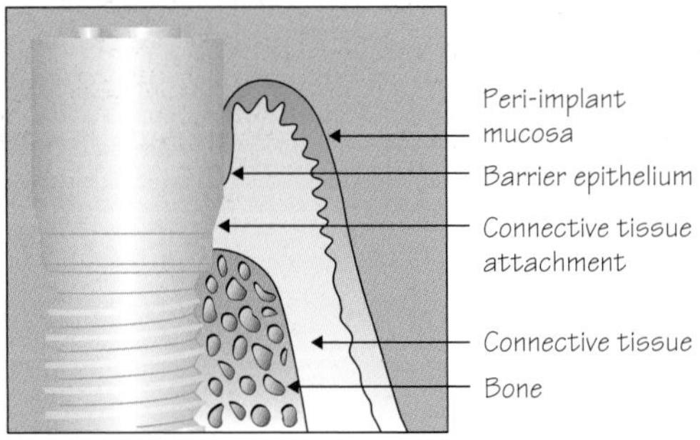

Peri-implant mucosa

Barrier epithelium

Connective tissue attachment

Connective tissue

Bone

Figure 28.6 Implant and peri-implant tissues.

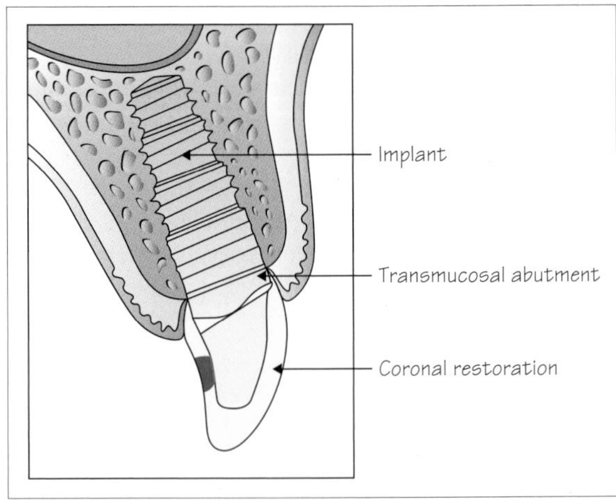

Figure 28.2 Implant with coronal restoration.

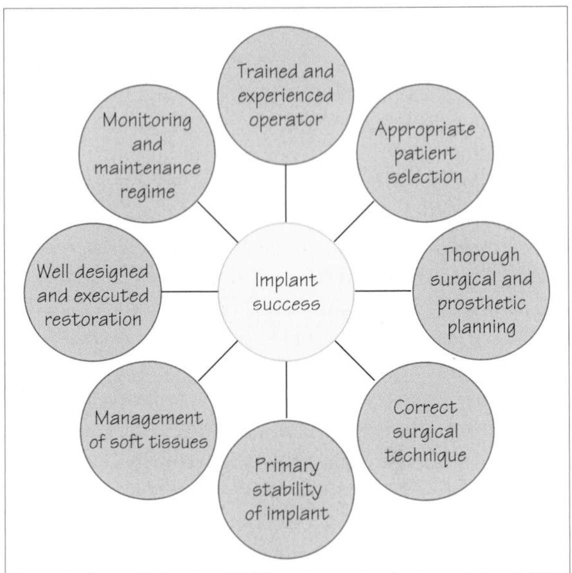

Figure 28.5 Factors in achieving implant success.

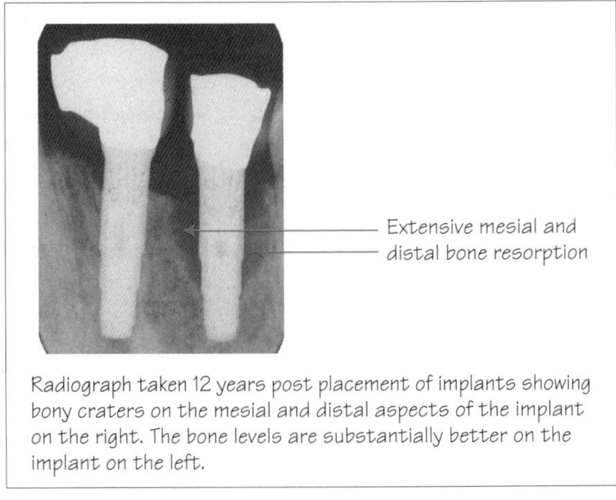

Radiograph taken 12 years post placement of implants showing bony craters on the mesial and distal aspects of the implant on the right. The bone levels are substantially better on the implant on the left.

Figure 28.7 Radiograph of a failing implant.

Dental implants give the clinician and patient a further option for restoring edentulous spaces. Implants may be used to replace teeth that have been lost because of periodontal disease. To improve the outcome of the procedure there are a number of things that should be addressed prior to the implant (Fig. 28.1). Final restoration of implants may be with single crowns (Figs 28.2, 28.3), bridges or overdentures. Implants are retained by osseointegration, the name given to the tight connection that develops as bone forms in close approximation to the implant surface.

The key parts of the implant-retained restoration are:

- An implant placed into bone.
- A component connected to the implant that projects through the mucosa into the mouth (transmucosal abutment).
- A coronal restoration.

A large number of implant systems are available, each with differing characteristics such as implant shape, lengths and widths, type of fixation of components and surface characteristics. Within each system there are components to aid planning before surgery, guide at the time of placement and to enable fabrication of temporary and final restorations. Planning often requires the use of specialist radiographs. There are various clinical considerations before implants are undertaken and many factors that influence their success (Figs 28.4, 28.5).

Osseointegration

Dental implants are made of titanium, a highly reactive and biocompatible metal, which forms a non-corrosive surface oxide layer in contact with the tissues. A large implant–bone interface is achieved by surface modifications, screw threads and perforations that allow forces to be transmitted over a wide area. Studies have shown that osteoblasts require a porous and rough surface in order to synthesise and lay down bone against the implant. A roughened implant surface is produced either by coatings (titanium-plasma spray coating or hydroxyapatite) or by grit blasting and etching. Osseointegration occurs around and within all these features.

Implant placement

When placing an implant a matched hole is prepared with precision low speed drills, which are irrigated to avoid damage to the bone. Drills are used in sequence to gradually widen a pilot hole and prepare it to the correct depth. The implant is placed in the prepared hole and screwed into its final position with a handpiece or driver. A good fit of the implant provides primary stability which will promote osseointegration.

A one- or two-stage technique can be used.

- The *two-stage method* involves placement of the implant and cover screw and coverage with the mucosal tissues while osseointegration occurs. This generally takes between 3 and 6 months depending on the implant location. The implant is then exposed, a gingival former (healing abutment) is placed to contour the soft tissues during healing, and the restoration is subsequently constructed.
- The *one-stage method* leaves the implant exposed but not loaded during the osseointegration period, and a gingival former is placed immediately after placement of the implant to allow soft tissue adaptation. Techniques have been described for early loading of the implant.

Guided tissue regeneration and bone grafts

Providing that primary stability is achieved, bony defects around the implant can be treated with guided tissue regenerative techniques. Where significant increases in bone width or height are required, more extensive surgical procedures such as block bone grafts or sinus lifts are needed. These require a high level of skill and an additional healing period prior to implant placement.

Peri-implant mucositis and peri-implantitis

The attachment of tissues around an implant is shown in Fig. 28.6. Bacterial plaque can form on implants and plaque retention can lead to inflammation of the peri-implant tissues. Good oral hygiene is therefore imperative for these patients.

Peri-implant mucositis is the term used to describe the reversible inflammation of the mucosa around an implant. This inflammation may spread into the supporting bone when it is known as peri-implantitis. The lesions tend to be less encapsulated than those around a tooth and can lead to loss of bone and increased probing depths. The clinical features of inflammation are similar to those of gingival inflammation: redness, swelling and bleeding. Peri-implantitis additionally is characterised by radiographic bone loss and the bone defects often appear crater-like (Fig. 28.7). Suppuration is also frequently seen. The implants may be stable but can show mobility when bone loss becomes severe. Implants should be monitored regularly by probing with a light probing force and using radiographs. In the presence of inflammation around an implant, the tip of the probe can pass beyond the apical cells into the connective tissue and almost to the bone crest.

Regular supportive therapy is required to reinforce and assist plaque removal around implants. Calculus removal is difficult as the titanium surface is easily damaged; plastic or carbon fibre instruments should be used. Peri-implant mucositis and incipient peri-implantitis lesions may be treated by conventional non-surgical therapy. Lesions of shallow pocketing may require the additional use of chlorhexidine as a mouthrinse or topically applied gel. More advanced lesions of peri-implantitis may also require surgical management, systemic antimicrobial therapy or local antimicrobial therapy.

Key points

- Dental implants are retained by osseointegration
- A soft tissue cuff similar to gingivae develops around the implant
- Successful implants will depend on appropriate patient selection and good planning
- Additional techniques such as guided tissue regeneration and bone grafting can augment bone at the implant site
- Regular supportive therapy is required to prevent plaque retention around implants that can lead to peri-implant mucositis and peri-implantitis

29 Periodontic–orthodontic interface

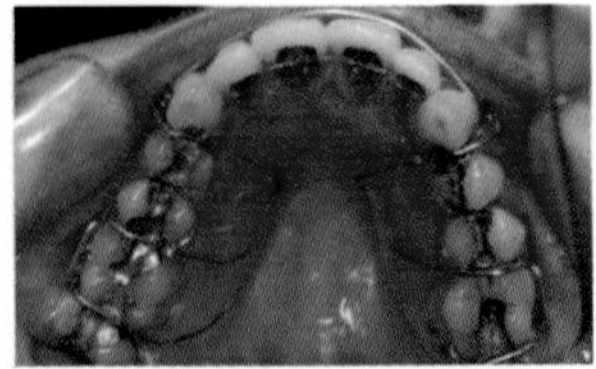

Figure 29.1 A Hawley retainer.

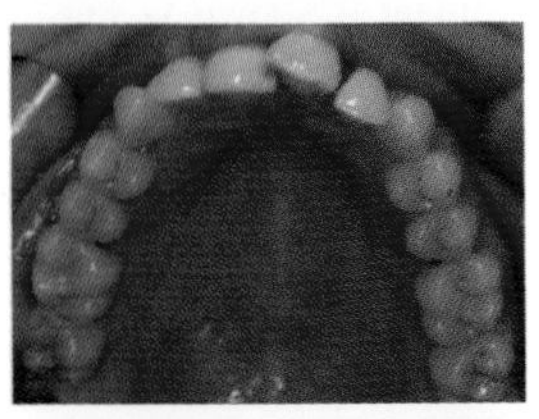

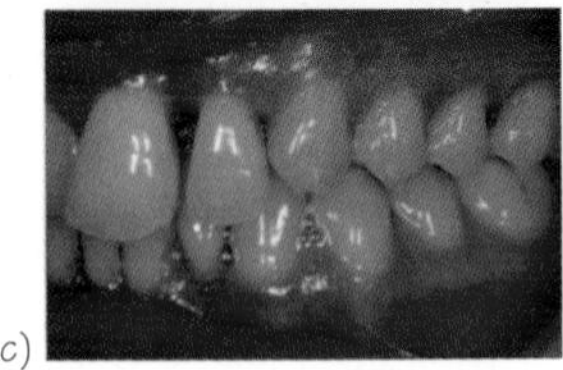

Figure 29.4 (a–c) A 28-year-old female patient (non-smoker) with a history of localised aggressive periodontitis, prior to periodontal therapy. Note inflammation around the lateral incisors, upper left central incisor and instanding lower left lateral incisor. Also note the position of the upper left central incisor which has drifted and dropped out of line of the arch and is rotated and tilted.

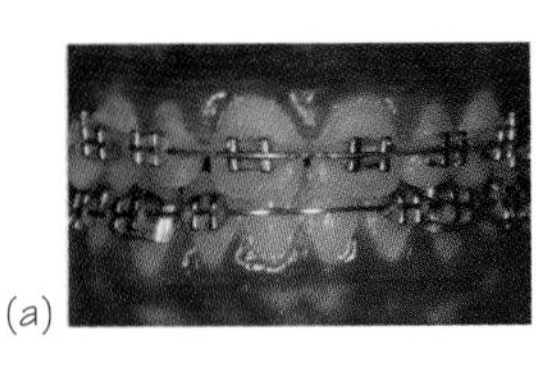

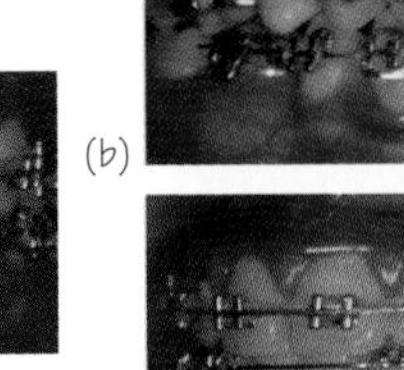

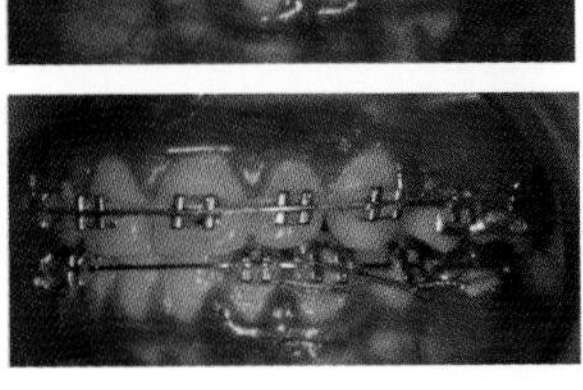

Figure 29.2 (a–c) Fixed orthodontic appliances in a 15-year-old Asian girl. Note the poor plaque control, gingival inflammation and swelling anteriorly and posteriorly.

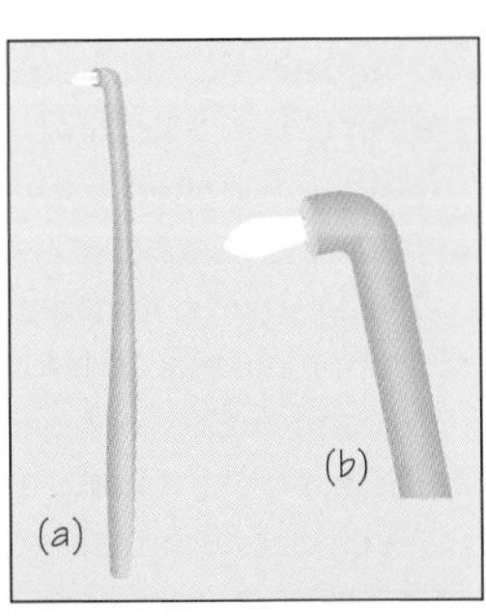

Figure 29.3 (a, b) Interspace brush with a single tufted head for cleaning around fixed appliance brackets, arch wires and elastics.

Adult orthodontics in periodontally compromised patients
• Adults who elect to have orthodontic treatment usually have the motivation to complete orthodontic treatment; increased compliance
• Medical, social and dental history can complicate orthodontics
• Lack of facial growth may inhibit orthodontic movements
• Less cellular activity, therefore takes longer before tooth movement occurs
• May experience more pain following arch wire adjustments, therefore lighter orthodontic forces needed
• Lack of periodontal support: • reduces resistance to unwanted tooth movement, creating anchorage problems – light forces are needed to avoid tipping or extrusion • increases risk of root resorption due to reduced available root surface area and decreased vascularity
• Reduced adaptation of periodontal fibres leads to requirement for stricter retention regime – permanent retention advocated

Figure 29.6 Adult orthodontics in periodontally compromised patients.

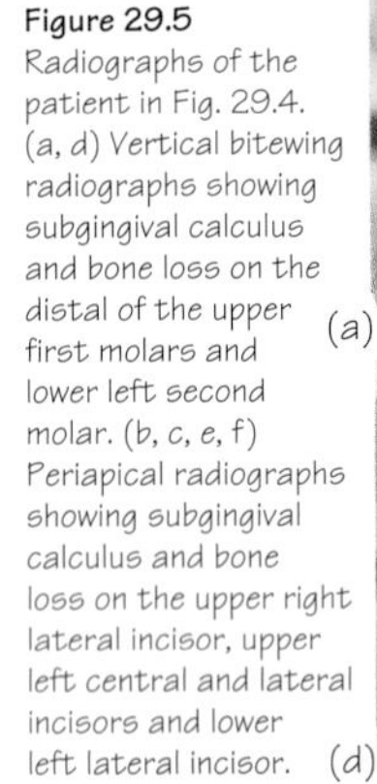

Figure 29.5 Radiographs of the patient in Fig. 29.4. (a, d) Vertical bitewing radiographs showing subgingival calculus and bone loss on the distal of the upper first molars and lower left second molar. (b, c, e, f) Periapical radiographs showing subgingival calculus and bone loss on the upper right lateral incisor, upper left central and lateral incisors and lower left lateral incisor.

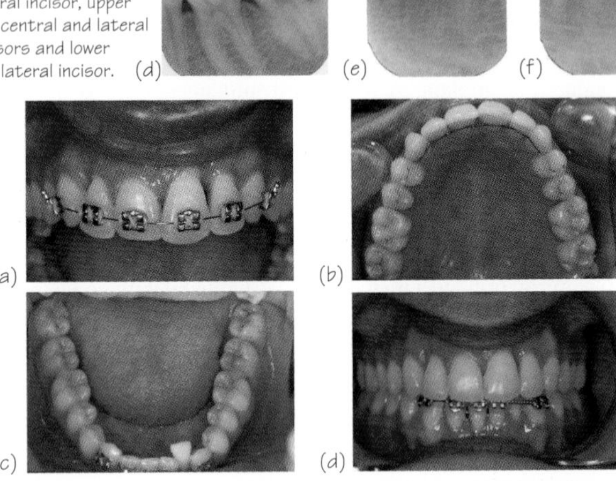

Figure 29.8 Stages of orthodontic treatment for the patient in Fig. 29.7: (a) fixed upper appliance; (b) bonded palatal upper retainer; (c) fixed lower appliance; and (d) aligned (permanently retained) upper anterior teeth and fixed lower appliance. There is improved aesthetics and spontaneous improvement in recession on the upper left central incisor following orthodontic tooth movement.

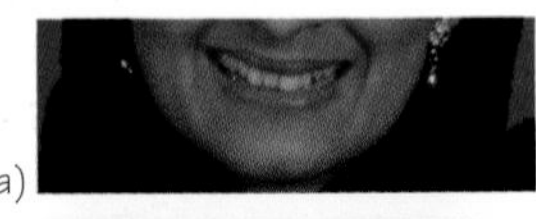

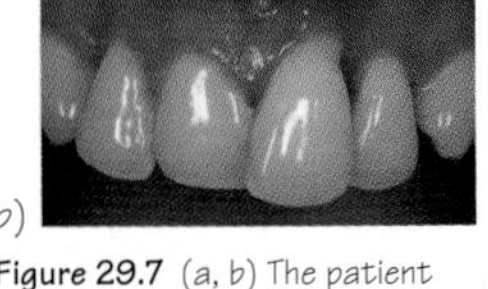

Figure 29.7 (a, b) The patient in Fig. 29.4 after periodontal therapy. The patient disliked the appearance and position of her upper left central incisor but wanted to retain the tooth if at all possible. Lip trapping occurs and localised recession.

Figure 29.9 (a) Pre-periodontal and orthodontic treatment of drifted upper central incisors in a female adult patient with chronic periodontitis. (b) After treatment. (c) Bonded orthodontic retainer.

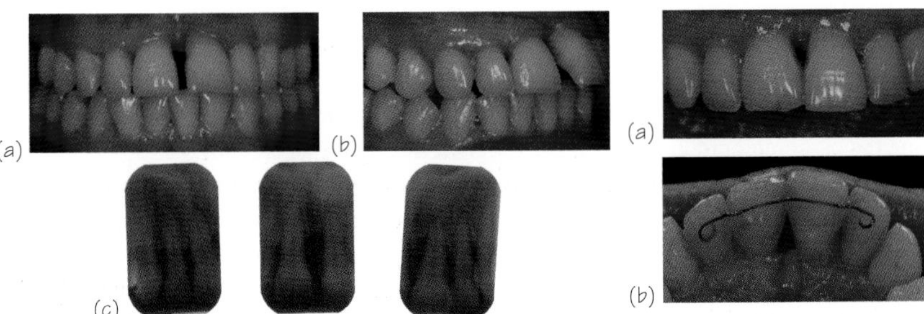

Figure 29.10 (a–c) Pre-periodontal treatment of a 33-year-old female patient with an aggressive form of periodontitis that led to drifting and proclination of the upper left central incisor, which had suffered recurrent periodontal abscesses. The prognosis of the tooth was deemed poor but responded to periodontal therapy, at the patient's request, and orthodontic treatment was instigated with an upper removable appliance.

Figure 29.11 Following orthodontic therapy of the patient in Fig. 29.10, the diastema closed (a) and a bonded retainer was placed (b). A 6-year follow up showed periodontal and orthodontic stability.

A dynamic two-way relationship exists between periodontics and orthodontics: (i) some patients undergoing orthodontic treatment experience secondary periodontal sequelae which can adversely affect their periodontal health unless appropriately managed; (ii) periodontal diseases can lead to incisor drifting, and aesthetic concerns that might subsequently be addressed by orthodontic treatment.

Orthodontic treatment and secondary periodontal sequelae

Orthodontic appliances can act as plaque retention factors, therefore optimum oral hygiene is essential during treatment. Traditionally, provision of orthodontic treatment has been deemed the domain of children, but the uptake of adult orthodontics has increased dramatically. The use of fixed appliances outweighs that of removable appliances nowadays.

Removable orthodontic appliances

The Adams clasps of the upper removable appliance (URA), whether active or passive (as a retainer), engage the undercut – usually of the maxillary first molar teeth (Fig. 29.1) – and impinge directly on the marginal interdental papilla and buccal gingivae. This can create local plaque retention problems leading to gingival inflammation and eventually, if unchecked, loss of attachment and alveolar bone loss.

Fixed orthodontic appliances

Plaque accumulation is a particular problem around fixed orthodontic appliances, which are renowned for:

- A hyperplastic gingival response to the plaque biofilm (Fig. 29.2).
- The potential for enamel demineralisation around the brackets and bonded attachments for the arch wires.

Plaque control

Exemplary oral hygiene is essential throughout treatment. For patients with fixed appliances, this can be achieved by small-headed manual brushes, interdental brushes, single tufted interspace brushes to get underneath the arch wires and around the brackets (Fig. 29.3), or powered brushes with orthodontic heads. The URA should be removed for toothbrushing, kept clean itself and then replaced.

The danger of inadequate plaque control is gingivitis, which although reversible with adequate plaque control, can, if unchecked progress to irreversible periodontitis.

Fluoride and diet

To prevent enamel demineralisation around the brackets and bonded attachments, in addition to optimum oral hygiene the patient should be provided with:

- Topical fluorides, especially fluoride mouthwash.
- Dietary advice to limit cariogenic intakes/acidic sweetened beverages.

Periodontal screening prior to orthodontic treatment

In view of the risks of periodontal disease from undergoing orthodontic treatment, it is critical to screen patients for periodontal diseases *prior* to commencing orthodontic treatment using the Basic Periodontal Examination (or Periodontal Screening and Recording) (Chapter 17) and to ensure periodontal review and supportive therapy are provided during treatment.

Other risks

- *Recession.* Providing teeth are orthodontically moved within the alveolar bone, there is little risk of gingival recession. If excessive proclination is anticipated, then connective tissue grafting can be undertaken to create keratinised gingiva prior to tooth movement.
- *Root resorption.* There is a risk of root resorption of 1–2 mm during orthodontic tooth movement, which leads to a shortened root length. Around 15% of patients may experience resorption of 2.5 mm or more which would have implications in a periodontally compromised patient.

Periodontal drifting

Periodontal drifting is a pathological migration of teeth that have reduced bone support and have lost clinical attachment as a consequence of periodontitis. Patients will usually complain of spacing appearing between their front teeth, incisor(s) dropping out of the line of the arch, and tipping or rotation (Figs 29.4, 29.5). It can occur relatively slowly in chronic periodontitis, but more rapidly in aggressive periodontitis or when risk factors are present. Occlusal factors are thought to play a role.

Usually the age group most affected will be adults, therefore prior to considering orthodontics, patients must be carefully assessed, counselled as to treatment options, the risks (see above) and benefits explained, and informed consent gained. Several differences exist between adults and children seeking orthodontic treatment (Fig. 29.6).

Periodontic–orthodontic management

The periodontic–orthodontic management involves a number of steps for a successful outcome (Figs 29.7–29.11):

- Initial and corrective periodontal treatment should be undertaken and completed and the periodontal condition should be stable. There should be no active pockets or residual inflammation (Fig. 29.7).
- Oral hygiene must be optimum.
- There should be assessment on an individual basis to check:
  - that there is adequate bone through which to move the drifted teeth and sufficient bone for post-orthodontic retention;
  - that there are sufficient teeth and bone and periodontal support for the fixed or removable orthodontic appliance to be functional.
- The patient should be aware of how long they will need to wear the orthodontic appliance(s), and the frequency of visits.
- The patient should be instructed how to care for their appliance(s).
- Appropriate fluoride supplements and diet advice should be provided to prevent demineralisation around the appliance(s).
- A periodontal maintenance programme should be in place during the orthodontic treatment (Fig. 29.8).
- The periodontally compromised patient should be aware of the need for permanent orthodontic retention following the completion of orthodontic treatment (Figs 29.8b, 29.9–29.11).

Key points

- To prevent periodontal sequelae due to orthodontic treatment:
  - periodontal screening should precede orthodontic treatment
  - oral hygiene must be optimum during treatment
  - fluoride supplements/diet advice are needed to prevent demineralisation
- Periodontal drifting may lead patients to seek orthodontic treatment
- There are differences between orthodontics in adults and children
- Risk-benefit should be advised and informed consent gained
- Periodontal–orthodontic management involves a number of steps for a successful outcome

30 Plaque-induced gingivitis

A. Dental plaque-induced gingival diseases*

1. **Gingivitis associated with dental plaque only**
   a. Without other local contributing factors
   b. With other local contributing factors
2. **Gingival diseases modified by systemic factors**
   a. Associated with the endocrine system
      1) puberty-associated gingivitis
      2) menstrual cycle-associated gingivitis
      3) pregnancy-associated
         a) gingivitis
         b) pyogenic granuloma
      4) diabetes mellitus-associated gingivitis
   b. Associated with blood dyscrasias
      1) leukaemia-associated gingivitis
      2) other
3. **Gingival diseases modified by medications**
   a. Drug-influenced gingival diseases
      1) drug-influenced gingival enlargements
      2) drug-influenced gingivitis
         a) oral contraceptive-associated gingivitis
         b) other
4. **Gingival diseases modified by malnutrition**
   a. Ascorbic acid-deficiency gingivitis
   b. Other

*Can occur on a periodontium with no attachment loss or on a periodontium with attachment loss that is not progressing

Figure 30.1 Classification of plaque-induced gingivitis from the 1999 International Workshop.

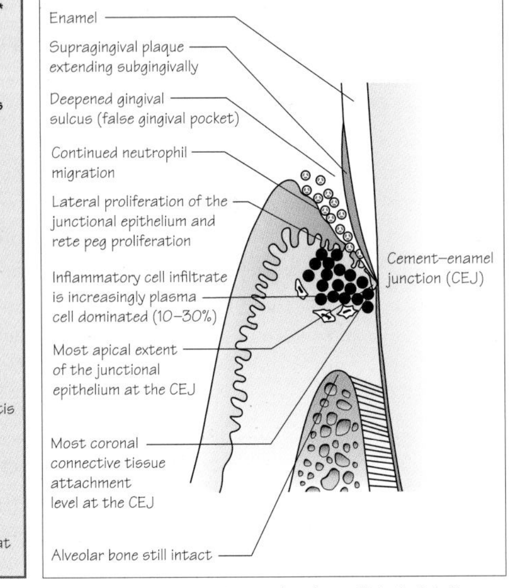

Figure 30.2 Section through a tooth with established, clinically evident, plaque-induced gingivitis.

Figure 30.3 Plaque-induced gingival inflammation. (a) Left and (b) right views showing plaque visible at the gingival margin, blunted papillae and red, swollen gingiva.

BPE code	Criteria	Management
0	Healthy periodontal tissues No bleeding after gentle probing	Maintain preventive measures
1	Bleeding after gentle probing Black band remains completely visible above gingival margin No calculus or defective margins detected	Oral hygiene instruction
2	Supragingival and/or subgingival calculus and/or other plaque retention factor Black band remains completely visible above gingival margin	Oral hygiene instruction Eliminate plaque retention factors Scale and polish
3	Shallow pocket (4 or 5 mm) Black band partially visible in the deepest pocket in the sextant	As above, but periodontal indices are needed; scaling/root surface debridement may take longer
4	Deep pocket (6 mm or more) Black band disappears in the pocket	As above but full periodontal indices and root surface debridement required
*	Furcation involvement Recession + probing depth = 7 mm or more	Periodontal indices and more complex treatment required

Figure 30.4 BPE codes, criteria and management. Plaque-induced gingivitis would typically be associated with a BPE code 1 or 2. Note that if the BPE code is 3, there is a need to differentiate between false gingival pockets and true periodontal pockets.

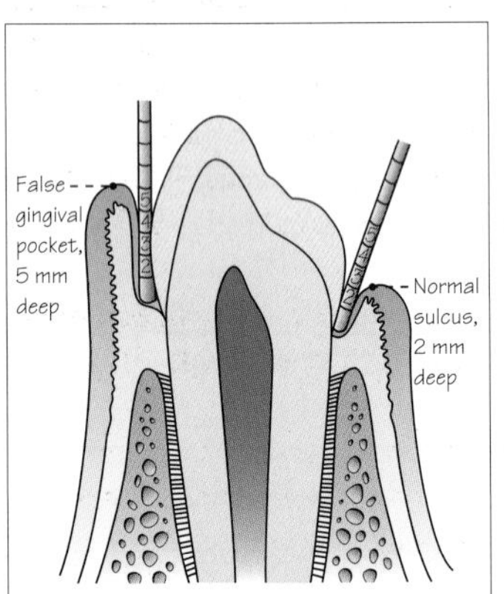

Figure 30.5 A false gingival pocket.

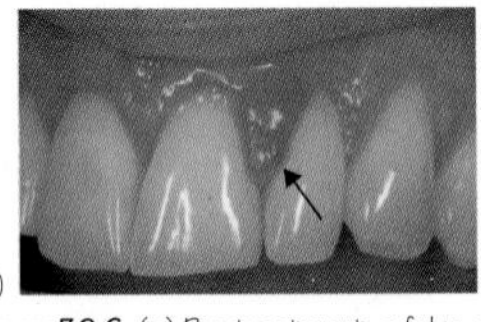

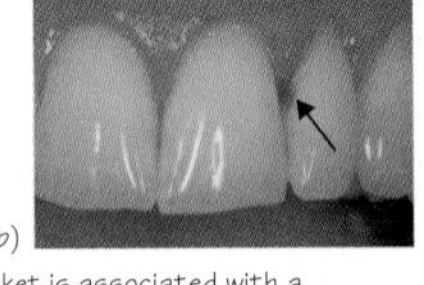

Figure 30.6 (a) Pre-treatment: a false pocket is associated with a subgingival cavity (arrow) and plaque retention on the mesial UL2. The papilla is swollen and red. (b) Post-treatment for gingivitis: the inflammation is diminished. The cavity on UL2 is now supragingival and accessible for restoration.

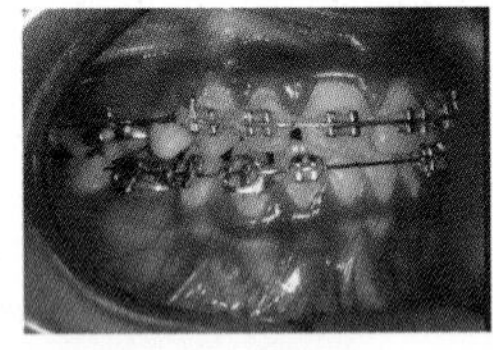

Figure 30.7 Plaque accumulation around a fixed orthodontic appliance in a 17-year-old female. There is gingival inflammation and a hyperplastic response to plaque.

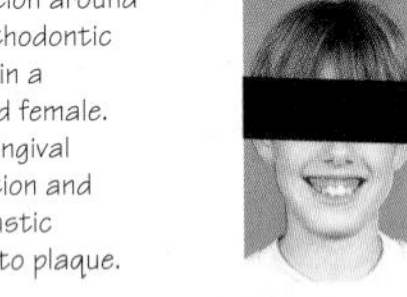

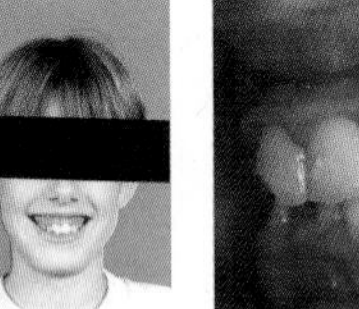

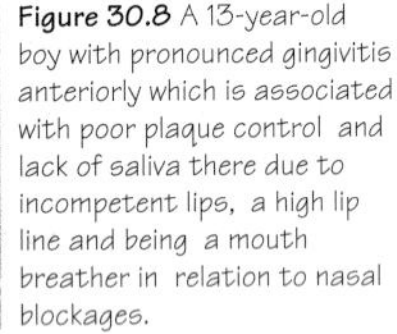

Figure 30.8 A 13-year-old boy with pronounced gingivitis anteriorly which is associated with poor plaque control and lack of saliva there due to incompetent lips, a high lip line and being a mouth breather in relation to nasal blockages.

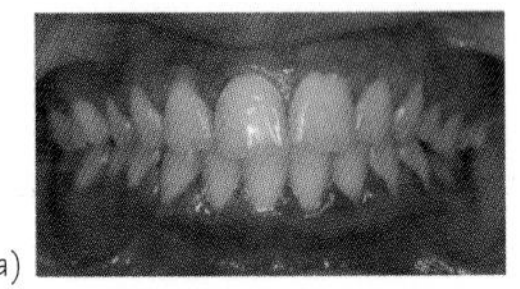

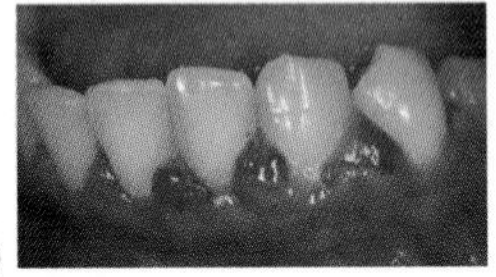

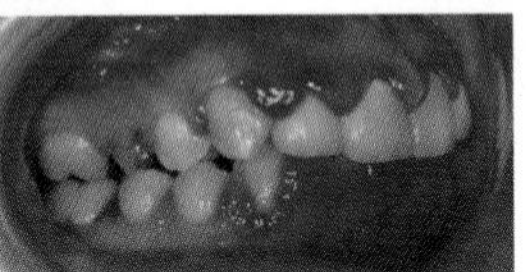

Figure 30.9 Pregnancy-associated gingivitis. (a) A 21-year-old pregnant patient with inflamed anterior gingivae, which bled on gentle probing. (b) A close up of the lower anterior gingivae which are inflamed and swollen. (c) A different pregnant patient with an even more marked response to plaque and severe gingival overgrowth, especially on the lower incisors.

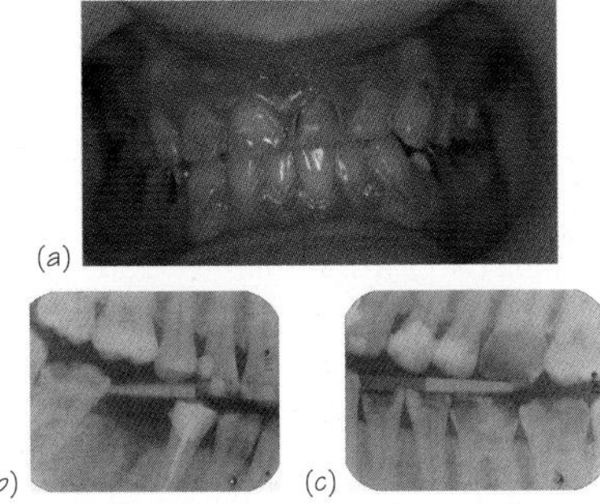

Figure 30.10 (a) Diabetes-associated gingivitis and uncontrolled caries in a young woman with poorly controlled type 1 diabetes mellitus. (b, c) Right and left bitewing radiographs showing caries but good bone levels. Courtesy of Mr P. J. Nixon.

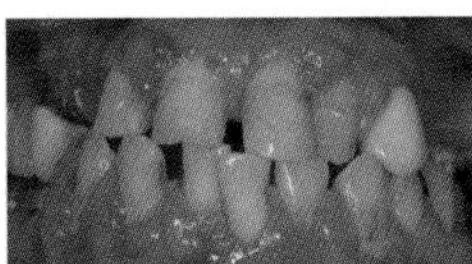

Figure 30.11 Drug-induced gingival overgrowth in an adult male patient with inadequate plaque control who was taking ciclosporin and a calcium channel blocker (nifedipine) following a renal transplant.

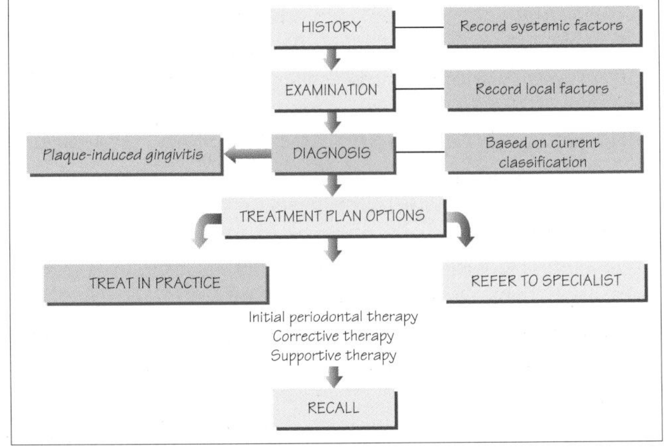

Figure 30.12 A flow diagram of the diagnosis and management of plaque-induced gingivitis.

There is considerable variation between subjects in susceptibility to the development of gingival inflammation. It is currently thought that gingivitis and periodontitis are a continuum of the same disease; however the interface is complex (Chapters 8, 9).

Classification

Different types of plaque-induced gingival disease were recognised in the 1999 International Workshop for the Classification of Periodontal Diseases and Conditions (Fig. 30.1). A correct diagnosis is reached after considering the findings of the history and examination and relies on knowledge of the classification.

Diagnostic features of plaque-induced gingivitis

There are many diagnostic features of plaque-induced gingivitis (Figs 30.2, 30.3):

- Change in colour of the gingiva.
- Marginal gingival swelling.
- Loss of contour (blunting) of the interdental papilla.
- Increased gingival crevicular and sulcular temperature.
- Bleeding from the gingival margin on probing or brushing.
- Plaque is present at the gingival margin, and there is an inflammatory infiltrate.
- There is no clinical attachment loss or alveolar bone loss.
- Basic Periodontal Examination (BPE) score is 1 or 2 (Fig. 30.4).
- The gingival sulcus measures 3 mm or less from the gingival margin to the base of the junctional epithelium, which is still at the cement–enamel junction (CEJ).
- False gingival pockets may be present in which the most apical extent of the junctional epithelium is still at the CEJ, but the sulcus is deepened to more than 3 mm due to gingival swelling.
- Clinical and histological changes are reversible on the removal of plaque.

Plaque-induced gingivitis on a reduced periodontium

The features of gingivitis as above may occur on a periodontium with reduced periodontal support in which loss of attachment and loss of alveolar bone are present but not progressing.

Modifying factors

Gingival diseases may be modified by the following factors.

Local contributing factors

- Supragingival or subgingival calculus.
- Subgingival restoration margins, overhangs or cavities (Fig. 30.6).
- Tooth anatomical factors, e.g. root groove or enamel pearl.
- Malocclusion or crowding.
- Fixed and removable prosthodontic or orthodontic appliances (Fig. 30.7).
- Incompetent lips or lack of lip seal, which compromise the protective benefits of saliva (Fig. 30.8).

Systemic factors

- Puberty: pronounced inflammatory response of the gingiva to plaque and hormones during the circumpubertal period.
- Menstrual cycle: pronounced inflammatory response of the gingiva immediately prior to ovulation.
- Pregnancy:
  - there is a pronounced inflammatory response of the gingiva to plaque and hormones during the second and third trimesters (Fig. 30.9);
  - pregnancy epulis is an exaggerated inflammatory response that typically presents interdentally as a mushroom-like mass with a pedunculated base from the gingival margin.
- Diabetes mellitus: inflammatory response of the gingiva to plaque which is aggravated by poorly controlled blood glucose levels (Fig. 30.10).
- Blood dyscrasias: gingivitis associated with abnormal function or number of blood cells (e.g. leukaemia, a malignant condition that can manifest with increased bleeding and purple-red, enlarged, spongy gingiva).

Medications

- Drug-influenced gingival enlargement, e.g. phenytoin (for epilepsy), ciclosporin (an immunosuppressant) or calcium channel blockers (commonly used for hypertension or heart problems) (Fig. 30.11; Chapter 33).
- Drug-influenced gingivitis, e.g. contraceptive pill.

Malnutrition

Vitamin C deficiency (scurvy) is uncommon in developed countries but in some parts of the world can lead to bright red, swollen, ulcerated gingivae which tend to bleed readily.

Management

Effective management of plaque-induced gingivitis requires the correct diagnosis and any local, systemic or contributing factors to be identified (Fig. 30.12). The suspicion of leukaemia requires urgent medical referral. Initial cause-related therapy is generally amenable to primary dental care and involves the disruption and removal of the plaque biofilm, with measures put in place to control the biofilm and prevent recurrence of the gingivitis:

- Plaque and marginal gingival bleeding indices: calculation of per cent surfaces free from plaque or bleeding is motivational.
- Oral hygiene instruction:
  - toothbrushing advice – manual or powered brush;
  - interdental cleaning advice – floss/tape or interdental brushes;
  - advice on toothpastes and mouthwashes.
- Smoking cessation advice.
- Manage modifiable systemic factors, e.g. liaise with diabetes care team to help improve diabetes control.
- Eliminate modifiable local plaque retention factors.
- Scale and polish by dental professional.
- Arrange caries management, endodontic treatment, extractions and immediate/transitional prosthodontic treatment.
- Review and monitor response to initial therapy.
- If there is inadequate plaque control and residual disease is present, then arrange additional (corrective) therapy.
- If there is adequate plaque control and resolution of disease, then arrange supportive therapy to prevent disease recurrence.

Key points

- There are different plaque-induced gingival diseases
- Diagnosis:
  - follows history and examination and use of the BPE
  - is aided by knowledge of the current classification
- Management:
  - relies on control/disruption of the plaque biofilm and the elimination of modifiable contributory factors
  - can generally be provided in the primary dental care setting

31 Non-plaque-induced gingival conditions and lesions

1. **Gingival diseases of specific bacterial origin**
   a. *Neisseria gonorrhoea-associated lesions*
   b. *Treponema pallidum-associated lesions*
   c. Streptococcal species-associated lesions
   d. Others
2. **Gingival diseases of viral origin**
   a. Herpes virus infections
      1) primary herpetic gingivostomatitis
      2) recurrent oral herpes (gingival, mucosal, labialis)
      3) varicella-zoster infections
   b. Others (e.g. Coxsackie viruses of childhood (hand foot and mouth, herpangina))
3. **Gingival diseases of fungal origin**
   a. Candida species infections
      1) generalised gingival candidosis
   b. Linear gingival erythema
   c. Histoplasmosis
   d. Others (e.g. other deep mycoses: geotrichosis, coccidiomycosis, aspergillosis)
4. **Gingival diseases of genetic origin**
   a. Hereditary gingival fibromatosis
   b. Others (e.g. sebaceous naevus of Jadassohn)
5. **Gingival manifestations of systemic conditions**
   a. Mucocutaneous disorders
      1) lichen planus
      2) pemphigoid
      3) pemphigus vulgaris
      4) erythema multiforme
      5) lupus erythematosus
      6) drug-induced lesions (e.g. erosive lesions)
      7) other (e.g. epidermolysis bullosa)
   b. Allergic reactions
      1) dental restorative materials (e.g. mercury, nickel, acrylic)
      2) reactions attributable to toothpastes, mouthrinses, chewing gum additives and food substances/additives
      3) others
6. **Traumatic lesions** (factitious, iatrogenic, accidental)
   a. Chemical injury
   b. Physical injury
   c. Thermal injury
7. **Foreign body reactions**
8. **Not otherwise specified (NOS)**

Figure 31.1 Classification of non-plaque-induced gingival conditions resulting from the 1999 International Workshop for the Classification of Periodontal Diseases and Conditions (Armitage, 1999).

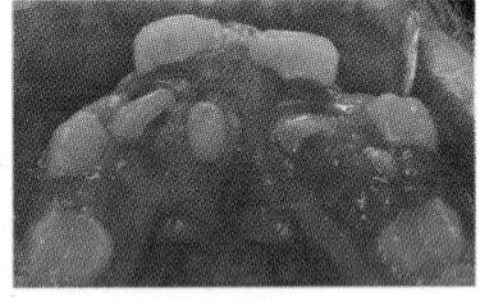
(a)
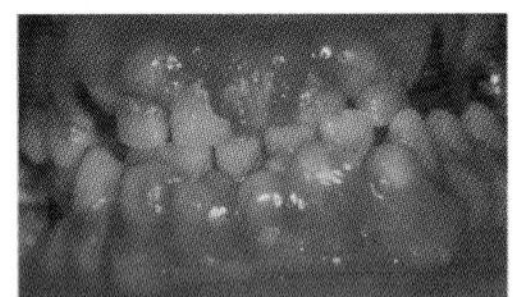
(b)

Figure 31.3 (a, b) Drug-induced gingival overgrowth.

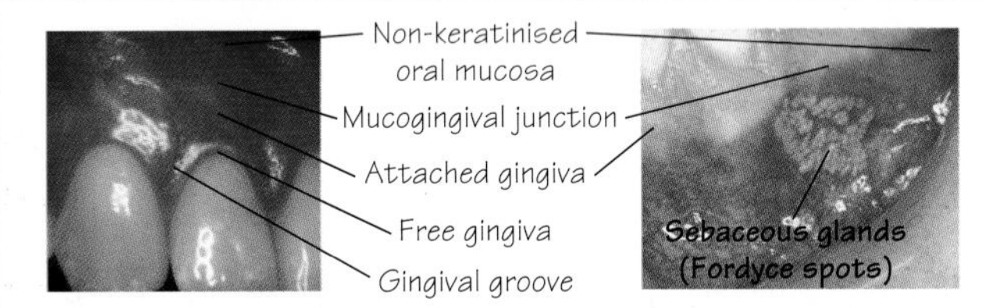

Figure 31.4 The normal gingival anatomy.

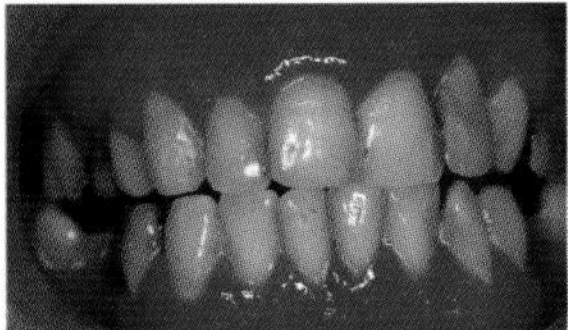
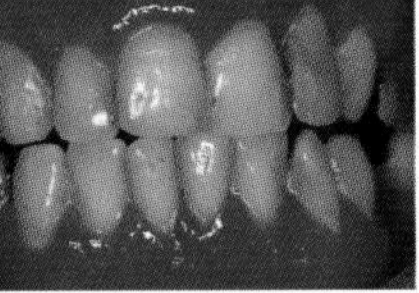

Figure 31.5 Sarcoidosis.

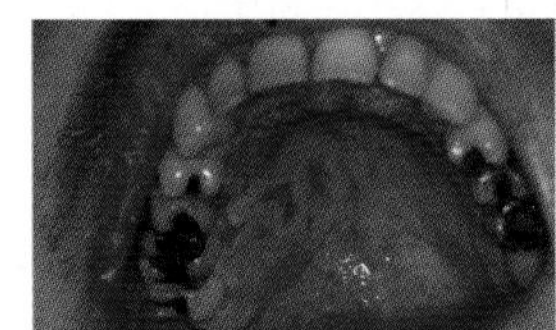

Figure 31.6 Varicella zoster.

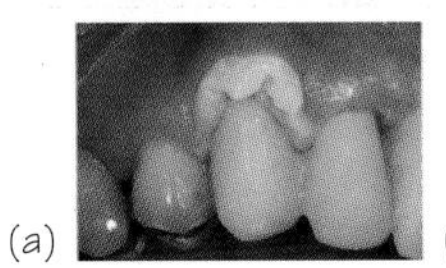
(a)
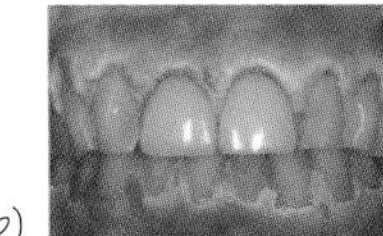
(b)

Figure 31.8 Leukoplakia: (a) localised veruccous leukoplakia; and (b) generalised homogenous leukoplakia.

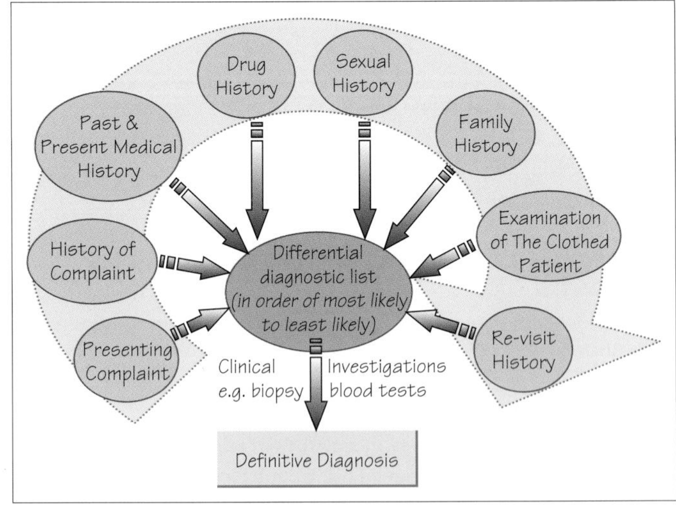

Figure 31.2 The surgical sieve: arriving at a correct differential diagnosis.

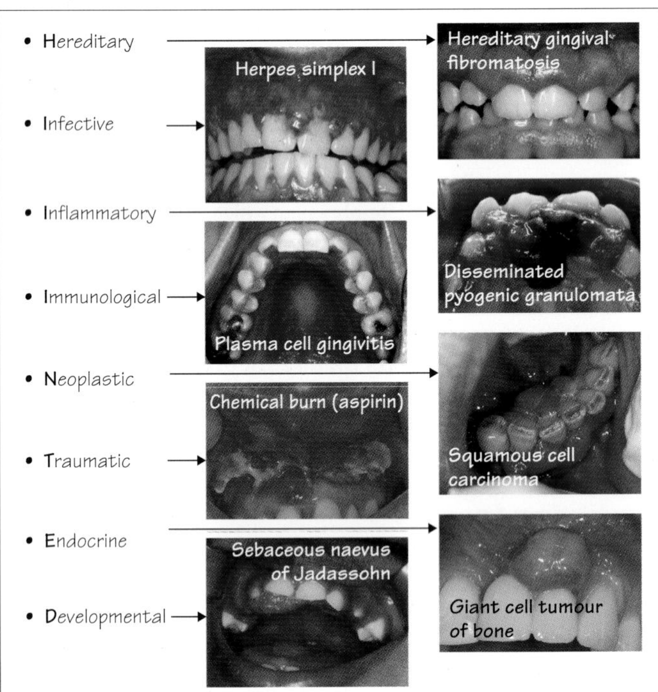

Figure 31.9 A surgical sieve utilising a mnemonic: 'HINTED'.

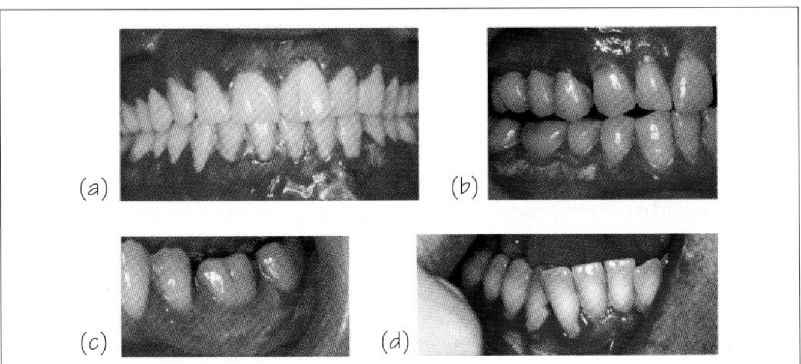

Figure 31.7 Lichen planus: (a) desquamative gingivitis; (b) plaque-like lichen planus; (c) reticular lichen planus; and (d) erosive lichen planus.

All slides are Courtesy of Professor I. L. C. Chapple.

Non-plaque-induced gingival conditions were classified for the first time in 1999 by an international workshop in periodontology (Fig. 31.1), but the system is by no means comprehensive. Given the heterogeneity of the constituent cells of the gingivae (epithelial, endothelial, fibroblasts, adipocytes, inflammatory-immune cells) and the various disorders associated with mixed tissues (ranging from immune-mediated to traumatic ulceration, to granulomatous inflammation, atopy and infections to tumour formation), it is estimated that well over 100 systemic or local non-plaque-induced conditions may involve the gingivae.

The diagnostic process

Establishing a differential diagnosis for such a large number of conditions is challenging and a procedural algorithm to approach this is illustrated in Fig. 31.2. It is important to:

- Adopt a forensic approach to history taking and examination procedures.
- Keep an open mind about potential causes.
- Use every piece of available information (visual and tactile).

It is important to take a detailed history:

1 *Presenting complaint*: this is often key to establishing a differential diagnosis. For example, gingival 'pain' or 'soreness' tends to indicate ulcerative or erosive conditions (viral or immune-mediated lesions are likely) such as lichen planus, pemphigoid or erythema multiforme.

2 *History of complaint*: this is extremely important in the diagnostic pathway. For example, the temporal relationship between the onset of symptoms and a patient commencing a course of medication could be the diagnostic key. Drug-induced pigmentation or ulceration, lichenoid drug reactions or drug-induced gingival enlargement (Fig. 31.3) are all examples. Gingival overgrowths have variable appearances, ranging from fibrous (e.g. dilantin therapy for epilepsy) to vascular (e.g. calcium channel blocking drugs with superimposed plaque-induced inflammation).

3 *Past or present medical history*: a positive medical history often leads directly or indirectly to a diagnosis. A history of atopy may indicate an allergic aetiology to the condition (e.g. plasma cell gingivitis). The presence of mucocutaneous diseases such as epidermolysis bullosa or lichen planus may explain oral blistering, erosions or scarring. Connective tissue diseases (e.g. systemic sclerosis) or inflammatory conditions (e.g. angioedema) may all present with gingival manifestations.

4 *Drug history*: prescription drugs can produce side effects following correct use (e.g. pigmentation with minocycline) or incorrect use (e.g. aspirin burns following topical application) and recreational drugs may cause ulcerative/necrotic lesions (e.g. cocaine).

5 *Sexual history*: this may be necessary if sexually transmitted diseases (herpes simplex 2 or syphilis) or human immunodeficiency virus (HIV) are suspected. This should only be taken where there is a high index of suspicion and should be done sensitively and in the presence of a chaperone.

6 *Family history*: may be important for conditions like hereditary gingival fibromatosis (autosomal dominant mutation of Son of Sevenless gene, 2p21-p22 or 5q13-q22).

7 *Extra-oral examination*: such an examination of clothed patients requires the oral physician to observe the face, neck, hands/arms and legs/shins for peripheral signs of lesions that may be relevant to the gingival pathology. Examples are: enlarged lymph nodes in infectious conditions; purple/pruritic lesions on the flexor surfaces of arms and shins in lichen planus; target lesions in erythema multiforme; telangectasia/spider naevi in liver disease or CREST syndrome (Calcinosis, Raynaud's, disease, Esophagitis, Sjögren's syndrome, Telangectasia), now called progressive systemic sclerosis.

8 *Intra-oral examination*: this should be systematic and thorough. The identification of non-gingival involvement may be essential in establishing a diagnosis. Definitive diagnosis may require a biopsy or assimilation of several strands of information from clinical tests. Always ignore the obvious pathology initially and return to it at the end of the examination, as patients may have multiple pathology. Good knowledge of normal gingival anatomy is essential (Fig. 31.4), as lesions involving attached and free gingiva are unlikely to be plaque induced. For example, the erythema in Fig. 31.5 crosses the mucogingival junction and deep biopsy revealed granulomata of sarcoidosis. Equally, consider nerve distributions carefully – some anti-retroviral drugs used in the management of HIV disease cause a painful trigeminal neuropathy. The ulceration in Fig. 31.6 is limited to the maxillary division of the trigeminal nerve and does not cross the midline (it was a varicella zoster infection).

9 *Re-visitation of a history*: issues highlighted by the examination process frequently necessitate a re-visitation of the clinical or medical history, e.g. primary biliary cirrhosis is associated with Sjögren syndrome and chronic active hepatitis may associate with lichen planus.

Clinical investigations

A differential diagnosis should always list the presumptive diagnoses in order of most likely to least likely. Clinical investigations such as a biopsy or blood tests then help establish a definitive diagnosis.

When and where to biopsy

Biopsies are generally necessary in the following situations:

- For the diagnosis of conditions or lesions that have variable clinical but classical histological features (e.g. lichen planus; Fig. 31.7).
- Where the consequences of a positive histological diagnosis have implications for other body systems (e.g. sarcoidosis, vesiculobullous diseases).
- Where a sinister lesion is suspected (Fig. 31.8). As gingival tissues always exhibit plaque-induced inflammation, which can mask classical histological features of other conditions, always try to biopsy non-gingival sites. This is essential in cases of 'desquamative gingivitis', where differential diagnoses may include lichen planus, pemphigoid, pemphigus or lupus (Fig. 31.7a).

The surgical sieve

A surgical sieve utilising a mnemonic (e.g. 'HINTED') may be helpful in stimulating thought processes towards formulating a differential diagnosis (Fig. 31.9).

Key points

- Adopt a forensic and systematic approach to questioning
- Keep an open mind throughout
- Use every piece of visual information available
- Consider links to existing medical conditions
- Consider the likelihood of multiple pathology
- Try to avoid gingival biopsies and utilise adjacent sites if possible
- If in doubt about a diagnosis, refer

32 Gingival recession

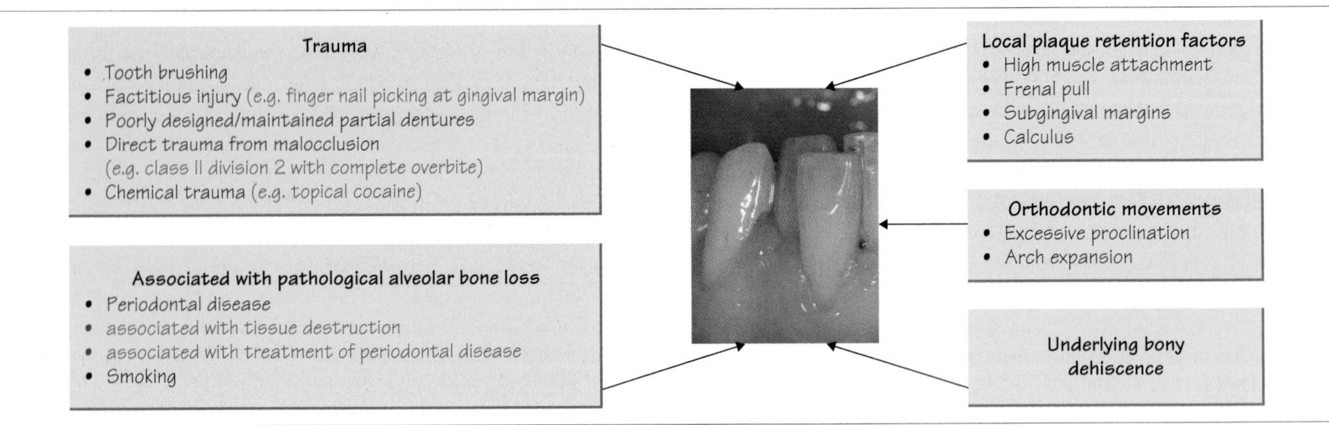

Figure 32.1 Aetiological factors associated with gingival recession.

Surgical root coverage techniques

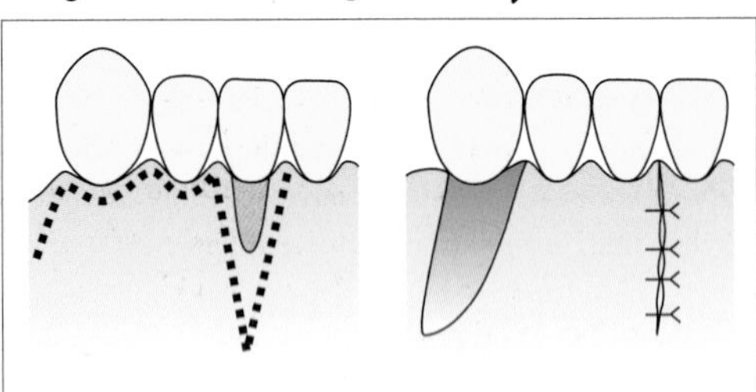

Figure 32.2 Pedicle grafts: laterally repositioned rotational flap. The flap is taken from an adjacent site to cover the localised area of recession.

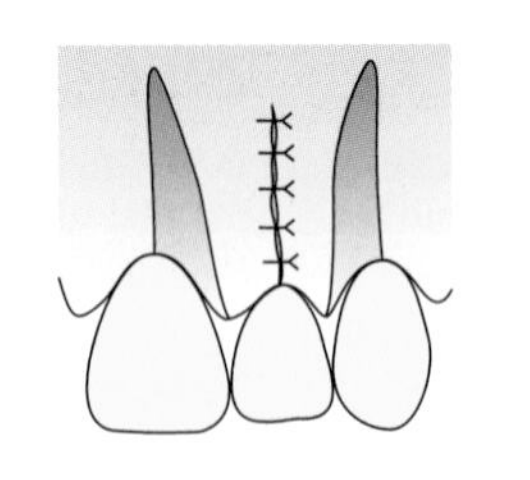

Figure 32.3 Pedicle grafts: double papilla rotational flap. Coverage is achieved from adjacent donor sites on either side of the area of recession.

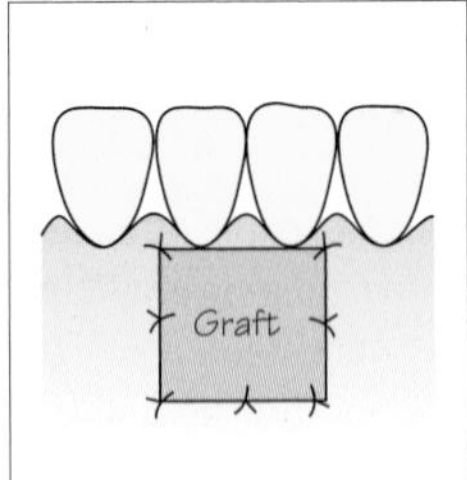

Figure 32.4 Free grafts: free epithelialised gingival graft. At the recipient site the epithelium and outer part of the connective tissue are removed by split dissection around and below the recession defect. The graft is taken from the remote donor site and sutured securely at the recipient site.

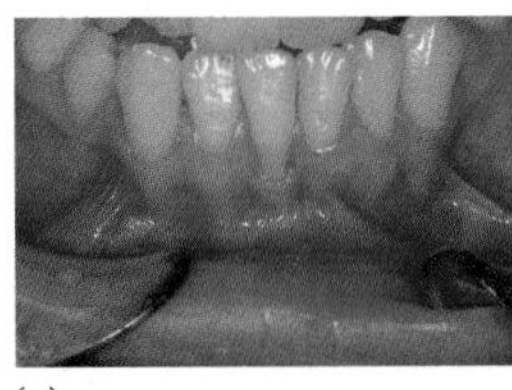

(a)

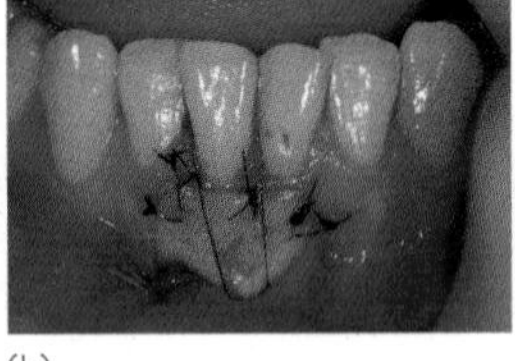

(b)

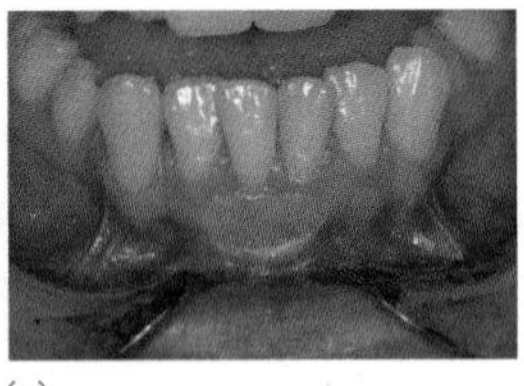

(c)

Figure 32.5 Free grafts: free epithelialised gingival graft. (a) Site shown preoperatively. (b) The tissue graft sutured in place. (c) The site shown 4 months' postoperatively. Courtesy of Mr P. J. Nixon.

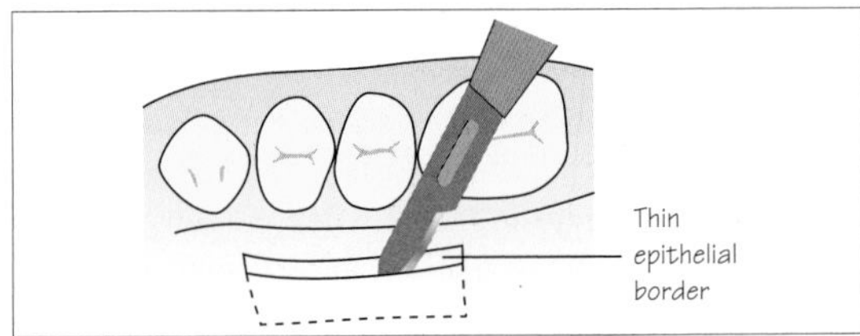

Figure 32.6 Free grafts: subepithelial connective tissue graft. A free graft is taken from the palate, removing underlying connective tissue with only a thin epithelial border. The tissue is sutured at the prepared recipient site. The graft is then covered by a flap (commonly a coronally advanced flap) so that the graft gains its nutrition from the underlying periosteum and deep connective tissue and the overlying flap.

Gingival recession is defined as the location of marginal tissue apical to the cement–enamel junction resulting in exposure of the root surface. Aetiological factors associated with gingival recession are shown in Fig. 32.1.

Consequences of gingival recession

Unlike many other oral problems, patients are very often aware of gingival recession. Patients may potentially experience the following problems associated with recession:

- Pain from exposed dentine.
- Aesthetic concerns.
- Plaque retention and gingival inflammation.
- Root caries.
- Tooth abrasion.

Management

A history and examination are carried out to identify aetiological factors and a diagnosis of gingival recession is made. Recession can be measured in millimetres with a periodontal probe; study models and photographs can be useful for records.

Management can be divided into the management of:

- Aetiological factors associated with recession.
- Consequences of recession.

Management of aetiological factors associated with recession

- Oral hygiene advice: advise an atraumatic brushing technique using:
  - manual toothbrushing;
  - electric toothbrushing.

- Smoking cessation advice.
- Advice relating to traumatic habits.
- Orthodontic treatment planning. If this is likely to create a dehiscence, review the volume of soft tissue at the site and consider grafting prior to unfavourable orthodontic movements.
- Partial denture design and restorations:
  - good support of dentures;
  - supragingival restorations where possible;
  - regular review and maintenance.
- Treatment of periodontal disease.

Management of consequences of recession

- Dentine hypersensitivity:
  - dietary advice;
  - antisensitivity dentifrices;
  - topical products for professional application: (i) containing fluoride (e.g. Duraphat®, Colgate-Palmolive, Guildford, UK), (ii) other (e.g. containing chlorhexidine and thymol), and (iii) sealants;
  - restorations.
- Root caries:
  - prevention: diet, oral hygiene instruction and fluoride application;
  - reshaping of shallow lesions;
  - restorations.
- Restoration of aesthetics:
  - gingival veneer: silicone mask to disguise interdental spaces (note this will act as a plaque retention factor);
  - restorations: these can camouflage the exposed root surface in some cases; pink porcelain or composite can try to disguise exposed roots;
  - root coverage by surgical techniques (see following section)

Recession can be monitored to ensure there is no further progression. In many cases where there are no consequences to the presence of the recession defect, sites are accepted and kept under review. In particular situations, root coverage to eliminate or reduce the recession defect may be appropriate.

Mucogingival surgery and the surgical management of gingival recession

Mucogingival surgery is a term used for surgical manipulation of the attached gingivae and vestibular tissues and so includes those techniques for management of gingival recession.

Several techniques have been developed to manage gingival recession and the factors that have been considered causative. Historically, many surgical techniques were developed to increase the width of the attached gingivae and deepen the sulcus. It is now known that these two factors are not significant in determining gingival health and therefore these techniques are mostly redundant.

Where frenal pull on a gingival margin is considered to be a factor in localised recession, then a frenectomy can be carried out. A high frenal attachment can also sometimes impede oral hygiene measures and a frenectomy may give greater access to the site for cleaning if local hygiene measures have failed.

Surgical root coverage

The main techniques are:

- Pedicle grafts:
  - rotational flaps: (i) laterally repositioned flap, and (ii) double papilla flap;
  - advanced flaps: coronally advanced flap.
- Guided tissue regeneration.
- Free grafts:
  - epithelialised gingival grafts;
  - subepithelial connective tissue graft.

Pedicle grafts

Rotational flaps

These are effective for covering small areas of gingival recession where a donor site is locally available. For the laterally repositioned flap (Fig. 32.2), a split thickness flap is created by sharp dissection at the donor site and advanced to the new location. Two flaps are raised in the double papilla flap technique (Fig. 32.3). Flaps gain nutrition from the wide base of the pedicle flap and from the prepared recipient site of periosteum surrounding the denuded area of root.

Advanced flaps

A mucosal flap can be raised beyond the mucogingival junction and moved coronally because of the elasticity of the tissue. Single or multiple defects can be covered and the technique can also be used in conjunction with enamel matrix derivative (Straumann® Emdogain). The principles of enamel matrix derivative are discussed in Chapter 26.

Guided tissue regeneration

The principles are discussed in Chapter 26 and the technique is used in conjunction with traditional flaps.

Free grafts

A free graft is taken from a remote site of keratinised tissue, usually the palate, to cover the area of recession (Figs 32.4, 32.5). A template can be used to take the correct amount of epithelialised graft tissue.

The subepithelial connective tissue graft is harvested from the palate by a 'trap door' approach (Fig. 32.6) and generally leaves a less invasive wound and gives a better aesthetic result. The recipient site must be prepared to receive the graft and the graft carefully stabilised with sutures.

Key points

- The aetiology of gingival recession is multfactorial and includes:
  - underlying bony anatomy
  - orthodontic movements
  - trauma
  - local plaque retention factors
  - association with pathological alveolar bone loss
- Management is directed at the:
  - aetiological factors associated with recession
  - consequences of recession
- Sites can be maintained and monitored for progression
- Surgical intervention and root coverage may be indicated

33 Gingival overgrowth

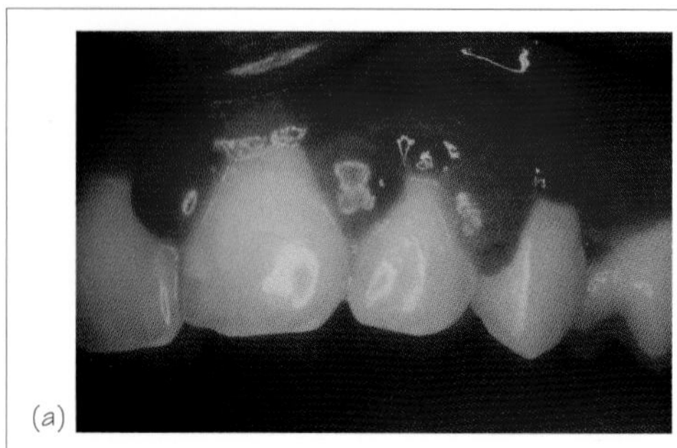
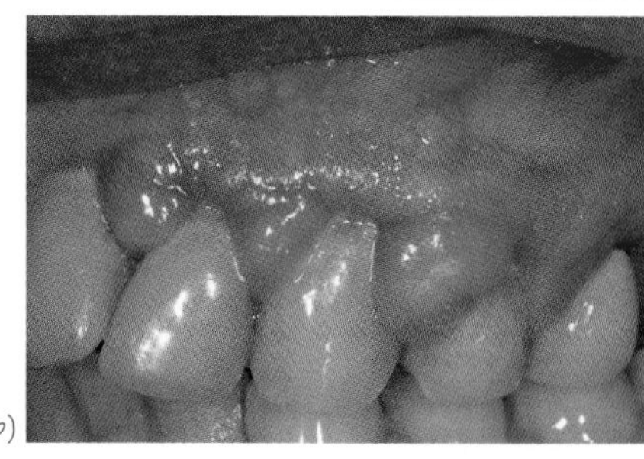

Figure 33.1 Gingival overgrowth. (a) Gingival overgrowth in a patient in the second trimester of pregnancy. The gingivae are very inflamed and bleed easily and are associated with the presence of generalised plaque deposits. (b) Gingival overgrowth associated with the calcium channel-blocking drug nifedipine. Note the enlarged interdental papillae and deposits of gingival plaque.

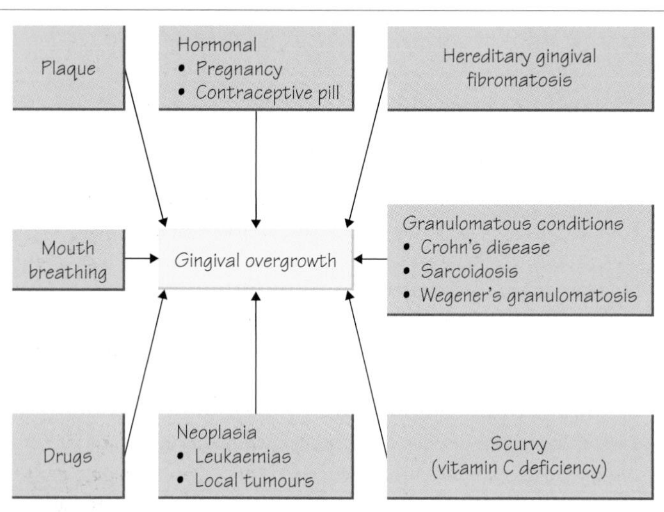

Figure 33.2 Causes of gingival overgrowth.

- Interdental areas
- Anterior gingivae more than posterior
- Labial more than lingual
- Mandible more than maxilla
- Dense, firm, lobulated
- Pseudo-pocketing
- Lobulated masses separated by grooves
- Minimal tendency to bleed if fibrous
- If plaque-induced inflammation is present:
  - bleeding
  - oedema
  - redness
- Higher prevalence in young age groups
- Onset within 3 months of drug use

Figure 33.4 Characteristics of DIGO. The features listed may be seen in DIGO but some also occur in gingival overgrowth related to other aetiological factors.

Phenytoin
Anticonvulsant:
- Epilepsy
- Prophylactic control of seizures after neurosurgery or head injury

Ciclosporin
Immunosuppressant:
- Renal and heart transplants
- Diabetes, Behcet's disease, multiple sclerosis
- Systemic lupus erythematosus, erosive lichen planus

Calcium channel blockers
Vasodilating agent:
- Angina
- Hypertension

Figure 33.3 The main drugs associated with DIGO.

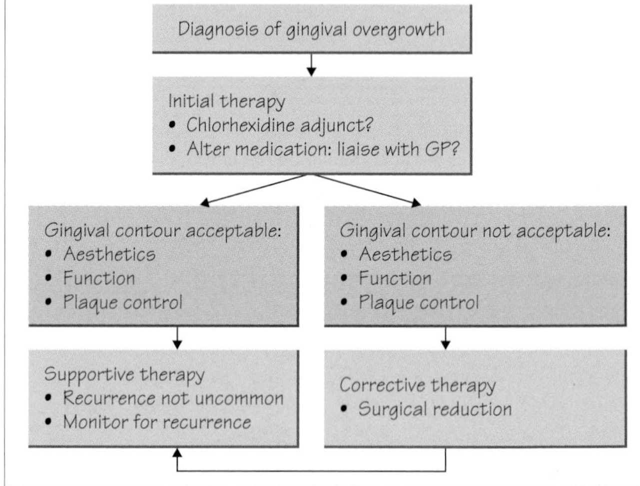

Figure 33.5 Management of gingival overgrowth.

Gingival overgrowth is a term given to the development of increased gingival bulk that can arise from a number of causes. In many cases there is associated plaque-related inflammation. This may be involved in the development of the overgrowth, but the enlarged tissue contour is difficult to clean and thus acts as a local plaque retention factor.

The appearance of the overgrowth varies. The tissue may be red, swollen and inflamed and tend to bleed easily, or it may be pink and fibrous if associated with increased collagen formation (Fig. 33.1). If the gingival tissue is invaded by neoplastic cells or granulomas then it may appear more solid but may still present with a superimposed inflammatory component. The clinical appearance cannot be considered as diagnostic of any particular aetiology.

Problems experienced by patients with gingival overgrowth are:

- The poor appearance of the gingivae.
- Functional discomfort if the overgrowth extends onto the occlusal surfaces.
- Difficulty in plaque removal.

Causes of gingival overgrowth

Readers are referred to textbooks in oral medicine for greater depth on this subject (Chapple and Hamburg, 2006). Drug-induced gingival overgrowth (DIGO) is covered in the following section, while the other main causes are listed below (Fig. 33.2).

Hormonal

This is most commonly associated with pregnancy:
- It is plaque related.
- It ranges in prevalence and severity.
- It commences in the second month, and peaks in the eighth month.
- Increased progesterone alters the microcirculation.
- Subgingival microflora may be altered.
- A pregnancy epulis can develop in some cases (marked swelling of the interdental papilla).

Leukaemias

In the leukaemias, white blood cells are abnormal:
- The white cells are unable to control infection at the gingival margins.
- The white cells infiltrate the gingival tissue, causing swelling.

Hereditary gingival fibromatosis

- This is associated with several hereditary disorders.
- The most common is an autosomal dominant syndrome: mental retardation.
- Gingival overgrowth can precede eruption or occur in childhood.
- Marked overgrowth can bury the teeth.

Crohn's disease

- This affects the ileocaecal region.
- Abdominal pain, constipation or diarrhoea can occur.
- Oral lesions may precede abdominal symptoms:
  - gingival swelling and reddening;
  - cobblestone thickening of the buccal mucosa;
  - lip swelling;
  - ulcers;
  - glossitis.

Wegener's granulomatosis

- This is characterised by granulomatous inflammation of the naso-pharynx, pulmonary cavitation and glomerulonephritis.
- The gingivae are swollen with a granular surface clasically described as 'strawberry gingivae'. Giant cells are seen histologically.

Sarcoidosis

- Non-caseating granulomas are found in the lungs, lymph nodes and other sites such as the mouth.
- The gingivae, lips, palate and buccal mucosa can be involved.

Scurvy

The gingivae are grossly enlarged in advanced disease.

Drug-induced gingival overgrowth

This is associated mainly with:
- Phenytoin.
- Ciclosporin.
- Calcium channel blockers:
  - nifedipine;
  - diltiazem;
  - amlodipine.

Figure 33.3 shows the main uses of these drugs. A wide range in the prevalence of the condition has been described for all of these drugs. Other drugs for which DIGO has been described as a side effect are sodium valproate and erythromycin.

Figure 33.4 lists the main characteristics of DIGO.

Role of plaque in DIGO

There is an association between oral hygiene and gingival inflammation and the severity of DIGO. However, it is not clear if plaque contributes or if it accumulates because of the marked tissue contour.

Risk factors

- There is an association between age and the severity of overgrowth for ciclosporin.
- Males seem to be more severely affected.
- There is an increased prevalence and severity of gingival overgrowth with combinations of the associated drugs:
  - ciclosporin and amlodipine;
  - ciclosporin and nifedipine.
- Other medication can affect severity:
  - there is reduced severity in transplant patients with prednisolone and azathioprine;
  - increased overgrowth is seen with phenytoin given with other anticonvulsants: phenobarbitone and carbamazepine.
- Genetic factors: HLA-B37 may protect from overgrowth.

Drug variables

- A threshold of drug is probably required to initiate overgrowth.
- Drug dosages are a poor predictor of gingival changes.
- The extent of overgrowth and dose are not always closely related.
- Other measures such as degree of drug protein binding or bioavail-ability may be appropriate.
- It is not clear if salivary concentrations of the drugs are correlated with the degree of gingival overgrowth.

Management

Chlorhexidine mouthrinse can be a useful adjunct in the management of gingival overgrowth (Fig. 33.5). In severe cases of DIGO, liaison with the general medical practitioner and any specialists may be appropriate to consider prescribing alternative drugs. Tacrolimus has been given to renal and cardiac transplant patients as an alternative to ciclosporin. It is not associated with gingival overgrowth and rapid resolution or substantial reductions of the ciclosporin-induced overgrowth have been reported following a change to tacrolimus. However, this drug does have several other non-oral side effects.

Recurrence of gingival overgrowth, particularly where it is drug induced, is not uncommon. Supportive therapy is important but repeated surgical reduction may be required.

Key points

- There are several causes of gingival overgrowth, although the clinical appearance is not generally diagnostic
- In most cases there is associated plaque-related inflammation
- Drug-induced gingival overgrowth is associated mainly with:
  - phenytoin
  - ciclosporin
  - calcium channel blockers
- Following the identification of aetiological factors, management is organised into:
  - initial therapy including control of plaque
  - corrective therapy including surgical reduction as required
  - supportive therapy including monitoring for recurrence

34 Chronic periodontitis

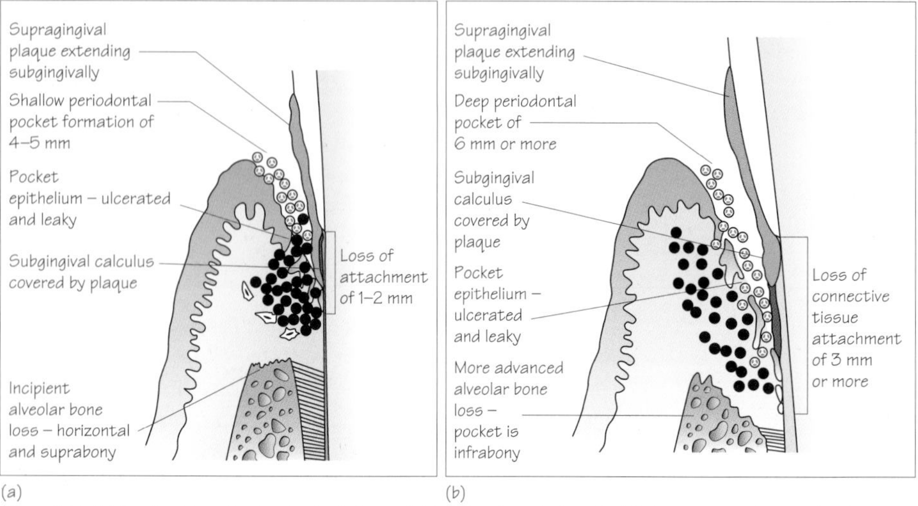

Figure 34.1 (a) Section through a tooth with incipient (initial) chronic periodontitis. (b) Section through a tooth with chronic periodontitis.

Figure 34.2 Incipient chronic periodontitis. (a) Calculus on mesiobuccal UR6 (arrow). (b) Anterior view. (c) Supragingival calculus on UL7 and subgingival calculus on mesiobuccal UL6 (arrows). (d) Right horizontal bitewing radiograph showing early crestal changes (slight horizontal bone loss) and calculus on mesiobuccal UR6 (arrow). (e) Left horizontal bitewing radiograph showing early crestal changes (slight horizontal bone loss) and calculus on mesiobuccal UL6 (arrow).

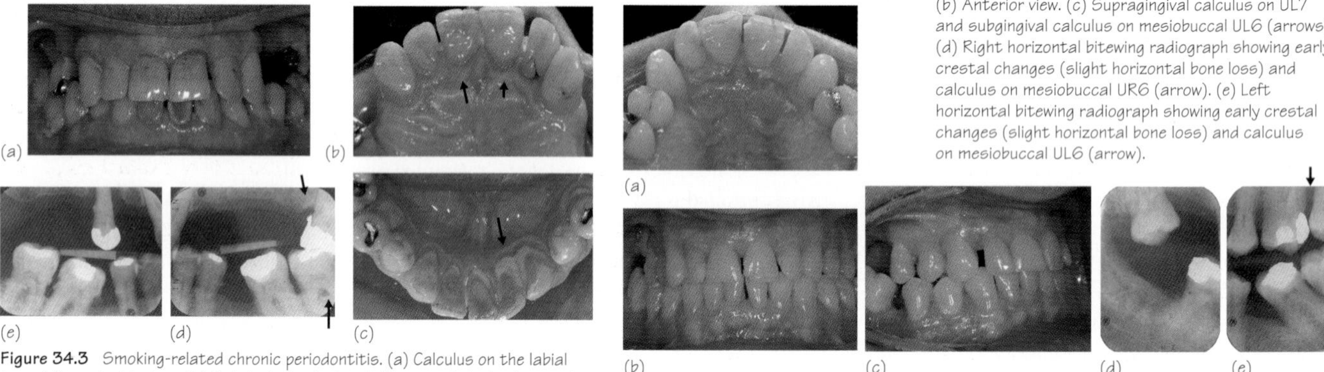

Figure 34.3 Smoking-related chronic periodontitis. (a) Calculus on the labial lower left central incisor. (b) Subgingival calculus visible as a dark shadow on the palatal upper incisors (arrows). (c) Supragingival calculus on the lingual lower anteriors (arrow). (d) Left horizontal bitewing radiograph showing a mesial overhang and vertical bone loss at UL8 (arrow), with furcation involvement at LL8 (arrow). (e) Right horizontal bitewing radiograph showing subgingival calculus.

Figure 34.4 (a–c) Slight drifting of incisors, with diastemas present between the upper incisors. (d) Right vertical bitewing radiograph. (e) Left vertical bitewing radiograph showing vertical bone loss between UL6 and UL7 (arrow).

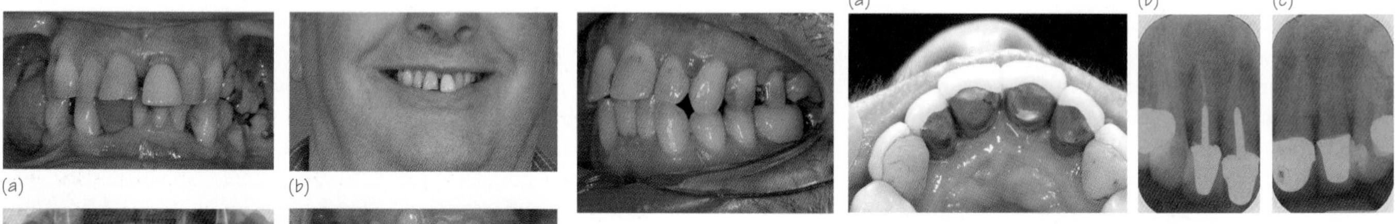

Figure 34.5 (a–c) Severe drifting of UL1 due to bone loss leading to lip trapping. (d) Scanora dentition only panoramic radiograph showing bone loss and periodontic–endodontic lesions on UL6 and LR2, which were both extracted.

Figure 34.6 Inflammation and blunting of papilla between UL2 and UL3.

Figure 34.7 Suppuration: (a) palatal suppuration, and (b, c) periapicals of crowned incisor teeth showing horizontal bone loss.

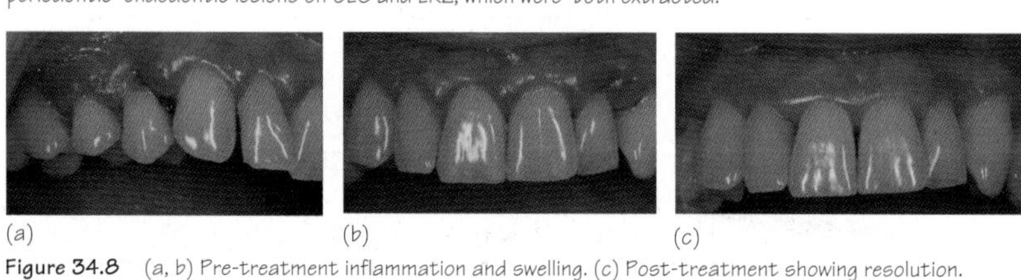

Figure 34.8 (a, b) Pre-treatment inflammation and swelling. (c) Post-treatment showing resolution.

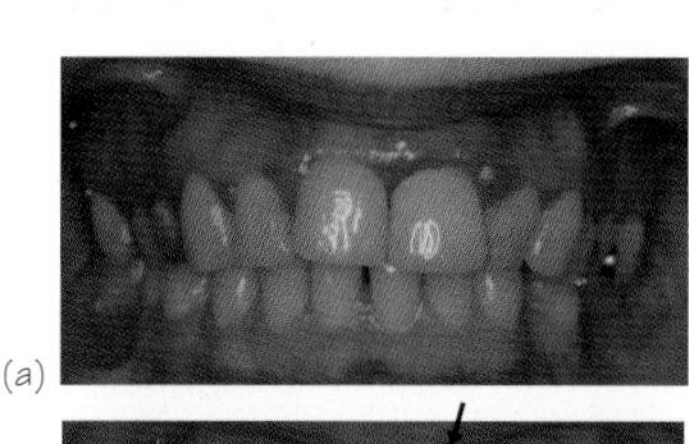

Figure 34.9 (a) Pre-treatment inflammation and swelling around the upper anterior teeth. (b) Post-treatment (non-surgical) resolution of inflammation with recession and exposure of the crown margin of UL1 which is now supragingival. Due to poor aesthetics, the crown could now be replaced (arrow).

Chronic periodontitis is the commonest form of periodontitis found in adults, but it can manifest in the incipient (initial) stages in teenagers. With increasing age, the cumulative effects of attachment loss, pocket formation and alveolar bone loss become more apparent and can affect a sizeable proportion of the adult population. The prevalence, extent, severity and rate of progression are variable and may be influenced by various periodontal risk factors. While microbial plaque is the key aetiological factor, the balance between the microbial challenge and the host defences is important in determining progression.

Features of chronic periodontitis

- Interproximal clinical attachment loss (CAL) (Fig. 34.1).
- True pocket formation of 4 mm or more.
- Screening by the Basic Periodontal Examination (BPE) or Periodontal Screening and Recording (PSR) gives a code of 3 or 4 (Chapter 17).
- Typically, there is a horizontal pattern of bone loss on radiographs (Figs 34.2, 34.7b);
  - vertical (infrabony) bone loss may be present on some sites (Figs 34.3, 34.4).
- Poor plaque control; supragingival and subgingival calculus are frequently found (Figs 34.2, 34.3).
- Possible (variable) presence of: drifting of incisors (Figs 34.4, 34.5); inflammation (Fig. 34.6); mobility; recession (Figs 34.3, 34.5); furcation defects (Fig. 34.3); suppuration (Fig. 34.7); halitosis.
- There is a variable subgingival plaque microflora.
- Usually progression is slow to moderate with exacerbations.
- Destruction is consistent with the presence of plaque and calculus; modifying local and systemic factors can exacerbate.
- Risk factors include tobacco smoking, stress and poorly controlled diabetes mellitus.
- Can further classify according to:
  - extent (localised, less than 30% sites are affected; generalised, more than 30% are affected);
  - severity (slight = 1–2 mm CAL; moderate = 3–4 mm CAL; severe ≥5 mm CAL).

Features in young people: incipient chronic periodontitis

- Age of onset can be during adolescence.
- An interproximal CAL of 1–2 mm will be found, commonly on maxillary first molars and mandibular incisors in the initial stages, but any teeth can become affected (Fig. 34.1a, 34.2).
- The prevalence, extent and severity of CAL increase slowly throughout the teens, in association with plaque and subgingival calculus.
- Concomitant true shallow pockets of 4–5 mm occur (Fig. 34.1a).
- Supragingival plaque and calculus are common.
- The severity and extent of the inflammation is variable.
- There is a variable subgingival plaque microbiota, including *Prevotella intermedia* and *Aggregatibacter actinomycetemcomitans*.
  - the presence of *Porphyromonas gingivalis* and *Tannerella forsythia* have been associated with subsequent CAL;
- Early crestal alveolar bone loss (around 0.5 mm) may be present (Fig. 34.2d, e) – best seen in serial bitewing radiographs over 18 months or longer.
- Bone loss typically shows a horizontal pattern.
- If the BPE = 4 or * in an adolescent, look for modifying factors or suspect an aggressive form of periodontitis (Chapter 40).

Features of smoking-related chronic periodontitis

Typical diagnostic features of patients who smoke (Fig. 34.3) are:

- The smoking habit often starts in teenage years.
- More severe CAL, pockets and radiographic bone loss are seen than in same-age peers with similar plaque levels.
- The gingiva are pale and fibrous.
- There is less tendency to bleed on probing due to fewer blood vessels and the vasoconstrictive effects of nicotine on the vasculature.
- Maxillary anterior and palatal surfaces are more adversely affected.
- Anterior recession may be a presenting feature.
- Nicotine staining is readily detectable.
- There is increased supragingival calculus formation.
- There is a poorer response to periodontal treatment; may be refractory.

Management

Management follows the usual three phases (Chapter 19):

Initial therapy

During the initial cause-related phase, pre-treatment periodontal indices are taken, followed by oral hygiene instruction and smoking cessation advice. Any modifiable plaque retentive factors are dealt with, such as removing restoration overhangs. A full mouth supragingival and subgingival scale and polish is undertaken plus root surface instrumentation of deep pockets, using local analgesia as necessary. Monitoring is 8–12 weeks after therapy (minimum 6 weeks), when initial healing has occurred, to evaluate the treatment response (Fig. 34.8). The provisional treatment plan might include endododontic treatment of non-vital teeth if the prognosis is favourable or extractions of teeth with hopeless prognosis (Fig. 34.5) and the provision of temporary 'immediate' partial dentures. The initial phase of therapy for chronic periodontitis is often amenable to the general dental practitioner unless additional complexities justify specialist referral.

Corrective therapy

The definitive treatment planning decisions would normally be made at the corrective phase of therapy, including further non-surgical periodontal therapy possibly with adjunctive local antimicrobials at carefully selected sites, periodontal surgery and orthodontics. Once the periodontal status has stabilised, removable or fixed prosthodontics can be arranged as required (Fig. 34.9).

Supportive therapy

Supportive periodontal therapy is crucial to prevent disease recurrence and involves continued patient motivation and compliance for home plaque control, maintenance of smoking cessation, and professional debridement as necessary. The general dental practitioner, hygienist or therapist can provide this care. Recall intervals are commonly 3 monthly, although, when stable, 6-monthly intervals may be appropriate to the individual patient's needs.

Key points

- Chronic periodontitis is the commonest form of periodontitis
- It can begin in adolescence
- It progresses into adulthood, with exacerbations
- Progress is usually slow unless modifying factors are present
- Treatment is amenable to initial, corrective and supportive therapy, much of which can be undertaken in primary dental care

35 Aggressive periodontitis

STAGES OF BACTERIAL PATHOGENICITY	Examples of A.a. virulence factors
1. Attachment to host tissues	Autotransporter proteins; fimbriae; PGA polysaccharide
2. Multiplication	Bacteriocins
3. Evasion of host defences	Chemotactic inhibition factors; leukotoxin; immunosuppressive factors to IgG, IgM
4. Penetration (invasion) of tissues	Cytolethal distending toxins
5. Tissue destruction	Activation of T-helper cells and B-cells; collagenases; lipopolysaccharide

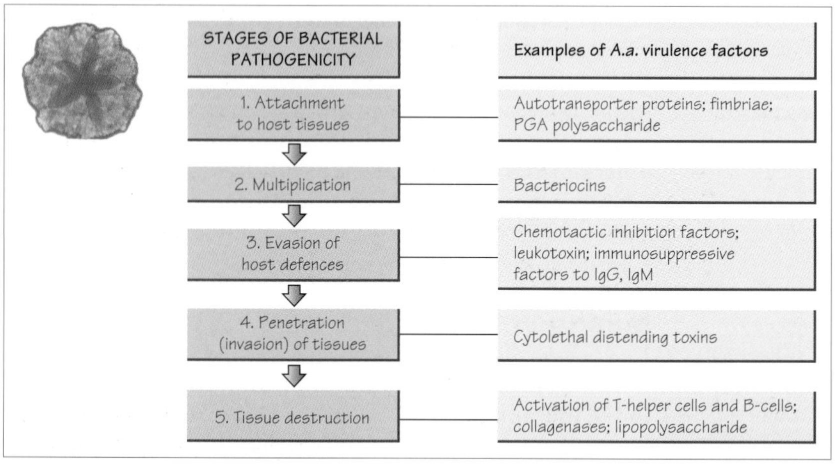

Figure 35.1 For *Aggregatibacter actinomycetemcomitans* (A.a.) to initiate periodontal destruction, it needs to undergo the following stages. (1) Attach to buccal cells, move to the tooth surface and progress from a supragingival to subgingival location. Adhesins and autotransporter proteins like Aae and EmaA have a role in attachment to epithelial cells and collagen; fimbriae are involved in autoaggregation, attachment and biofilm formation; and PGA (poly-N-acetyl-glucosamine) polysaccharide may be involved in autoaggregation and is resistant to phagocytosis and antimicrobial peptides. (2) Multiply. Bacteriocins inhibit beneficial species, thereby allowing pathogens to multiply. (3) Evade host defences. A.a.'s leukotoxin is a powerful virulence factor that destroys neutrophils and macrophages; A.a. also produces factors that inhibit neutrophil chemotaxis and are immunosuppressive to immunoglobulin G (IgG) and IgM. (4) Penetrate (invade) tissues (only a few bacteria have this property) – possibly via cytolethal distending toxins and ApiA (an outer membrane protein produced by A.a.). (5) Destroy tissue. A.a. activates T-helper cells and B-cells to incite bone loss and produces collagenases that degrade collagen and periodontal ligament; lipopolysaccharide (endotoxin) activates the host to secrete mediators that lead to bone resorption.

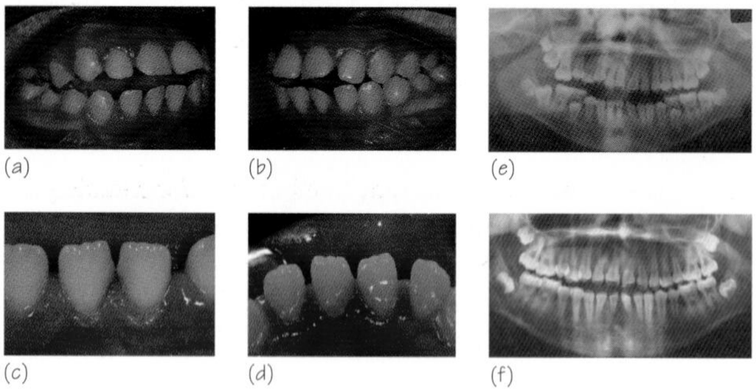

(a) (b) (e) (c) (d) (f)

Figure 35.2 A black African girl, aged 12 years, with localised aggressive periodontitis. (a, b) Right and left clinical views. (c) Labial and (d) lingual of the lower incisors showing some plaque, supragingival calculus, subgingival calculus and inflammation. (e) Panoramic radiograph of the patient aged 11 years, when still in the mixed dentition stage, and (f) aged 12 years. The radiographs show characteristic bone loss around the first molars (bilaterally symmetrical, arc-shaped defects with furcation involvement) and angular bone loss around the incisors. Although oral hygiene was unsatisfactory, the levels of plaque are inconsistent with the severe amount of bone loss found in this child.

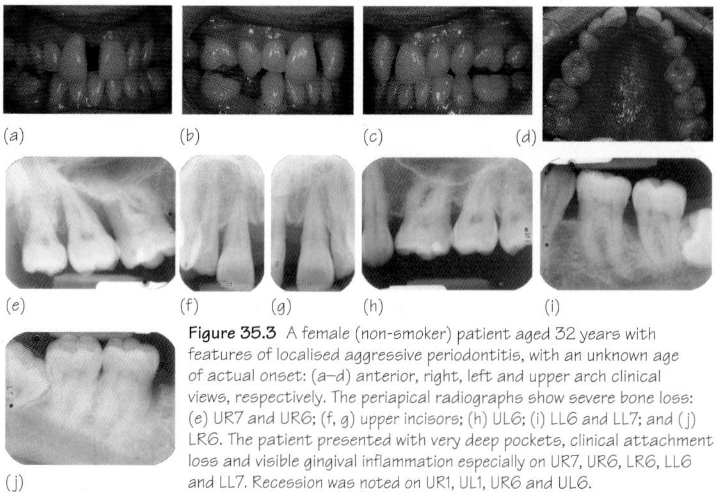

(a) (b) (c) (d) (e) (f) (g) (h) (i) (j)

Figure 35.3 A female (non-smoker) patient aged 32 years with features of localised aggressive periodontitis, with an unknown age of actual onset: (a–d) anterior, right, left and upper arch clinical views, respectively. The periapical radiographs show severe bone loss: (e) UR7 and UR6; (f, g) upper incisors; (h) UL6; (i) LL6 and LL7; and (j) LR6. The patient presented with very deep pockets, clinical attachment loss and visible gingival inflammation especially on UR7, UR6, LR6, LL6 and LL7. Recession was noted on UR1, UL1, UR6 and UL6.

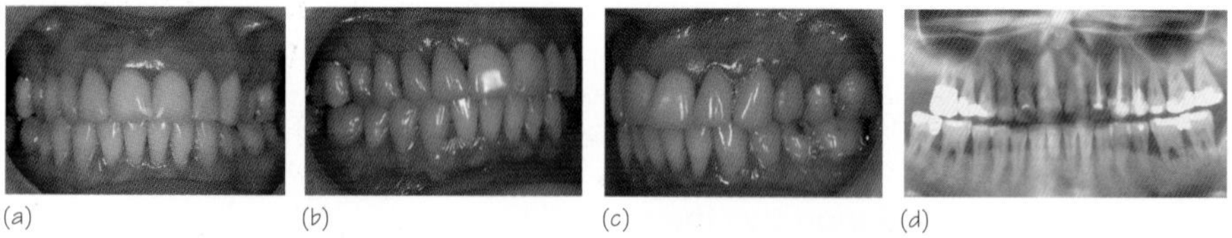

(a) (b) (c) (d)

Figure 35.4 A female (non-smoker) patient aged 35 years with generalised aggressive periodontitis: (a–c) anterior, right and left clinical views in occlusion, respectively. (d) A panoramic radiograph showing generalised advanced alveolar bone loss. Generalised mild gingival inflammation is visible, but a relatively small amount of plaque is present which is inconsistent with the severity of destruction, deep pocketing and clinical attachment loss present.

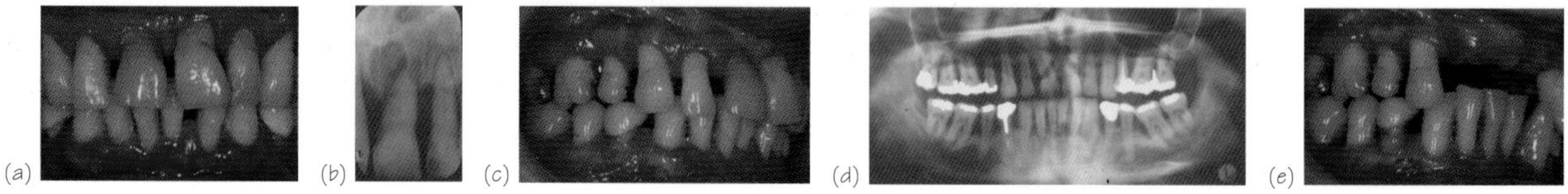

(a) (b) (c) (d) (e)

Figure 35.5 A male (non-smoker) patient aged 29 with generalised aggressive periodontitis. (a) Anterior clinical view showing marked inflammation, drifting of the incisors and suppuration on UL1 and UL2. (b) A periapical radiograph showing advanced bone loss, apical radiolucency and resorption on UL1 and apical radiolucency on UL2. (c) A right view showing generalised inflammation and loss of attachment. (d) A panoramic radiograph showing generalised advanced bone loss. (e) A right view following the preliminary periodontal treatment and extraction of UR2, UR1, UL1 and UL2.

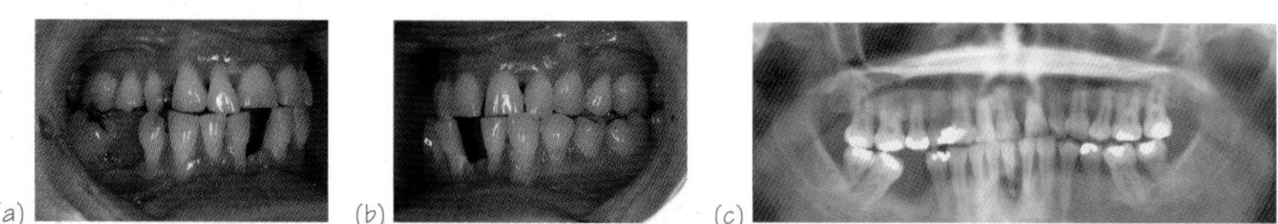

(a) (b) (c)

Figure 35.6 A female (non-smoker) patient in her early thirties with poorly controlled type 1 diabetes and generalised aggressive periodontitis. (a, b) Right and left clinical views in occlusion, showing mild gingival inflammation, recession, relatively little plaque and localised supragingival calculus on LR1 and LL2. (c) A scanora dentition only panoramic radiograph showing generalised advanced bone loss and a periodontic–endodontic lesion on LL2 – this tooth exfoliated spontaneously prior to the clinical photographs. Generalised deep pockets and clinical attachment loss were present.

Aggressive periodontitis is a rapidly destructive but less common form of periodontitis than chronic periodontitis. The aetiology is multifactorial, including the constituents and virulence of the microbial plaque, host defence defects and genetic elements. The consensus statement on aggressive periodontitis from the 1999 International Workshop for the Classification of Periodontal Diseases and Conditions designated a localised and a generalised form which replace earlier classifications that placed too much emphasis on age of presentation. Instead, the focus is on clinical, radiographic, historical and laboratory findings.

Epidemiological data show ethnic variation in aggressive periodontitis in the 11–25-year-old age group: 0.1–0.2% Caucasians; 0.4–1.0% Asians; 0.5–1.0% Hispanics and South Americans; 1.0–3.0% Africans and Afro-Americans.

Features of aggressive periodontitis

Common features

The three common features of aggressive periodontitis are:

- Patients are healthy except for the periodontitis.
- There is rapid attachment loss and bone destruction.
- Familial aggregation.

Inheritence may be due to Mendelian genes inherited due to an autosomal dominant pattern and specific genes may differ in different populations and ethnic groups. Further research is needed.

Secondary features

The five secondary features generally but not always present in both types of aggressive periodontitis are:

- The amounts of microbial deposits are inconsistent with the severity of periodontal tissue destruction.
- There are elevated proportions of *Aggregatibacter* (formerly *Actinobacillus*) *actinomycetemcomitans*, and in some populations levels of *Porphyromonas gingivalis* may be raised.
- Phagocyte abnormalities are found.
- There is a hyperresponsive macrophage phenotype, including elevated levels of prostaglandin E 2 (PGE-2) and interleukin-1β (IL-1β).
- The progression of attachment loss and bone loss may be self-limiting.

Specific features

Localised aggressive periodontitis

- Circumpubertal onset.
- Robust serum antibody response to the infecting agent A. *actinomycetemcomitans*.
- Localised first molar/incisor presentation: interproximal attachment loss on at least two permanent teeth, one of which is a first molar, and involving no more than two teeth other than first molars and incisors.

A. actinomycetemcomitans is considered a true infectious agent and possesses various determinants of virulence and pathogenic potential (Fig. 35.1). It has five serotypes, a–e, of which serotype b is most common in aggressive periodontitis.

A 2-year longitudinal study found there was an 18-fold risk of attachment loss in 12-year-olds in Morocco with the JP2 clone of *A. actinomycetemcomitans*, which belongs to serotype b, in contrast to those with the non-JP2 clone in which the risk was three-fold.

Generalised aggressive periodontitis

- Usually affects people younger than 30 years, but they may be older.
- There is a poor serum antibody response to infecting agents.
- There is a pronounced episodic nature of the destruction of periodontal attachment and alveolar bone.
- Generalised interproximal attachment loss affects at least three permanent teeth other than first molars and incisors.

Presentation

The tissues may look relatively normal or only mildly inflamed until periodontal examination or radiographs reveal the severity and extent of the problem (Figs 35.2–35.4). In other cases the appearance can show obvious clinical evidence of disease (Fig. 35.5). The amount of plaque is typically inconsistent with the severity and extent of periodontal destruction found. The amount of subgingival calculus can vary but studies have shown subgingival calculus is associated with subsequent attachment loss, therefore it is important to locate and remove it. Where modifying factors are present, additional descriptors can be applied, such as aggressive periodontitis related to cigarette smoking, stress or poorly controlled diabetes (Fig. 35.6).

Management

Screening using the Basic Periodontal Examination (BPE) or Periodontal Screening and Recording (PSR) would typically yield codes of 4 or *. Successful management and prognosis are dependent on early diagnosis, the ability to suppress or eradicate infecting organisms, and providing an intra-oral environment conducive to maintenance.

Initial therapy

The initial cause-related phase of therapy reflects that for chronic periodontitis (Chapter 34). However, the corrective and supportive phases may differ. Non-surgical therapy may not eradicate virulent organisms like *A. actinomycetemcomitans* and *P. gingivalis*, which have a propensity to invade tissues and evade host defences.

Corrective therapy

Following monitoring of the tissue response, if a number of active deep sites with bleeding on probing persist, adjunctive systemic antibiotics may be indicated, with either non-surgical or surgical therapy. Microbial or antibiotic sensitivity testing can be undertaken. Various regimes have been supported in the literature (tetracycline 250 mg × 4 per day for 14 days; doxycycline 200 mg loading dose, then 100 mg daily for 13 days), but the following has particular efficacy against *A. actinomycetemcomitans*:

- Metronidazole 250 mg (UK either 200 or 400 mg available) + amoxicillin 375 mg (UK either 250 or 500 mg available) × 3 per day for 7 days.

Supportive therapy

Vigilance is required to detect any relapse. Frequent recall is therefore indicated according to an individually tailored treatment plan.

Key points

- Aggressive periodontitis:
  - is relatively uncommon but rapidly destructive
  - has common and secondary features
  - can be localised or generalised, each with specific features
- Management differs from chronic periodontitis particularly in the corrective and supportive phases
- Key aetiological factors include microbial virulence (*A. actinomycetemcomitans*, *P. gingivalis*), host defence defects and genetic elements

36 Periodontal management of patients who smoke

(a)

Cancers due to smoking
- Lung
- Oral
- Throat
- Oesophagus
- Bladder
- Kidney
- Stomach
- Pancreas
- Leukaemia

(b)

Other diseases
- Chronic obstructive pulmonary disease
- Pneumonia
- Heart disease, angina
- Cerebrovascular disease
- Osteoporosis
- Infertility, impotence
- Skin wrinkling
- Macular degeneration (retina)
- Low birth weight baby
- Periodontal disease, necrotising ulcerative gingivitis
- Passive smoking effects

Figure 36.1 Health problems related to cigarette smoking.

(a)

Clinical appearance in smoker
- Fibrotic 'tight' gingiva, rolled margins
- Less gingival redness and bleeding
- More severe, widespread disease than same age non-smoking control
- Anterior, maxilla, palate are worst areas affected
- Anterior recession, open embrasures
- Nicotine staining
- Calculus

(b)

Clinical characteristics of smoker
- Relatively earlier onset
- Rapid disease progression
- Greater severity and extent of disease (pockets, clinical attachment loss, bone loss)
- More tooth loss
- Poorer response to non-surgical therapy
- Recurrence within 1 year of surgery
  – ?avoid surgery
- Increased % are refractory to treatment

Figure 36.2 Details of clinical appearance and characteristics in a smoker.

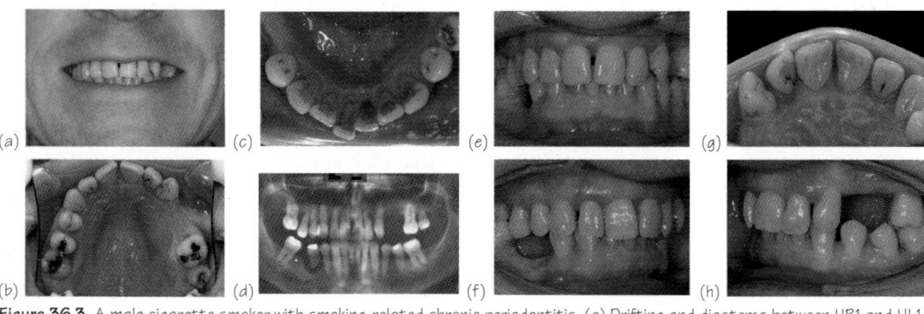

Figure 36.3 A male cigarette smoker with smoking-related chronic periodontitis. (a) Drifting and diastema between UR1 and UL1. (b) Palatal effects of smoking. (c) Nicotine-stained supragingival calculus on the lingual of the lower incisors. (d) A panoramic radiograph showing generalised bone loss and a periodontic–endodontic lesion on LR5 which was extracted. (e) Anterior view showing fibrotic, pale gingiva. (f) Right view following extraction of LR5. (g) Upper palatal surfaces showing nicotine staining and inflamed, rolled gingival margins. (h) Left side showing recession and nicotine staining.

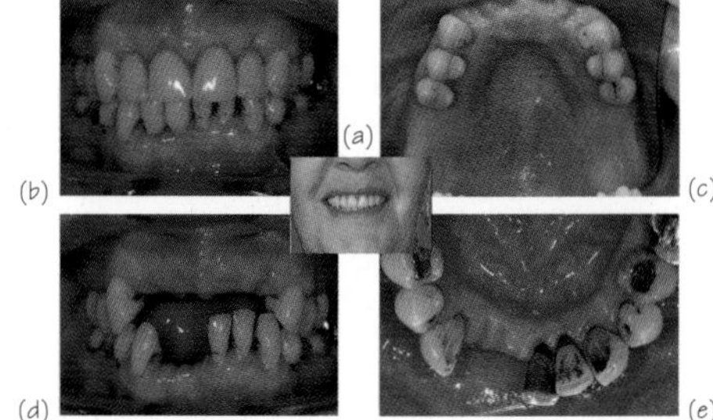

Figure 36.4 (a) A female cigarette smoker with smoking-related chronic periodontitis. (b) Anterior view with the upper and lower partial dentures in place; note the staining and generalised recession. (c) Palatal view showing a shortened dental arch following several extractions and also denture-related stomatitis. (d) Marked recession/loss of attachment anteriorly. (e) Heavily nicotine-stained supragingival calculus on the lingual of the lower incisors.

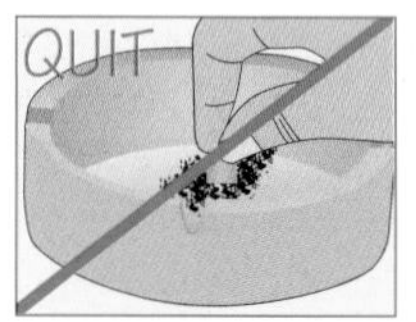

Figure 36.5 Quit smoking!

(a)

The five 'A's for the dental professional
- Ask about tobacco use at every visit
- Advise all smokers to quit
- Assess readiness to quit
- Assist with a quit plan
- Arrange follow up visits

(b)

ASK
- Ask all patients about their smoking status and record information in the clinical notes
  – Current, former, never smoker
- If current smoker, record:
  – How many cigarettes smoked daily/how much tobacco smoked
  – How many years smoked; if any quit attempts
  – Pattern of smoking, e.g. on waking or socially

(c)

ADVISE
- Use clear, strong and personalised language
- Highlight oral health effects of tobacco
- Emphasise benefits of quitting

(d)

ASSESS
- Assess readiness to quit
- Ask if patient wants to quit, record reply in the notes
  – If no, help motivate patient to quit:
    - identify reasons to quit
    - build confidence to quit
    - make a note to ASK again at next visit
  – If yes, provide resources and ASSIST

(e)

ASSIST
- Set a quit date, ideally within 2 weeks
- Remove tobacco products from environment
- Encourage to get support
  – From family, friends, colleagues
- Identify reasons to quit and benefits
- Give advice on successful quitting
  – Review past quit attempts
- Encourage nicotine replacement therapy or medication (unless contra-indicated)
- Provide resources

(f)

ARRANGE
- Arrange follow-up visits to review progress
- If relapse, repeat quit attempt
  – Review reasons for failure
  – Review medication
  – Refer for help to quit line or intensive smoking cessation programme
    - four times more likely to succeed with such support (http: //smokefree.nhs.uk)

Figure 36.6 The five 'A's: ask, advise, assess, assist and arrange.

1. PREPARING TO STOP
   – Set quit date
     - Vital to want to stop
   – List and re-read the benefits of stopping
2. STOPPING
   – Aim to get through the first day without smoking
   – Have strategies to relieve craving
     - e.g. Deep breaths until craving gone, chew sugar-free gum
3. STAYING STOPPED
   – Be aware that most people need several attempts to stop
     - Should not give up trying to quit
   – It can take up to 3 months to become a non-smoker
     - Usually takes less time
   – Physical craving often disappears in less than a week
     - Psychological dependence can last longer

Figure 36.7 Three steps to stop smoking.

UK
- Free NHS Smoking Helpline 0800 169 0 169 for local NHS Stop Smoking Services
- Website for free materials http://smokefree.nhs.uk
- Website for National Institute for Health and Clinical Excellence (NICE) www.nice.org.uk
- NHS Direct 0845 4647 / www.nhsdirect.nhs.uk for questions

USA
- Free National Quitline 1-800-QUIT NOW (784-8669) for state-based quitline services
- Websites for free materials
  – www.ahrq.gov/path/tobacco.htm (US Department of Health and Human Services, Agency for Healthcare Research and Quality)
  – www.smokefree.gov

Figure 36.8 Resources and support to stop smoking in the UK and the USA (all websites accessed 14 April 2009).

Table 36.1 Direct benefits of stopping smoking.

Time after cessation	Direct benefits
2days	Sense of taste and smell improved
1 month	Skin clearer, more hydrated
3 months	Improved breathing, no cough or wheeze Improved lung function (up to 10%) Risk of mouth and throat cancer reduced
6 months	Most smoking-related oral white patches will have disappeared
1 year	Gingival circulation improved
10 years	Risk of heart attack reduced to half that of a smoker
15 years	Risk of lung cancer reduced by half Risk of heart attack same as never smoker

Table 36.2 Indirect benefits of stopping smoking.

Reasons to stop	Indirect benefits
Passive smoking	No longer causing harm to others through passive smoking, especially babies/children: – Sudden infant death syndrome – Asthma, ear and chest infections
Children	Less likely children will go on to smoke – Children of smokers are three times more likely to smoke
Unborn baby	Limiting harm to unborn baby – Most harmful effects in second and third trimester; risk of low birth weight baby – Quitting in first 3 months reduces risk to normal
Costs	Savings from not buying cigarettes

Tobacco smoking is a major cause of death and morbidity (Fig. 36.1) throughout the world. According to the World Health Organisation in 2002, smoking-related diseases killed one in ten adults globally, accounting for 4 million deaths, with daily sales of 15 billion cigarettes. In 2006, in the UK, approximately 23% of men and 21% of women smoked cigarettes; on average men smoked 15 cigarettes daily, while women smoked 13 (Office of National Statistics). In the USA in 2005, an estimated 25.9 million men (23.9%) and 20.7 million women (18.1%) smoked (National Health Interview Survey). Although the prevalence of smoking has declined in the UK and USA, it is rising in developing countries.

Nicotine

Tobacco smoke contains around 4000 chemicals including nicotine (which is highly addictive), tar (which deposits in the lungs and contains carcinogens), carbon monoxide (which binds to haemoglobin in the blood thus preventing carriage of sufficient oxygen) and oxidant gases (which make the blood more likely to clot and increase the risk of heart attack or stroke). Nicotine increases the heart rate, and causes a rise in noradrenaline and dopamine in the brain, which in turn creates a positive mood swing. When the nicotine effects begin to wear off, this is accompanied by feelings of irritability, anxiety and craving for another cigarette. Nicotine causes dehydration of the skin and can increase certain forms of high blood pressure.

Smokeless tobacco

There are over 30 types of smokeless products including dry chewing tobacco (part of 'betel quid' or 'paan') and sucked and inhaled tobacco (nasal snuff). Many forms are highly carcinogenic and almost all types cause oral cancer. They contain at least as much nicotine as smoked tobacco and so are highly addictive.

Clinical periodontal management

As well as the general health risks, tobacco smoking is associated with a greater risk of periodontitis (Chapters 10, 11), necrotising ulcerative gingivitis and oral cancer. The effects are thought to be both local and systemic (Chapter 8). The level of risk relates to the number of pack years (i.e. packs of cigarettes smoked daily multiplied by the number of years smoked). Periodontal diseases manifest at an earlier age in smokers, are more severe and exhibit several characteristic clinical features (Figs 36.2–36.4).

Management follows the basic principles of initial, corrective and supportive therapy. However, periodontal diseases have been found to be more refractory to treatment in smokers than non-smokers.

Use of local antimicrobials may provide small adjunctive clinical benefits over and above root surface instrumentation for the management of chronic periodontitis, however, clinical improvement is less than in a non-smoker. Some clinicians prefer not to undertake periodontal surgery or implant provision in smokers due to compromised clinical outcome. It is imperative that:

- Patients are advised about the risks of smoking and are encouraged to quit.
- The provision of smoking cessation advice is recorded in the treatment notes for medicolegal reasons.

Smoking cessation

The National Institute for Health and Clinical Excellence (NICE) in the UK and the Department of Health and Human Services, Agency for Healthcare Research and Quality (AHRQ) in the USA advocate the delivery of brief smoking cessation interventions for every patient who smokes. Health care personnel, including the dental practitioner, hygienist, therapist, dental nurse and oral health educator, have a key role in this. Around one in 40 patients receiving such advice will stop (Fig. 36.5), so this strategy can make an impact at population level.

The five 'A's

The five 'A's (**a**sk, **a**dvise, **a**ssess, **a**ssist, **a**rrange) have been widely advocated for professionals to help patients quit smoking (Fig. 36.6). The New Zealand Smoking Cessation Guidelines also supported an 'ABC' memory aid to prompt health care workers to (i) **a**sk about smoking status, (ii) give **b**rief advice to stop smoking, and (iii) provide **c**essation support to those who want to quit.

Stopping smoking

There are three important steps for the patient (Fig. 36.7):

- Preparing to stop.
- Stopping.
- Staying stopped.

The patient should remember the benefits of quitting (Tables 36.1, 36.2) and use all available resources (Fig. 36.8).

Nicotine replacement therapy

Due to nicotine's highly addictive properties, nicotine replacement therapy (NRT) is the commonest form of smoking cessation treatment. There are various formulations but a key aspect of NRT is to achieve a sufficient dose, often by regular topping up, for a recommended 8–12-week period.

- Transdermal patches that release nicotine for either 16 hours (15, 10 or 5 mg strength) or 24 hours (21, 14 or 7 mg strength).
- Chewing gum (2 or 4 mg strength).
- Tablets and lozenges (1, 1.5, 2 and 4 mg strength).
- Inhalators or nasal sprays (single strength).

Side effects are mainly due to local reactions, sleep disturbances, gastrointestinal problems, dizziness or headaches, which may be alleviated by using a different dose or formulation. Some find alternative remedies useful, e.g., hypnosis and acupuncture.

Medication

Bupropion and Varenicline are drugs available on prescription from a medical practitioner to help stop smoking in patients who want to quit and have a date for doing so:

- Bupropion may work on the brain pathways involved with addiction and withdrawal.
- Varenicline aids smoking cessation by binding to nicotine receptors in the brain that are implicated in nicotine addiction, thus easing cravings and reducing the pleasurable effects of nicotine.

Both drugs can cause drowsiness. There are various contraindications and side effects that must be taken into account when prescribing. NICE and AHRQ guidance has been issued for each.

Key points

- Tobacco smoking is a major risk factor for general and oral health problems, including periodontitis, necrotising ulcerative gingivitis and oral cancer
- Patients should be advised of the risks of smoking and this should be recorded in the notes for medicolegal purposes
- Smoking cessation advice should be offered
- Helpful approaches include:
  - the five 'A's (ask, advise, assess, assist, arrange)
  - 'ABC' (ask, brief advice, cessation support)
  - nicotine replacement therapy or medication

37 Periodontal management of patients with diabetes

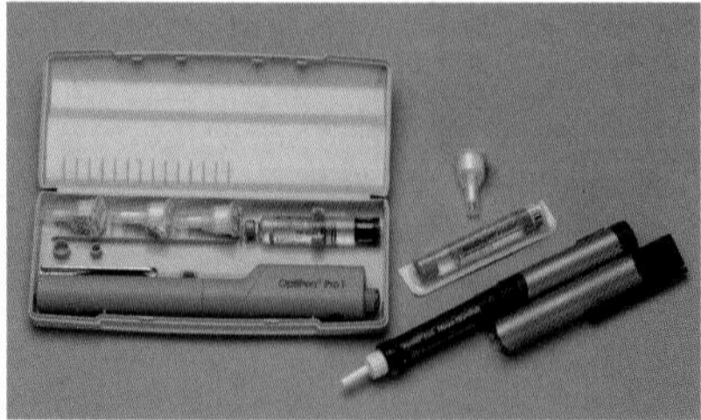

Figure 37.1 Examples of insulin pens, cartridges and disposable needles for insulin injections. The Optipen® (Sanofi-Aventis) in the case is used to deliver a long-acting basal insulin; the Novopen® (Novo-Nordisk) is used to inject quick-acting insulin prior to meals.

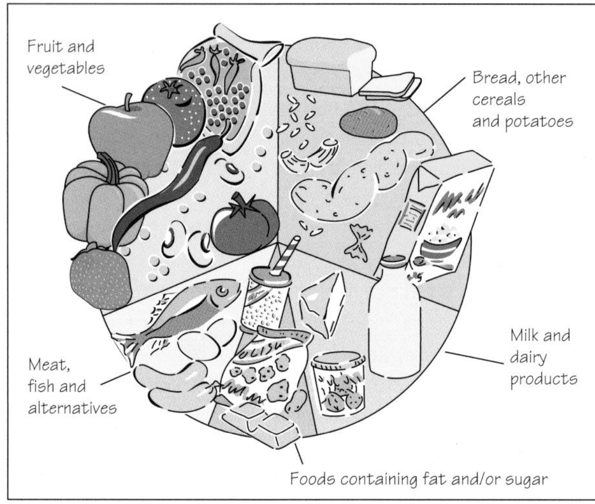

Figure 37.2 A healthy plate of food for people with diabetes: five daily portions of fruit and vegetables are recommended; bread, other cereals and potatoes should make up the bulk of the diet as they are usually low in fat and high in fibre; milk and dairy products should be eaten in moderation as they are often high in fat; foods containing fat and sugar should be limited to avoid obesity and caries; meat, fish and alternatives can be consumed in moderation as a good source of protein.

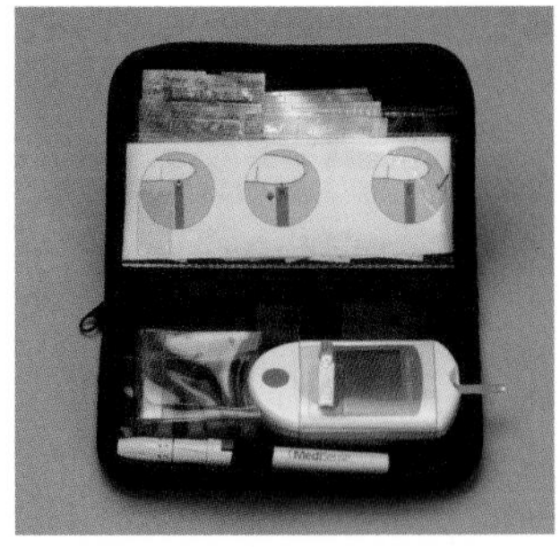

Figure 37.3 Glucose monitor for home testing. A small drop of blood is obtained from the finger tip using the automatic lancet device and applied to the test strip. The blood glucose reading appears in the window of the monitor in a few seconds.

Macrovascular complications
- Cardiovascular disease (major cause of death) and peripheral vascular disease (amputations)
- Cerebrovascular disease and stroke

Microvascular complications
- Retinopathy (blindness)
- Nephropathy (renal failure)
- Neuropathy (painful nerve damage)

Figure 37.4 Possible complications which are more likely to develop if diabetes is poorly controlled or undiagnosed. Periodontal disease has been suggested to be the sixth complication of diabetes.

(a) (b) (c) (d) (e) (g)

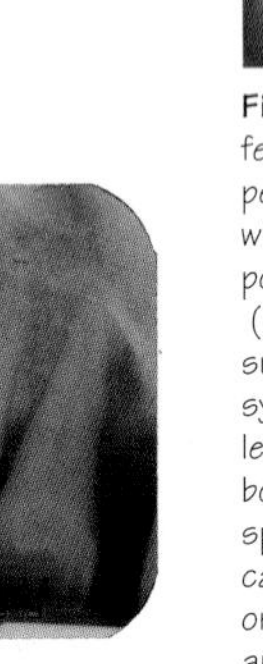

(f)

Figure 37.5 A 35-year-old male with chronic periodontitis who was a smoker and had poorly controlled type 1 diabetes (HbA1C >8.5%). Note the poor oral hygiene, calculus on the labial lower central incisors, drifting of the upper anterior teeth and diastema between the upper incisors (a–e), horizontal bone loss (c), suppuration on the upper right central incisor (e) and vertical bone loss (f), and nicotine-stained supragingival calculus on the lingual lower anterior teeth (g).

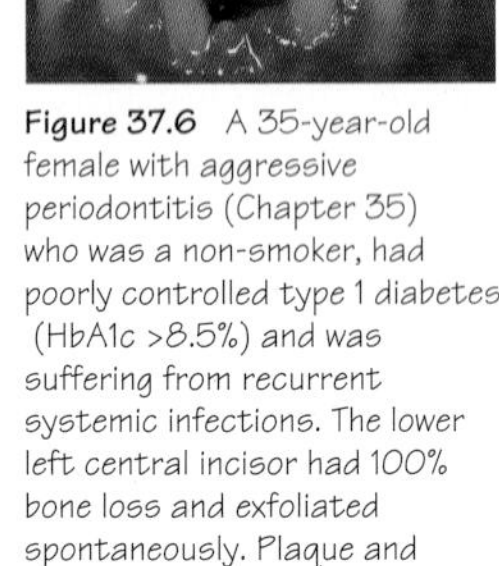

Figure 37.6 A 35-year-old female with aggressive periodontitis (Chapter 35) who was a non-smoker, had poorly controlled type 1 diabetes (HbA1c >8.5%) and was suffering from recurrent systemic infections. The lower left central incisor had 100% bone loss and exfoliated spontaneously. Plaque and calculus deposits are visible on the remaining lower anteriors, but plaque levels are generally inconsistent with the severity of the periodontal destruction. See Fig. 35.6 for more views of this patient.

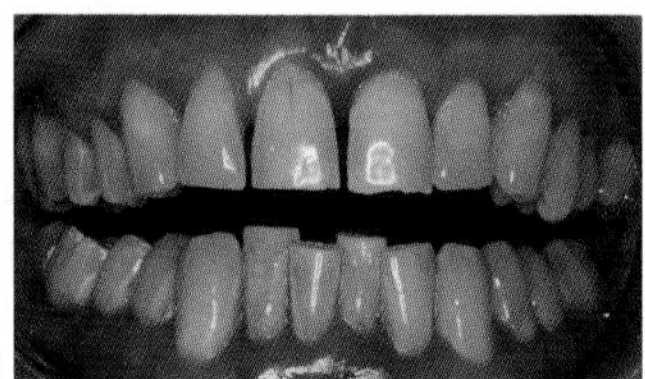

(a)

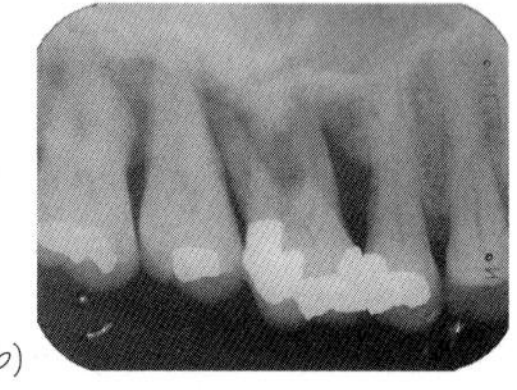

(b)

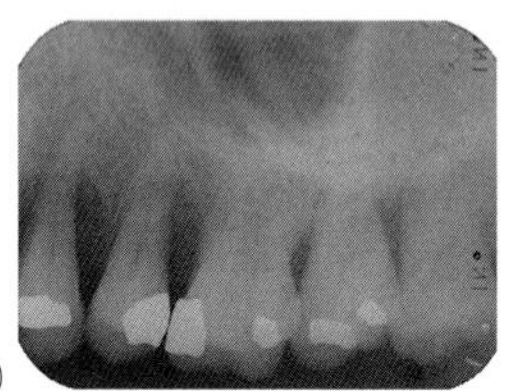

(c)

Figure 37.7 A 45-year-old male with chronic periodontitis who had poorly controlled type 2 diabetes and was on an oral hypoglycaemic drug. Home blood glucose checks were persistently >10 mmol/l. (a) Inflamed, purplish-red gingivae can be seen with poor oral hygiene and generalised subgingival calculus. (b, c) Advanced bone loss is seen on periapicals of the maxillary posterior teeth. Courtesy of P. Gregory.

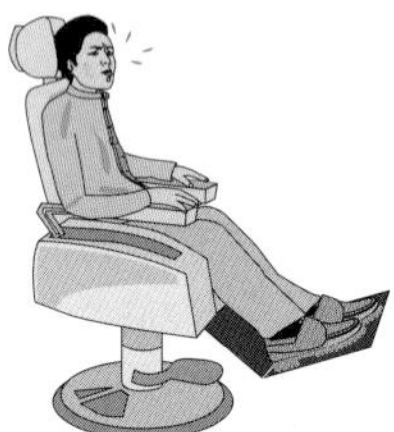

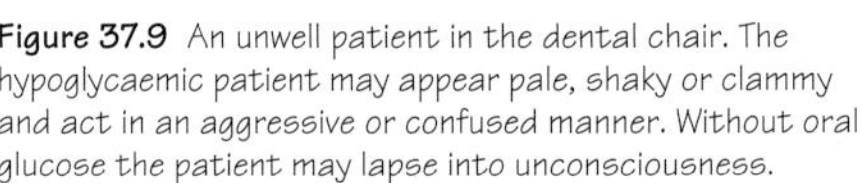

Figure 37.9 An unwell patient in the dental chair. The hypoglycaemic patient may appear pale, shaky or clammy and act in an aggressive or confused manner. Without oral glucose the patient may lapse into unconsciousness.

Hypoglycaemia
- Blood glucose <4 mmol/l
- Patient may be pale, shaky, clammy, sweating, aggressive or confused
  - more likely to occur in type 1 diabetes patient
- Give 10–20 g glucose tablets (3–6 × 3 g tablets)
- Alternatively, give glucose drink (e.g. Lucozade® 100 ml, or glass of water with 20 g glucose powder or glucose gel sachet)

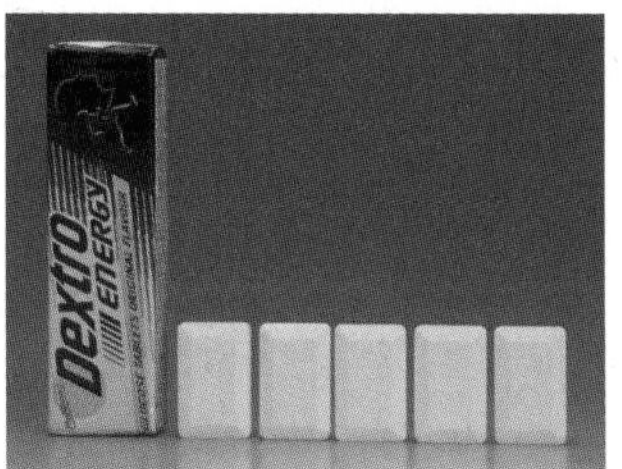

Pack of glucose tablets, 3 g of glucose per tablet

Figure 37.8 Glucose tablets.

Severe hypoglycaemia, loss of consciousness.
- Inject glucagon 1 mg for adult or 0.5 mg for child under 8 years or <25 kg (subcutaneous, intramuscular or intravenous)
  - Give glucose and oral carbohydrate on recovery
- If no recovery in 10 minutes and still unconscious, will need intravenous glucose 20% × 100 ml or 50% × 50 ml
  - Call an ambulance

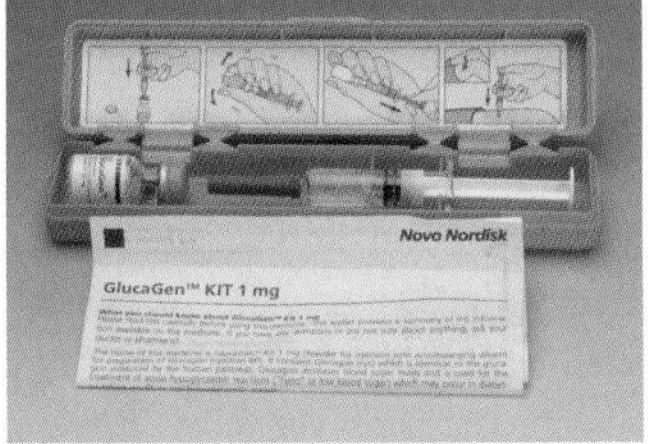

Glucagon for injection

Figure 37.10 Glucagon injection.

Diabetes mellitus is a common group of metabolic disorders characterised by chronic hyperglycaemia that results from insulin deficiency or impaired utilisation of insulin (insulin resistance). When poorly controlled, diabetes is a recognised risk factor for periodontal diseases and it has been hypothesised that a two-way relationship may exist (Chapters 10–12).

Diagnosis

Diagnosis of diabetes is based on the clinical symptoms (polyuria, polydipsia and unexplained weight loss) *plus*: (i) A random plasma glucose concentration of ≥11.1 mmol/l (200 mg/dl) or (ii) A fasting plasma glucose of ≥7.0 mmol/l (126 mg/dl) (normal level is <5.6 mmol/l or <100 mg/dl) or (iii) A 2-hour post-load glucose of ≥11.1 mmol/l (200 mg/dl) after 75 g anhydrous glucose in a glucose tolerance test.

Classification

Classification has four categories:

- Type 1 diabetes (formerly called insulin-dependent diabetes mellitus).
- Type 2 diabetes (formerly non-insulin-dependent diabetes mellitus).
- Gestational diabetes, diagnosed during pregnancy, which may be transitional.
- Other specific types, e.g. genetic defects of β-cell function (formerly called maturity onset diabetes in the young).

Type 1 diabetes

Type 1 diabetes affects 5–10% of cases and usually manifests in children or adolescents in whom it can present acutely. It is characterised by autoimmune-mediated destruction of the pancreatic β-cells which produce insulin.

Treatment is by daily insulin injections using a combination of short/medium/long-acting formulations (Fig. 37.1) or pump therapy. Islet cell transplants have been used successfully in a few individuals and inhaled insulin has been on trial. The key to success is a healthy diet balancing the dietary carbohydrate intake to injected insulin to achieve as normal a blood glucose as possible (Fig. 37.2). Blood glucose levels can be checked using home testing kits (Fig. 37.3). The target range for adults is 4–7 mmol/l (72–126 mg/dl) before meals and no more than 9 mmol/l (162 mg/dl) after meals.

Type 2 diabetes

This is associated with a defect in the β-cells, lack of insulin production and the phenomenon of insulin resistance. It generally manifests in mid-life in obese individuals with a sedentary life style and constitutes 90–95% of cases. Genetic predisposition is likely, but not well understood. Certain ethnic groups (e.g. Asians) seem more susceptible. The onset can be insidious by which time macrovascular and microvascular complications may already have occurred. Management is by diet (Fig. 37.2), exercise and, in some cases, oral hypoglycaemic drugs or even insulin injections to boost insulin levels.

Diabetes control/HbA1c

Although not universally available, medical practitioners/diabetes specialists usually arrange for a glycated haemoglobin (HbA1c) blood test. This measures the proportion of glucose bound to the haemoglobin in the red blood cells and indicates diabetes control over the last 8–10 weeks.

In the UK, the target set by the National Institute for Health and Clinical Excellence (NICE) is <7.5%, yet only 60% of adults and 16.6% of children/adolescents achieved this in the 2005–06 National UK Diabetes/Paediatric Diabetes Audits.

Complications of poor control

Macrovascular and microvascular complications are associated with poor diabetes control (Fig. 37.4). Periodontal disease has been suggested as a sixth complication.

Prevalence

- UK figures (2007) show 2.3 million (3.7% of the population) have diabetes, and it is estimated that another 750 000 may have undiagnosed type 2 diabetes.
- In the USA (2005–06), 14.6 million (4.9%) were diagnosed with diabetes and another 6.2 million were estimated to have undiagnosed type 2 diabetes.
- Worldwide, in 2000, 171 million people were affected. Global data indicate that diabetes prevalence, especially type 2, is rising dramatically, with highest incidence rates in Scandinavia and Sardinia.
- There are significant health care and cost implications.

Clinical periodontal management

Therapy

Well-controlled diabetes is not a significant risk factor for periodontal disease. If the diabetes is not well controlled, patients may present with a more severe, extensive form of periodontal disease than a non-diabetes affected peer with similar plaque levels. Poorly controlled diabetes is a systemic periodontal risk factor for chronic and aggressive periodontitis (Figs 37.5–37.7). Diabetes-associated gingivitis is a specific entity following the 1999 classification (Chapter 2). Clinical periodontal care follows the principles of initial, corrective and supportive therapy (Chapter 19).

At the start of initial therapy, enquiries should be made to the patient and their diabetes practitioner or specialist about the patient's diabetes control, and if available, the HbA1c sought. Some patients, medical practitioners and members of the diabetes care team may not be very well informed about: (i) the adverse effects of poor diabetes control on periodontal health; and (ii) the potential for some types of periodontal therapy to improve glycaemic control. Therefore education and advice of this two-way relationship should be offered where appropriate.

As new clinical trials are reported, evidence-based decisions can be made about the role of periodontal therapy and the potential value of adjunctive systemic antibiotics such as doxycycline in the periodontal management of diabetes cases (Chapter 12).

Medical emergencies

The dental team should recognise the signs and symptoms of hypoglycaemia and be prepared to treat (Figs 37.8–37.10). Hyperglycaemia may lead to ketoacidosis, but because of the time it takes to develop, it is less likely to present as an acute emergency; nevertheless, it is a serious condition needing medical intervention.

Key points

- Prevalence of diabetes is increasing worldwide
- Poorly controlled diabetes is a risk factor for periodontal diseases
- Periodontal infection can adversely affect diabetes control
- Periodontal treatment may improve diabetes control
- The dental team should know how to manage hypoglycaemia if it occurs during treatment

38 Necrotising periodontal diseases

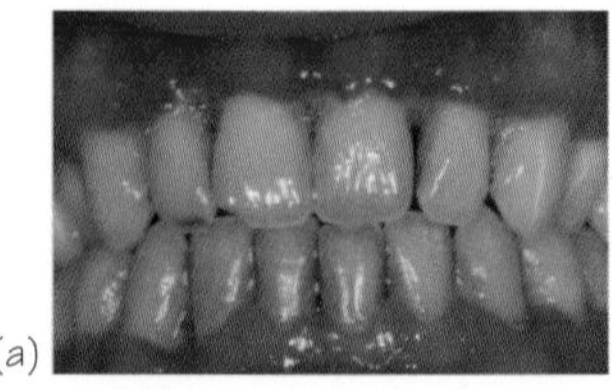
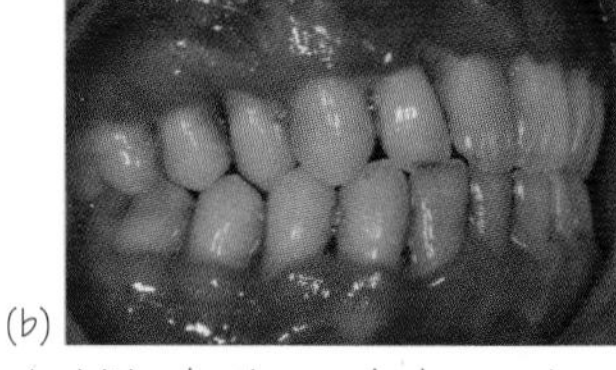
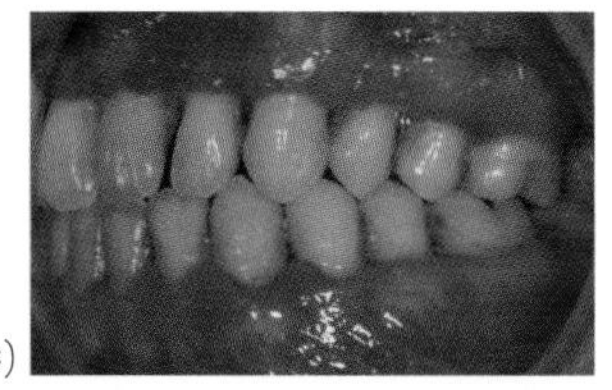

Figure 38.1 (a–c) Necrotising ulcerative gingivitis showing marked necrosis and typical punched out interdental papillae between the maxillary incisors and between the mandibular right lateral and canine.

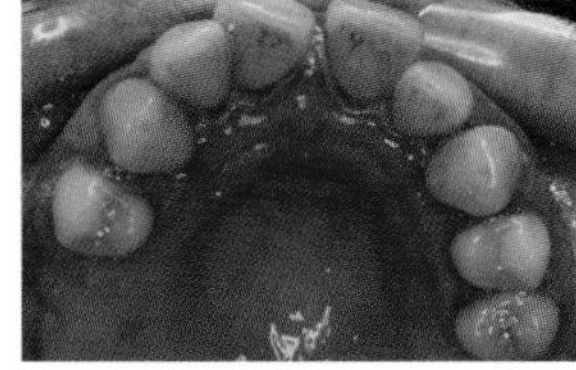

Figure 38.2 Sloughing and pseudomembrane interdentally in the maxillary incisor region.

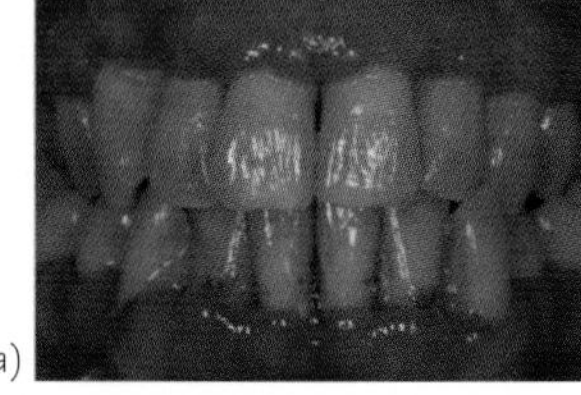
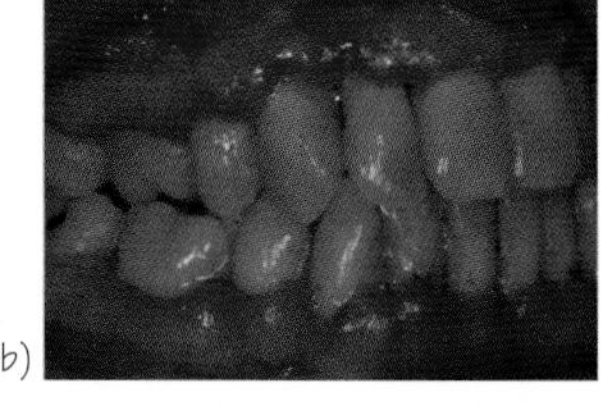
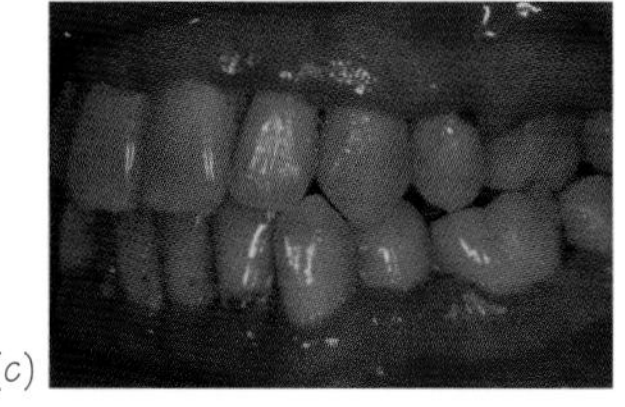

Figure 38.3 (a–c) Following the acute phase, the symptoms have settled down in this 27-year-old male smoker, but there is evidence of: (i) interdental necrosis and punched out papillae in the maxillary and mandibular anterior regions; (ii) gross deposits of subgingival calculus which are now located supragingivally due to apical migration of the gingivae; and (iii) detachment of the buccal gingiva from the mandibular incisors, indicating clinical attachment loss has occurred (i.e. destruction of the periodontal ligament. This indicates a transition from NUG to NUP.

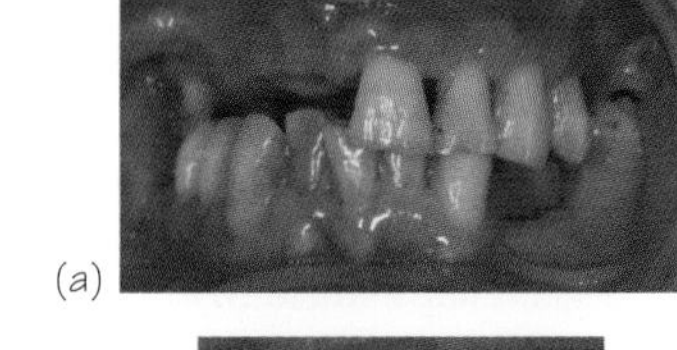
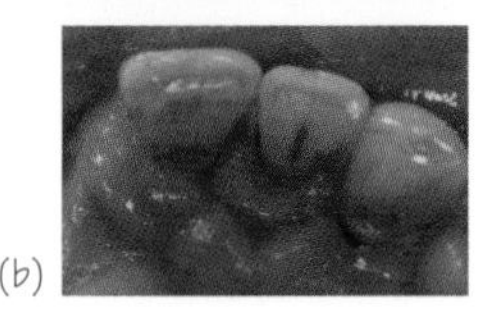

Figure 38.4 (a, b) A male patient with HIV/acquired immune deficiency syndrome (AIDS), and NUP leading to necrosis of the palatal tissue on the maxillary central incisor exposing the underlying palatal alveolar bone.

	Necrotising ulcerative gingivitis	Primary herpetic gingivostomatitis
Aetiology	Fusiform/spirochaete bacterial complex Predisposing factors include: immunosuppression (possibly HIV), stress, smoking, poor diet, poor oral hygiene	Herpes simplex virus 1
Age of onset	Young adults: late teens to early twenties	Often in children
Site	Interdental papillae	Gingiva and any part of oral mucosa
Distinctive symptoms	Painful, bleeding gingivae; necrotic punched out interdental papillae Pseudomembranous slough Fever, malaise and lymphadenopathy may occur Foetor ex ore	Prodromal (incubation) period 10–14 days Very inflamed, swollen gingivae Viral vesicles (yellow centre, red halo) on gingiva or oral mucosa Fever, malaise and lymphadenopathy are classic Foetor ex ore
Duration	A few days if treated. Possible role of antibiotics (metronidazole)	1–2 weeks; takes its course with supportive home care
Contagious	No	Yes, very contagious
Healing	Destruction of periodontal tissue remains	Full healing, no permanent destruction

Figure 38.6 Differential diagnosis between NUG and primary herpetic gingivostomatitis.

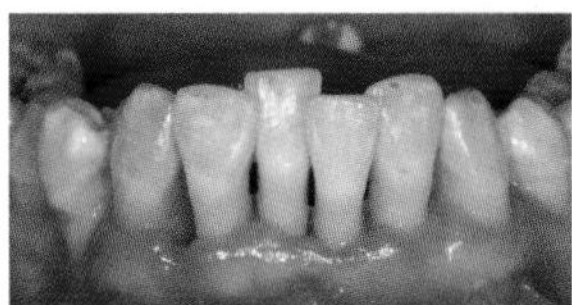

Figure 38.5 Necrotising ulcerative periodontitis-like lesions on the lower incisors in a 15-year-old girl who used cocaine orally. Local application to the gingival tissue causes inflammation, recession, necrosis of the underlying bone and, in due course, recession. Courtesy of Professor I. L. C. Chapple.

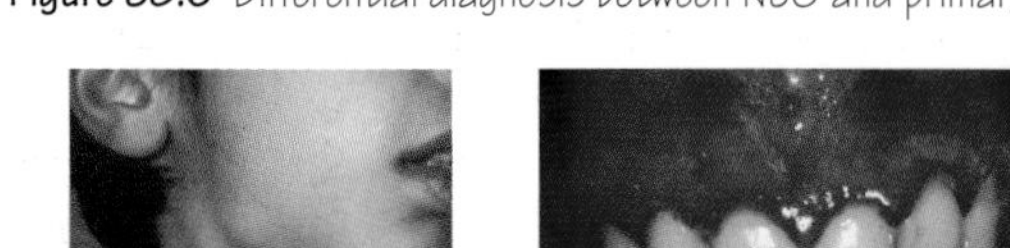
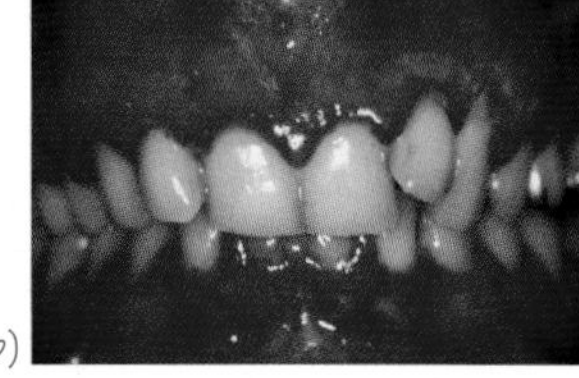

Figure 38.7 (a) Lymphadenopathy in child with primary herpetic gingivostomatitis. (b) Fiery red gingival inflammation and swelling plus herpetic viral vesicles on the margin of the gingiva.

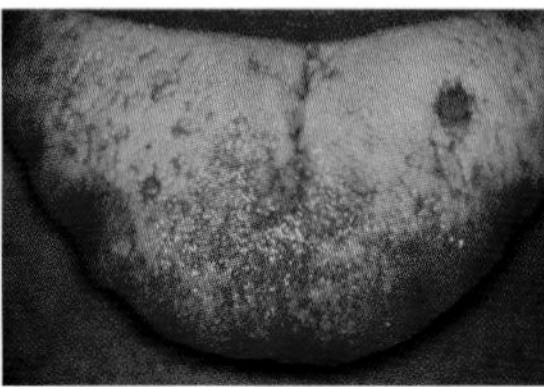

Figure 38.8 Herpetic vesicles on the tongue.

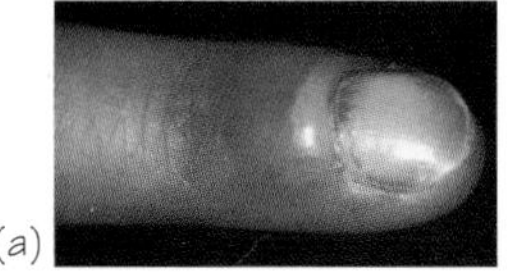
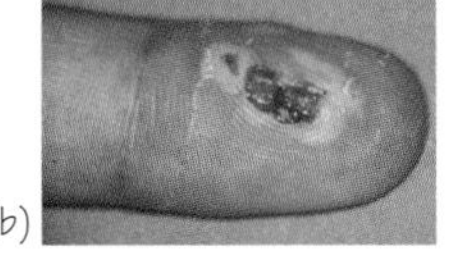

Figure 38.9 (a, b) Herpetic whitlow on a finger due to transmission of herpes simplex virus 1 from the mouth to a finger.

Following the 1999 International Workshop for the Classification of Periodontal Diseases and Conditions, it was recommended that necrotising ulcerative gingivitis (NUG) and necrotising ulcerative periodontitis (NUP) should be collectively called the necrotising periodontal diseases (NPDs). It was acknowledged that they may be different stages of the same infection. Necrotising stomatitis is thought to be an extension of the process below the mucogingival junction.

Necrotising ulcerative gingivitis

NUG has several distinctive features that distinguish it from plaque-induced gingivitis. It is characterised by its rapid (acute) onset, and painful, ulcerated, necrotic gingivae which bleed with little provocation (Fig. 38.1). The necrotic ulcers affect the interdental papillae and have a 'punched out' appearance. They may be covered by a pseudomembranous grey slough, comprising fibrin, necrotic tissue, leukocytes, erythrocytes and bacteria (Fig. 38.2). Patients often present with a characteristic marked halitosis ('foetor ex ore'). Some may also have lymph nodes involvement.

Microbiology

NUG has a specific fusiform/spirochaete bacterial aetiology. Four zones have been identified in the gingival lesion, the latter three of which are unique to NUG:

- Bacterial zone.
- Neutrophil-rich zone.
- Necrotic zone.
- Spirochaetal infiltration zone.

The predominant cultivable flora comprises: *Prevotella intermedia*, *Fusobacteria* spp., *Selenomonas* spp. and *Treponema* spp. Knowledge is limited about the pathogenic mechanisms by which the bacterial flora produce the destructive lesions in NPD. Both spirochaetes and fusiforms can invade the tissues and liberate endotoxins, producing tissue destruction by: (i) direct toxic effects; and (ii) indirect effects from activating and modifying the host responses.

Predisposing factors

Certain factors predispose individuals to NUG:

- Immune suppression including human immunodeficiency virus (HIV) infection.
- Smoking.
- Stress.
- Inadequate sleep.
- Poor diet or malnutrition.
- Heavy alcohol consumption.
- Pre-existing gingivitis, poor oral hygiene and previous history of NUG.

NPD was reported to be relatively common during World War II but nowadays it is unusual to find NPD in industrialised communities – overall prevalence has been reported to be 0.5% or even less. When it does occur, NUG tends to develop in young adults in their early twenties, in whom the prevalence has been reported to be around 3%. However, it can affect other age groups especially in the presence of predisposing factors. NUG is more common in developing countries, and has been reported in children, particularly if they are malnourished or following viral/protozoal infections. Whilst the acute nature of NUG means there is no 'chronic' form, recurrence and progression can be a feature.

NUG may present in HIV-positive individuals who are unaware of their status. If the history suggests this, the patient should be referred to their medical practitioner or specialist for further investigation and counselling.

Management

The painful nature of NUG usually drives patients to seek treatment.

Local measures

- The removal of gross deposits of plaque and calculus, using local analgesia where necessary:
  - an ultrasonic scaler is useful, due to its flushing action;
  - removal of the sloughed material will often reveal ulcerated, bleeding tissue.
- Gentle oral hygiene plus a chlorhexidine digluconate mouthwash (0.2% × 10 ml for 1 minute twice daily) to aid plaque control and help prevent secondary infection.
- Oxidising mouthwash (3% hydrogen peroxide with equal volume of warm water) to target the microbial flora.
- Review after 1–2 days.

Systemic measures

Due to the specific microflora and when there is lymph node involvement, systemic antimicrobials are effective:

- Metronidazole 200 mg (or 250 mg) three times per day for 3 days.

After the acute phase

Appropriate non-surgical periodontal therapy should be undertaken: oral hygiene instruction; smoking cessation advice; thorough scaling and root surface instrumentation; professional medical advice on stress management; dietary advice; and counselling on recreational drug use. Some regeneration of the papillae can occur. Surgical soft tissue recontouring (gingivectomy) may correct the soft tissue craters and deformities. Flap surgery may be needed for deep defects.

If inadequately treated, the acute phase may subside, but recurrences can occur leading to progressive tissue destruction and a shift from NUG to NUP (Fig. 38.3) particularly if the predisposing factors persist or in the presence of immunosuppression.

Necrotising ulcerative periodontitis

NUP is characterised by necrosis of the periodontal ligament and alveolar bone and may be a feature of HIV-infected patients (Fig. 38.4). NUP-type lesions can be seen in patients using oral recreational drugs (Fig. 38.5). Noma (called cancrum oris in Africa) is a fulminating, disfiguring condition that may follow on from NUP and necrotising stomatitis in developing parts of the world.

Necrotising stomatitis

Where the necrotising process extends more than 10 mm beyond the gingival margin, or below the mucogingival junction, this is classified as necrotising stomatitis. Specialist management is needed, involving broad surgical excision of the involved necrotic area and bone (usually maxilla) and extraction of affected teeth with packing of the defect and healing by secondary intention.

Differential diagnosis

NUG can sometimes be mistaken for primary herpetic gingivostomatitis (PHG), although the presentation and management differ due to the herpes simplex virus 1 aetiology of PHG (Figs 38.6–38.9).

Key points

- Necrotising periodontal diseases (NPDs) comprise necrotising ulcerative gingivitis (NUG) and necrotising ulcerative periodontitis (NUP)
- NUG is characterised by:
  - ulcerated, necrotic gingivae and punched out interdental papillae
  - bleeding
  - pain
- Only type of gingivitis for which antibiotics may be indicated
- Differential diagnosis: primary herpetic gingivostomatitis
- NUG predisposing factors include, stress, smoking, poor diet, pre-existing gingivitis, poor oral hygiene and HIV infection
- NUP is thought to be an extension of NUG
- Necrotising stomatitis may be a late stage development of NPD

39 Periodontal abscess and periodontic–endodontic lesions

- Vital pulpal response of affected tooth
- Pain is common symptom, easy to localise it to tooth
- Tooth generally tender to pressure or percussion
- Tooth may be slightly extruded from its socket and feel 'high' on the bite
- Patient may feel wants to bite down or grind tooth
- Swelling usually seen
- Mobility is common feature

- Pre-existing periodontal pocket(s), clinical attachment loss present on the affected tooth
- May be furcation involvement if affected tooth is a molar
- Generally see clinical evidence of periodontal involvement and radiographic evidence of bone loss in the mouth
- May possibly be a radiographic radiolucency in the alveolar bone on lateral border of root of affected tooth

Figure 39.1 Common features of periodontal abscesses.

(a)
- Redness and swelling of gingiva on affected tooth
- Swelling may be diffuse and not well localised yet
- Pus not draining through the pocket or through the swelling yet – no sinus tract
- Pain may be severe, constant, localised to tooth

(b)
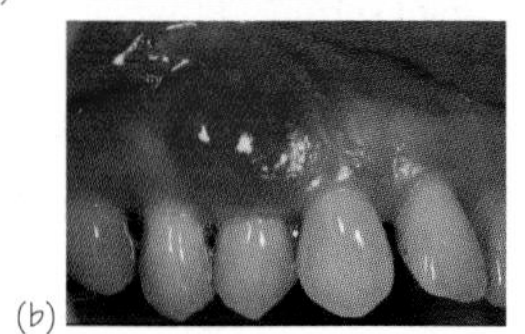

Figure 39.2 (a) Features of early periodontal abscess formation, where pus is not draining. (b) Periodontal abscess with pus not draining through the pocket and not yet ready to point.

(a)
- Gingiva is red and swollen
- Swelling usually becomes more localised
  - ovoid elevation of gingiva on lateral aspect of root
- Pus may be expressed from pocket on gentle pressure (suppuration) anywhere around the tooth
- Pus may point and drain through a fistula
  - sinus tract may form
- Pain and discomfort ease when pus discharges

(b) Periodontal abscess LR5, ready to point

(c) Periapical pathology UL5; Associated bone loss distal LR5; Periodontic–endodontic lesion LL6 distal root

Figure 39.3 (a) Features of a periodontal abscess with pus to drain. (b) Periodontal abscess with pus to drain by LR5. The swelling was fluctuant and pus discharged when the swelling was incised. (c) Panoramic radiograph showing vertical bone loss distal to LR5; note the generalised horizontal and vertical bone loss throughout the mouth. A periodontic–endodontic lesion can be seen on the LL6 distal root and periapical radiolucency on UL5.

(a)
- Occasionally see evidence of associated systemic involvement
- Extraoral swelling on affected side of mouth
- Lymphadenopathy
- Rarely cellulitis
- Malaise
- Raised temperature

(b)
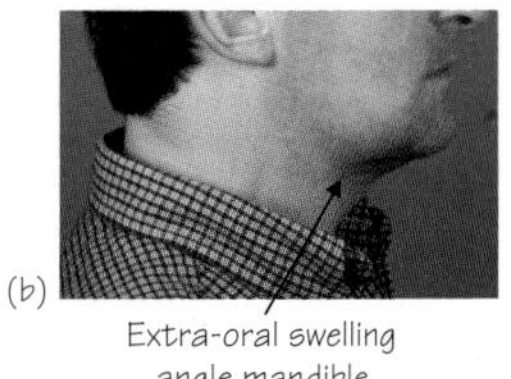

Figure 39.4 (a) Features of a periodontal abscess with systemic involvement. (b) An extra-oral swelling on the lower right angle of the mandible.

(a)
- Localised purulent infection that involves the marginal or interdental papilla
  - Localised, painful and rapidly expanding
  - Acute inflammatory response to foreign agents
  - Red, shiny and smooth
  - Fluctuant within 24–48 hours
  - Points and discharges spontaneously

(b)
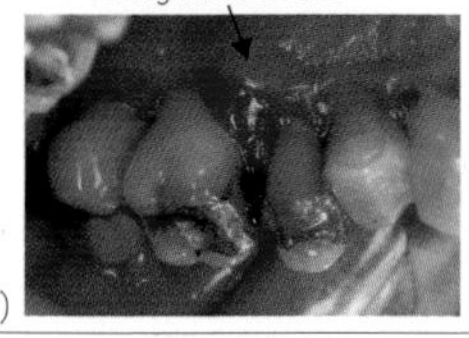

Figure 39.5 (a) Features of a gingival abscess. (b) An abscess on the mesiopalatal marginal gingiva of UR6.

- Localised purulent infection within the tissues surrounding the crown of a partially erupted tooth
  - Mandibular third molar common site
  - Red and swollen gingival flap
  - Infection may spread
  - Possible systemic involvement

Figure 39.6 Features of a pericoronal abscess.

(a)
- Pulpal necrosis e.g. carious pulpal involvement on heavily restored tooth
- Non-vital (confirm with pulp test)
- Periapical tissues involved
  - Periapical radiolucency may become visible on radiograph, but may not be present initially
- Periodontal tissue involvement is *not* a key feature
- Tooth very tender to percussion
- Severe, sharp, intermittent pain, can be difficult to localise

(b) Sinus

(c) Gutta percha inserted through sinus

(d)

(e) Gutta percha through sinus

Figure 39.7 (a) Features of a periapical lesion. (b) The buccal sinus at UR6. (c) A diagnostic gutta percha point inserted into the sinus to track the source of infection. (d) A periapical radiograph showing periapical radiolucency around the apices of a root canal treated at UR6. (e) A gutta percha inserted through the buccal sinus extends into the periapical area, indicating that the source of infection is from an endodontic origin not a periodontic origin.

(a)
Aetiology may be:
- Primary periodontal, secondary endodontic (i.e. necrotic pulp as consequence of periodontal involvement)
  - Often poor prognosis if periodontal involvement involving loss of attachment extends to apex of tooth
- Primary endodontic, secondary periodontal (i.e. periodontium is involved after pulpal necrosis)
  - Often good prognosis if endodontic treatment is carried out followed by periodontal therapy
- However, classification disregards aetiology and the lesion is called a combined periodontic–endodontic lesion

(b)
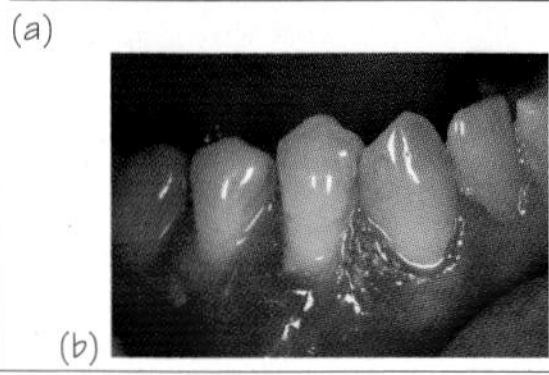

(c)
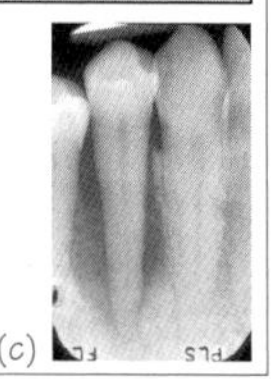

Figure 39.8 (a) Features of a combined periodontic–endodontic lesion. (b) Periodontic–endodontic lesion at LR4 showing a localised but quite large buccal swelling and pus discharging through the pocket. (c) A periapical radiograph showing typical radiographic features of a periodontic–endodontic lesion with vertical bone loss extending to the apex of the tooth and merging with periapical radiolucency due to non-vital pulp.

(a)
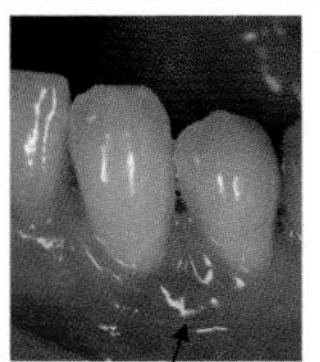
Before endodontic treatment and periodontal therapy

(b)
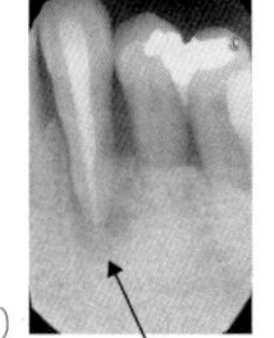
This radiolucency healed over the next few months after endodontic and periodontal treatment

(c)
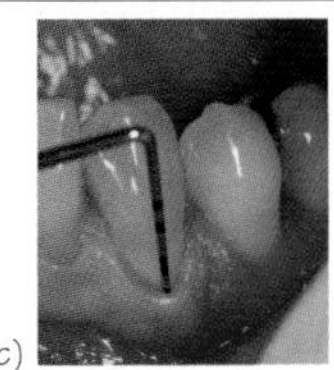
Healing after endodontic treatment and periodontal therapy

Figure 39.9 Before and after successful endodontic and periodontal treatment of a periodontic–endodontic lesion at LL3. (a) A localised, small, buccal swelling at LL3 (a deep but narrow pocket was detected on periodontal probing distobuccally). (b) A periapical radiograph after obturation of the root canal of LL3. The periapical radiolucency reduced over subsequent months, indicating some healing. (c) Healing of the pocket following successful endodontic and periodontal treatment.

Periodontal abscess

A periodontal abscess is a localised purulent infection within the tissues adjacent to the periodontal pocket that can lead to destruction of the periodontal ligament and alveolar bone. It can present as an acute infection that interrupts the scheduled treatment plan and requires emergency management.

Aetiology

There are a number of hypothesised causes.

• *Pocket occlusion*, due to: (i) incomplete removal of calculus; (ii) impaction of food or a foreign body; (iii) bacterial invasion after instrumentation.

Occlusion of the pocket orifice leads to reduced clearance of bacteria and an accumulation of host cells; infection spreads into the supporting tissues and is localised. Tissue damage occurs due to lysosomal enzymes released from neutrophils taking part in host defences.

• *Furcation involvement*: abscesses commonly occur in furcations or in relation to anatomical defects in the furcation area such as enamel pearls.

• *Systemic antibiotic therapy*: in patients with untreated periodontitis, superinfection with opportunistic organisms may occur following systemic antibiotics.

• *Manifestation of systemic disease*: multiple or recurrent abscesses can occur where a patient is immunocompromised and may alert the clinician to an underlying or undiagnosed medical condition (e.g. undiagnosed or poorly controlled diabetes, chronic lymphocytic leukaemia).

Microbiology

Streptococcus viridans is the most commonly isolated aerobic microorganism from abscesses, but bacteria are mainly Gram-negative anaerobes. High frequencies have been reported in the literature of *Porphyromonas gingivalis*, *Prevotella intermedia*, *Tannerella forsythia*, *Peptostreptococcus micros*, *Fusobacterium nucleatum*, *Aggregatibacter actinomycetemcomitans*, *Campylobacter rectus*, *Capnocytophaga* spp. and spirochaetes. The bacterial profile resembles that reported in deep periodontal pockets.

Features

Although there are some common features (Fig. 39.1), features of a periodontal abscess may vary according to the stage of development:

• Early (Fig. 39.2).
• Pus ready to drain or draining (Fig. 39.3).
• Systemic involvement (Fig. 39.4).

Differential diagnosis

It is important to consider the differential diagnosis, which includes:

• Gingival abscess (Fig. 39.5).
• Pericoronal abscess (pericoronitis) (Fig. 39.6).
• Periapical periodontitis (Figs 39.3c, 39.7).
• Periodontic–endodontic lesion (Figs 39.3c, 39.8, 39.9).
• Other pathology, e.g. cyst, tumour or osteomyelitis.

Confirmation of the diagnosis is reached after a thorough history and examination, consideration of the clinical and radiographic features and the results of any special tests.

Management

Acute phase

Treatment should be directed at relief of pain and controlling the acute infection to avoid destruction of vital periodontal tissues.

1 *Early stage of abscess formation, pus not draining*:

(i) Relieve occlusion: grind opposing tooth.

(ii) Advise hot salt mouthwashes to encourage drainage: half a teaspoon of salt in a cup of hot water; rinse for 1 minute and repeat until the cup is empty; repeat several times daily for 2–3 days or as needed.

(iii) Advise pain killers, e.g. ibuprofen (200 mg × 2 every 4–6 hours, maximum of six per 24 hours) or paracetomol (500 mg × 2 every 4–6 hours, maximum eight per 24 hours).

(iv) If it is not possible to achieve drainage, severe pain is present and there is a risk of spread of infection, systemic antibiotics may be prescribed, for example:

- metronidazole 200 mg three times per day for 5–7 days; *or*
- penicillin V 250 mg four times per day for 5–7 days; *or*
- tetracycline 250 mg four times per day for 10–14 days; *or*
- doxycycline 200 mg loading dose, then 100 mg daily for 5–7 days.

(v) Review after a few days. Consider prognosis, treatment options.

2 *Pus draining*:

(i) Follow steps as in 1(i),(ii),(iii),(v), plus achieve drainage through:

- local gentle debridement through pocket, being cautious to avoid further damage to vital periodontal ligament cells;
- incision and drainage through the swelling.

Although there is no consensus, it is *not* generally appropriate to prescribe antibiotics if drainage has been achieved and there is no evidence of systemic involvement or spread of infection.

3 *Systemic involvement*:

(i) Follow steps as in 1(i),(ii),(iii),(iv), plus incision and drainage if appropriate.

(ii) Systemic antibiotics – ideally determine antibiotic sensitivity from the culture of a pus sample.

(iii) Prescribe antibiotics as above unless there is very severe infection in which case a powerful antibiotic combination is metronidazole (200 mg) and amoxicillin (250 mg) three times a day for 5–7 days.

(iv) If there is no resolution, an appropriate antibiotic can be prescribed when the results of antibiotic sensitivity are known.

(v) Review.

After the acute phase, the prognosis of the tooth should be reviewed and a decision taken about whether non-surgical or surgical periodontal therapy is needed.

Periodontic–endodontic lesions

There are many channels of communication between periodontal and pulpal tissues via lateral and accessory canals or the apical foramina. The combined periodontic–endodontic lesion is a lesion where there is any coalescence of periodontic or endodontic lesions, irrespective of the primary origin of the lesion (Fig. 39.8).

Each case must be evaluated on its own merits and a treatment plan drawn up. Endodontic treatment is carried out first. Success depends on the ability to eliminate the bacteria in the root canal and gain a good coronal seal (Fig. 39.9). The outcome of periodontal therapy depends on the severity, extent and complexity of the periodontal involvement and can often influence the overall prognosis of the tooth.

Key points

• Periodontal abscess can occur as an acute infection requiring emergency management
• A thorough history and examination are needed to reach the diagnosis after consideration of differential diagnosis
• Management depends on the stage of development
• The outcome of a periodontic–endodontic lesion depends on its primary aetiology

40 Periodontal diseases in children and adolescents

- Gingival diseases
- Chronic periodontitis
- Aggressive periodontitis
- Periodontitis as manifestation of systemic disease
- Necrotising periodontal diseases
- Abscesses of periodontium
- Periodontitis associated with endodontic lesions
- Development of acquired deformities and conditions

Figure 40.1 Classification of periodontal diseases and conditions for children and adolescents. From Armitage (1999).

- Simplified BPE
  - Index teeth (WHO partial recording for adolescents) UR6, UR1, UL6 LR6, LL1, LL6
- BPE codes 0, 1, 2 ages 7–11 years (mixed dentition stage)
- Full range BPE codes 0, 1, 2, 3, 4,* ages 12+ years (permanent teeth erupted)

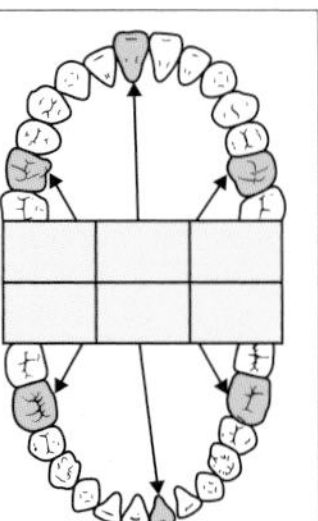

Figure 40.2 Simplified Basic Periodontal Examination (BPE) screening in children and adolescents. WHO, World Health Organisation. From Ainamo *et al.* (1984); see also Clerehugh (2008).

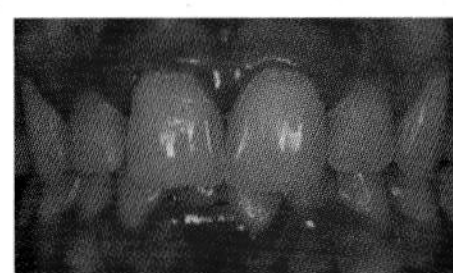

Figure 40.3 Plaque-induced gingivitis in a 16-year-old girl.

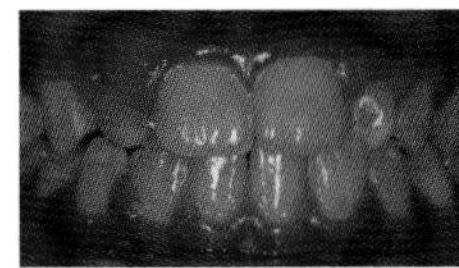

Figure 40.4 Plaque-induced gingivitis in a 15-year-old Asian girl.

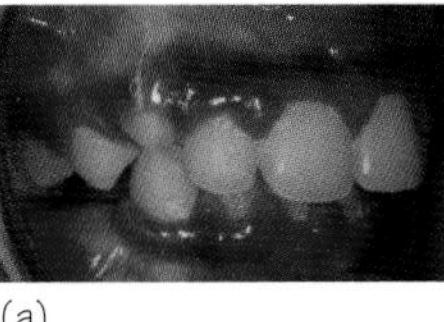

(a)

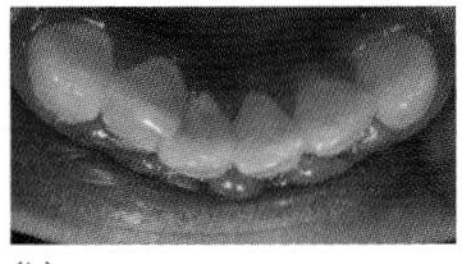

(b)

Figure 40.5 (a) Plaque-induced gingivitis and supragingival calculus on the labial of the lower incisors in a 10-year-old Asian girl. (b) Lingual lower anteriors with supragingival calculus.

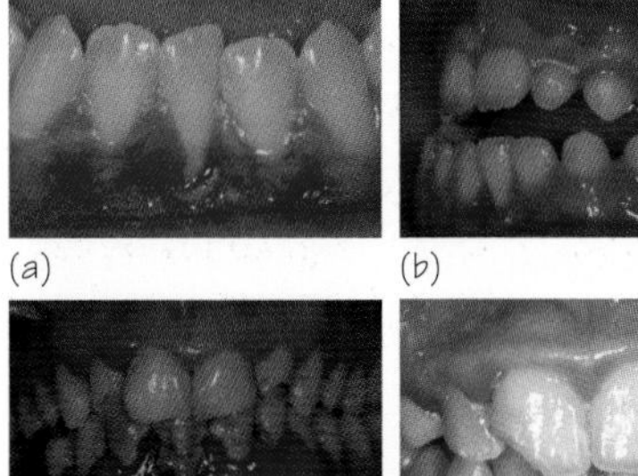

(a) (b) (c) (d)

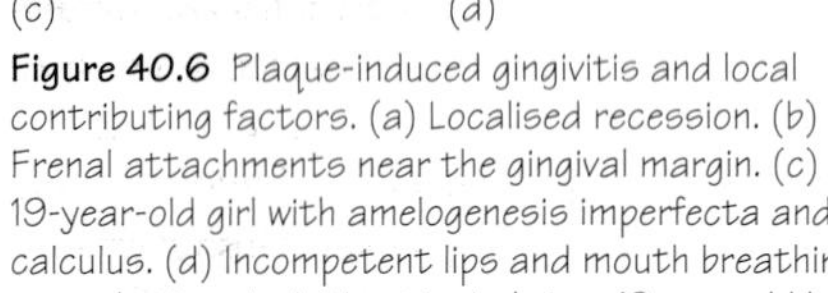

Figure 40.6 Plaque-induced gingivitis and local contributing factors. (a) Localised recession. (b) Frenal attachments near the gingival margin. (c) A 19-year-old girl with amelogenesis imperfecta and calculus. (d) Incompetent lips and mouth breathing exacerbating gingivitis anteriorly in a 12-year-old boy.

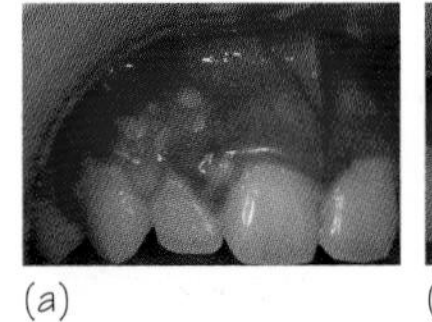

(a) (b)

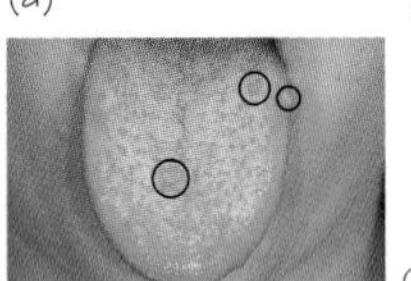

(c)

Figure 40.7 Non-plaque-induced gingival condition: primary herpetic gingivostomatitis. Herpes simplex virus 1 vesicles on the gingiva (a, b) and tongue (c). Courtesy of Dr S. Kindelan.

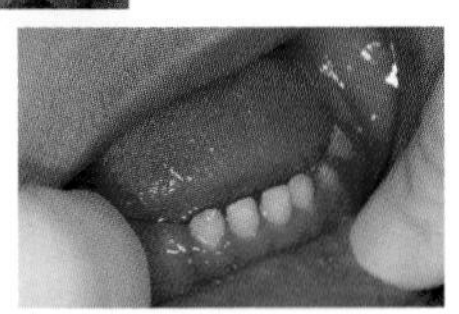

Figure 40.8 Non-plaque-induced gingival condition: neutropenia in a young child with severe gingival inflammation and mobile primary incisors. Courtesy of Dr S. Kindelan.

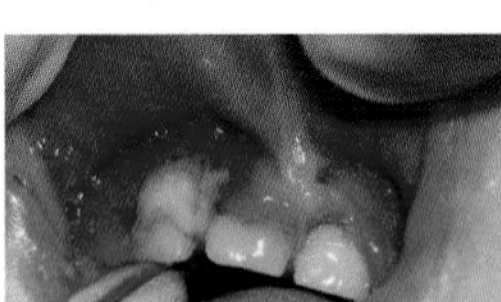

Figure 40.9 Non-plaque-induced gingival condition: histoplasmosis in a young, severely immunocompromised child with bone marrow rejection. There is a fungal infection, deep mycoses and histoplasma capsulatum. Courtesy of Professor I. L. C. Chapple.

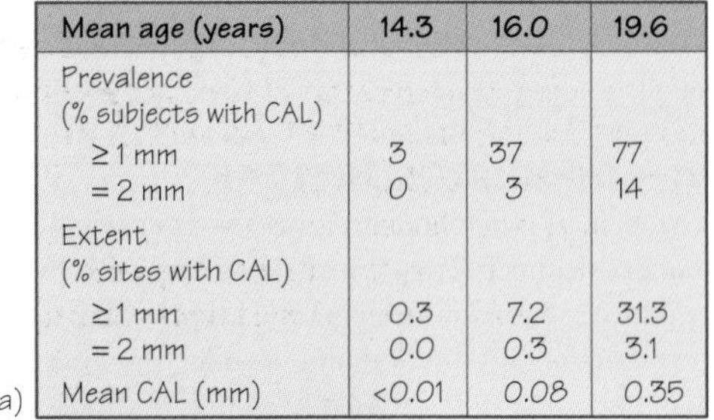

(a)

Mean age (years)	14.3	16.0	19.6
Prevalence (% subjects with CAL)			
≥1 mm	3	37	77
= 2 mm	0	3	14
Extent (% sites with CAL)			
≥1 mm	0.3	7.2	31.3
= 2 mm	0.0	0.3	3.1
Mean CAL (mm)	<0.01	0.08	0.35

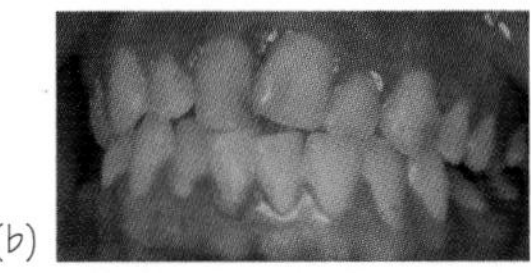

(b)

Figure 40.10 (a) The results of a 5-year study of clinical attachment loss in 14–19-year-old adolescents in Rochdale, UK. (b) Incipient chronic periodontitis in a 19-year-old. From Clerehugh *et al.* (1990).

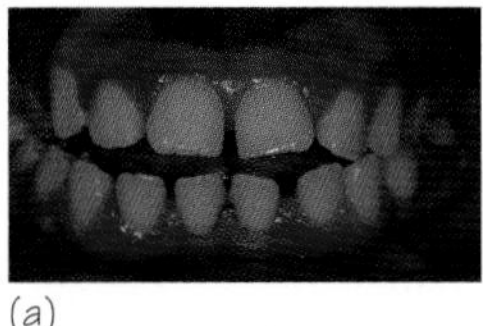

(a)

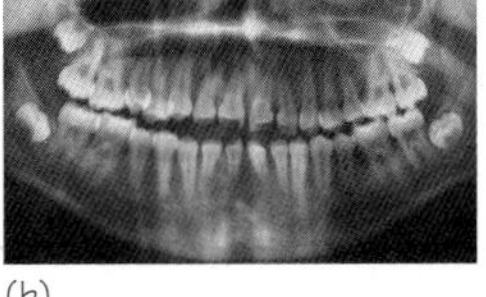

(b)

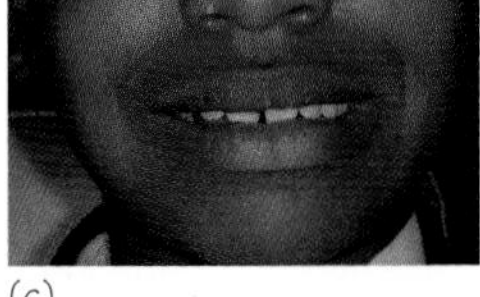

(c)

Figure 40.11 (a–c) Localised aggressive periodontitis in a 12-year-old black girl of African origin.

Diagnosis of aggressive periodontitis
Incipient chronic periodontitis not responding to treatment
Systemic medical condition associated with periodontal destruction
Medical history that significantly affects periodontal treatment or requiring multidisciplinary care
Genetic conditions predisposing to periodontal destruction
Root morphology adversely affecting prognosis
Non-plaque-induced conditions requiring complex or specialist care
Cases requiring diagnosis/management of rare/complex clinical pathology
Drug-induced gingival overgrowth
Cases requiring evaluation for periodontal surgery

Figure 40.13 When to consider referral to a specialist in young age groups.

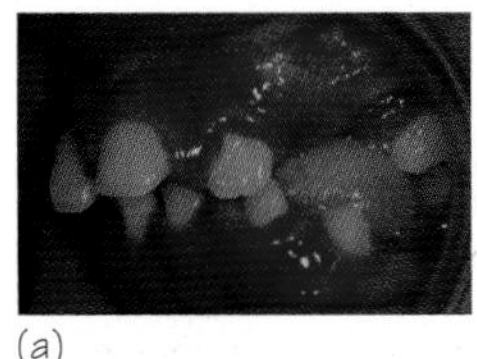

(a)

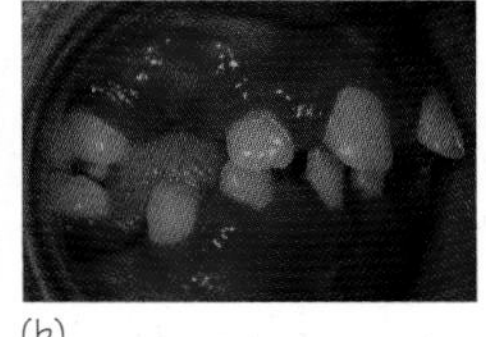

(b)

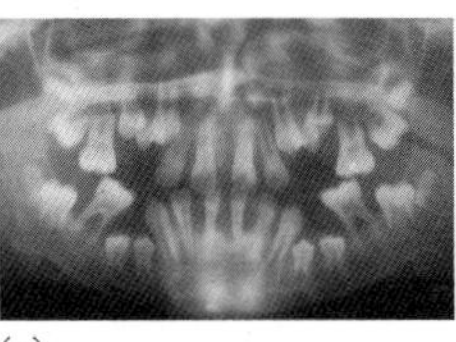

(c)

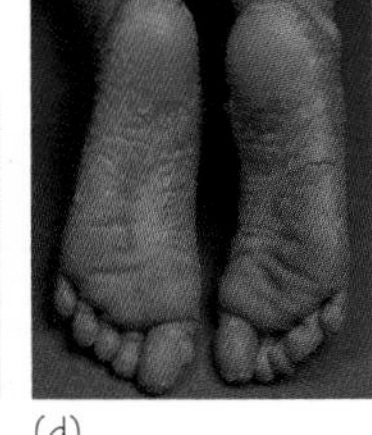

(d)

Figure 40.12 Papillon–Lefèvre syndrome in a 9-year-old boy with (a, b) acutely inflamed gingiva, and (c) severe periodontal destruction and bone loss of the permanent dentition, having lost all the primary dentition already. (d) Hyperkeratosis on the soles of the feet – the hands, knees and elbows are also affected.

Many different periodontal problems manifest in children and adolescents (Clerehugh *et al.*, 2004) and all of the categories of periodontal diseases and conditions that apply to adults from the 1999 International Workshop for the Classification of Periodontal Diseases and Conditions also apply to the younger age groups (Fig. 40.1). Periodontal screening is an important prerequisite in the dental examination of the child (Clerehugh, 2008) (Fig. 40.2; Chapter 17).

Gingivitis

Data from the 2003 UK Dental Survey (Pendry *et al.*, 2004; White *et al.*, 2006) support previous global findings that plaque-induced gingivitis is very common in the younger age groups (Figs 40.3, 40.4, 40.5). This survey was based on a representative sample of children aged 5, 8, 12 and 15 years of age attending government-maintained and independent primary and secondary schools in the UK (Table 40.1).

Table 40.1 Gingival condition in 5–15-year-olds in the 2003 United Kingdom Dental Health Survey (n = 10 381, with 1993 data in parentheses).

Age years	% with visible gingival inflammation		% with gingival bleeding on any index teeth		% with plaque		% with calculus	
	2003	(1993)	2003	(1993)	2003	(1993)	2003	(1993)
5	32	(26)	–	–	50	(45)	6	(5)
8	63	(58)	–	–	76	(70)	23	(16)
12	65	(60)	–	–	73	(68)	30	(20)
15	52	(52)	43	(45)	63	(57)	39	(32)

Local contributing factors

Various local contributing factors can influence the prevalence, severity and extent of plaque-induced gingivitis in the young (Fig. 40.6). Plaque-induced gingivitis can usually be treated readily in the primary dental care setting (Chapters 14, 30).

Non-plaque-induced gingival lesions

Non-plaque-induced gingival lesions (Figs 40.7–40.9) may be less common in the younger age groups and more difficult to diagnose and treat, in which case referral is indicated (Chapter 31).

Periodontitis

Incipient chronic periodontitis

Although study methodology has varied, data from the UK, USA and other countries support the conclusion that chronic periodontitis can begin to develop and progress in adolescents (Chapter 34). A 5-year longitudinal study in the UK (Clerehugh *et al.*, 1990) showed that 3% of 167 14-year-old adolescents had incipient clinical attachment loss (CAL) of 1 mm or more on the mesiobuccal surface of at least one first molar, premolar or central incisor tooth, rising to a prevalence of 37% at age 16 years and 77% at age 19 years (Fig. 40.10).

A simplified Basic Periodontal Examination (BPE) code of 3 is consistent with true shallow pockets of 4 or 5 mm and would be expected in an individual with incipient chronic periodontitis, especially on the proximal surfaces of first molars and incisors. Confirmation of true pockets is by CAL measures and, where appropriate, alveolar bone loss especially on serial bitewing radiographs. The presence of subgingival calculus has been found to be associated with subsequent development of CAL in adolescents (Clerehugh *et al.*, 1990). Periodontal pathogens typical of adults are also found in the subgingival plaque in adolescents (Clerehugh *et al.*, 1997): *Porphyromonas gingivalis*, *Prevotella intermedia* and *Aggregatibacter actinomycetemcomitans*. The presence of *Tannerella forsythia* (formerly *forsythensis*) has been associated with subsequent CAL in a 3-year longitudinal study in adolescents (Hamlet *et al.*, 2004).

Localised aggressive periodontitis

A BPE code of 4 should flag the possibility of localised aggressive periodontitis (Chapter 35). The localised form affects incisors and first molars and can present around puberty. The disease has a multifactorial nature, including a genetic element. Usually less than 1% of the population is affected, but an increased prevalence occurs in African/black ethnic groups (Fig. 40.11). The JP2 clone of *A. actinomycetemcomitans* may be important in the initiation of CAL in adolescents. Early detection and treatment, often with adjunctive systemic antibiotics, improves prognosis.

Periodontitis as manifestation of systemic disease

In youngsters, a small number may present with periodontitis as a manifestation of haematological disorders (acquired neutropenia, leukaemia) or genetic disorders including: i) Down syndrome (characterised by: trisomy chromosome 21; destructive periodontitis; primary and permanent dentitions affected; tendency for shortened roots; early tooth loss possible; neutrophil defects; abnormal T-cell function; abnormal collagen synthesis); ii) Papillon-Lefèvre syndrome (Fig. 40.12) (features include: loss of function mutations in Cathepsin C gene; palmar-plantar hyperkeratosis; periodontitis occurs pre-pubertally; autosomal recessive gene; treatment complex; poor success rates); iii) Chediak-Higashi syndrome (rare autosomal recessive condition; neutrophil and monocyte function affected; severe inflammation and periodontal destruction); iv) Ehlers-Danlos syndrome (types IV & VIII, features: autosomal dominant disorder; generalised aggressive periodontitis; defective collagen synthesis; skin hyperextensibility, joint mobility; excessive bruising due to fragile blood vessels); v) Hypophosphatasia (childhood form, features include: defect in alkaline phosphatase; premature loss of primary teeth due to cementum hypoplasia/aplasia). Early referral is indicated.

Other classifications

Various other periodontal conditions may affect youngsters and the key features of their diagnosis and management are covered in the following chapters of the book and also elsewhere (Clerehugh *et al.*, 2004):

- Necrotising periodontal diseases: Chapter 38.
- Abscesses of the periodontium: Chapter 39.
- Periodontitis associated with endodontic lesions: Chapter 39.
- Development of acquired deformities and conditions: Chapters 15, 32, 33.

Treat or refer the child?

This depends on the practitioner's experience, the patient and the complexity of the case (Fig. 40.13).

Key points

- Many periodontal diseases can occur in children/adolescents within the 1999 International Classification
- Periodontal screening using index teeth is important
- Plaque-induced gingivitis is common and local contributing factors may apply
- Non-plaque-induced gingival conditions are less common
- Incipient chronic periodontitis may develop in adolescence
- Vigilance for aggressive periodontitis is essential
- The decision to treat or refer depends on the practitioner and patient-centred factors and the complexity of the case

41 Periodontal management of the older adult

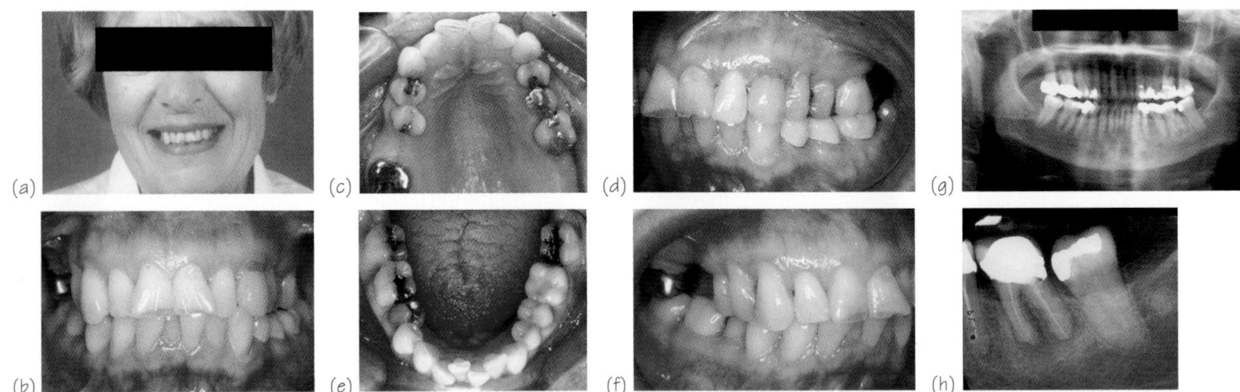

Figure 41.1 (a-f) A 'biologically young' patient aged 73 years, with a restored mouth, minimum gingival or periodontal problems, some recession and tooth wear (attrition, abrasion), especially in the upper incisors. (g) Orthopantomogram radiograph age 68 years prior to extraction of UR6 an UL7. Root caries and apical pathology LL6 prior to root filling. (h) Periapical radiograph showing the bone level and apical pathology on root-filled LL6. Courtesy of Dr M. Kellett.

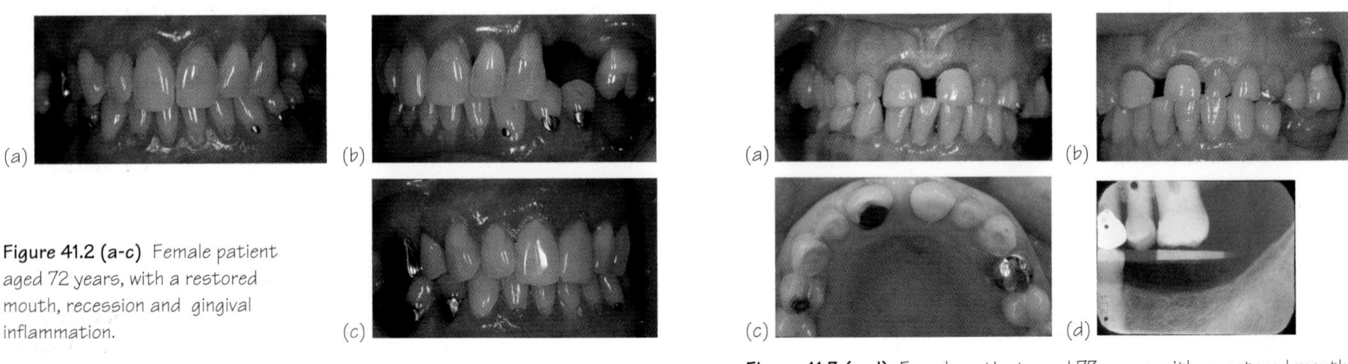

Figure 41.2 (a-c) Female patient aged 72 years, with a restored mouth, recession and gingival inflammation.

Figure 41.3 (a-d) Female patient aged 73 years, with a restored mouth, a history of chronic periodontitis, calculus on the lower anteriors, generalised slight recession and erosion due to a lemon-sucking habit.

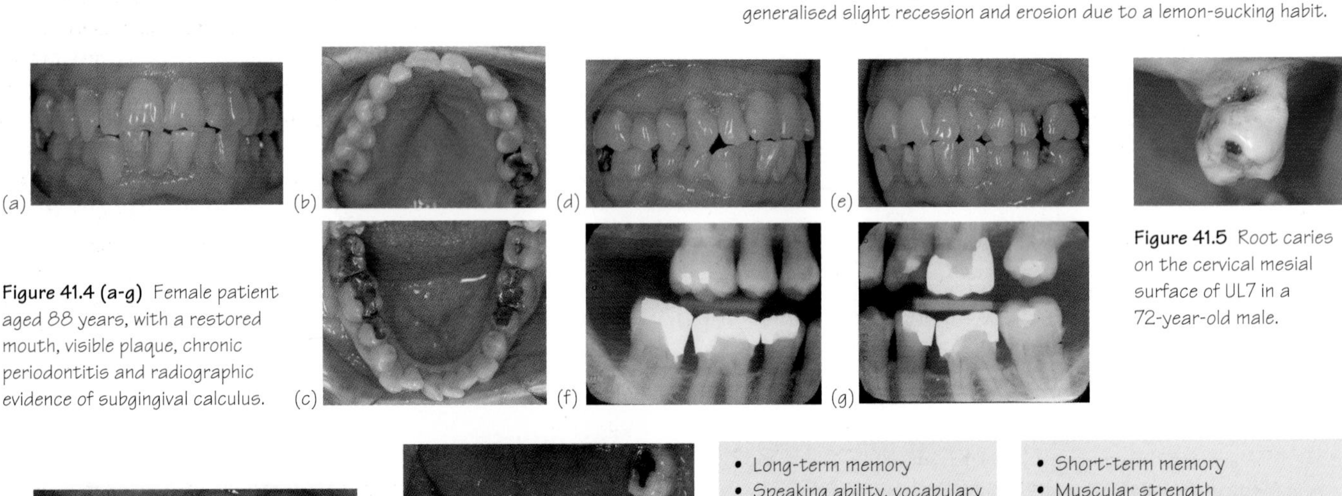

Figure 41.4 (a-g) Female patient aged 88 years, with a restored mouth, visible plaque, chronic periodontitis and radiographic evidence of subgingival calculus.

Figure 41.5 Root caries on the cervical mesial surface of UL7 in a 72-year-old male.

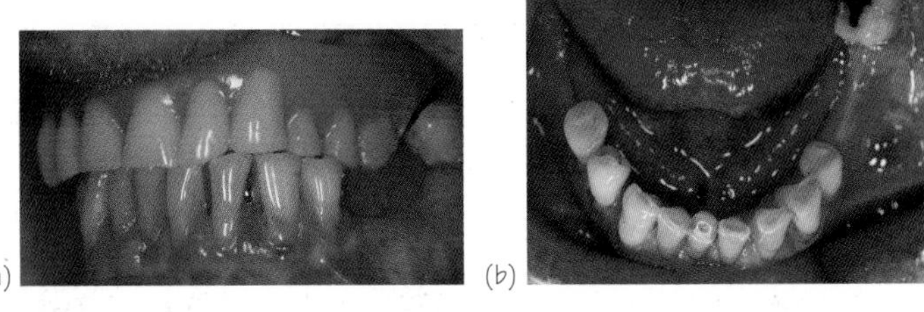

Figure 41.6 (a, b) Male patient aged 90 years, with an upper complete denture, lower teeth with occlusal wear, some marginal gingival inflammation, and root caries on the LL3 buccal cervical margin.

- Long-term memory
- Speaking ability, vocabulary
- Experience
- Positive attitude
- Reliability
- Stability
- Simple learning skills
- Ability to discriminate

Figure 41.7 Attributes that may be unaffected or enhanced in older adults.

- Short-term memory
- Muscular strength
- Coordination
- Visual, auditory, taste perception
- Adaptability
- Complex learning skills
- Immune status, host resistance, medical well being

Figure 41.8 Attributes that may be reduced in older adults.

The definition of the 'older adult' varies in different countries and cultures. In developed, westernised communities it is commonly taken as the age of retirement from work. Currently in the UK, up until 2010, eligibility for a state pension is at age 65 years for men and 60 years for women, but between 2010 and 2020 this is changing to 65 years for women too. From 2024 to 2046, it is planned that the age of eligibility will rise to age 68 years for men and women, reflecting the longer life expectancy and work potential of the population. However, the biological age of the patient can vary from their actual chronological age. Patients well into their 80's and beyond may be spritely, active and young at heart in spite of their advancing years.

Epidemiology of periodontal diseases

Some age changes occur in the epithelium, periodontal ligament and connective tissues, and the prevalence of periodontal diseases increases with age. Accordingly, it has been questioned whether:

- The worsening periodontal condition is an inevitable consequence of getting older (i.e. age related).

Or:

- The worsening periodontal condition is associated with other factors or characteristics in older adults (i.e. age associated).

A review of 14 cross-sectional and eight longitudinal studies of older adults from 1971 to 1995 at the 1996 World Workshop in Periodontics supported the view that periodontal disease progression is age associated (Beck, 1996).

Risk factors for progression included: smoking; oral hygiene habits (irregular flossing); length of time since last dental visit (more than 3 years); presence of periodontal pathogens (including *Porphyromonas gingivalis* and *Prevotella intermedia*); educational status; financial status; and health (depression).

A systematic review of 47 studies from 1965 to 2004 reported at the Fifth European Workshop on Periodontology in 2005 concluded that socioeconomic variables associated with periodontal diseases were of less importance than smoking, but in non-smokers, educational status could have an impact on periodontal diseases (Klinge & Norlund, 2005). Literacy issues have also been flagged (Jones & Wehler, 2005). The Elders' Oral Health summit in Boston, USA in 2004 encompassed the fact that the elderly are an ever increasing proportion of Americans and, by 2050, approximately one in five will be age 65 years or older (Dolan *et al.*, 2005; Jones & Wehler, 2005). Although the oral health of older adults has improved in recent decades, access to dental care will be an ongoing concern for the future.

The UK Adult Dental Health Survey in 1998 (Kelly *et al.*, 2000) showed that:

- 30% of 65–74-year-olds and 10% of those aged 75 years or older had 21 or more of their own teeth.
- 42% of those aged 75 years or older still had some of their own teeth.

Because of increased tooth retention, maintaining periodontal health is an increasing issue for people aged 65 years or older as data show:

- 85% had loss of attachment of 4 mm or more.
- 31% of people aged 65 years or older had clinical attachment loss of 6 mm or more.
- 67% had shallow pockets of 4 mm or more.
- 23% of teeth had shallow pockets of 4 mm or more.

Periodontal problems in older adults

Adults who have retained their teeth into old age must have maintained a reasonably favourable balance between host defences, bacterial challenge and an ecologically conducive oral environment. Therefore, they can be assumed to have a degree of resistance to periodontal diseases, unless some new periodontal risk factor or upset in the balance occurs.

Periodontal problems likely to be seen in the older adult (Figs 41.1–41.6) include:

- Plaque-induced gingivitis.
- Chronic periodontitis.
- Loss of attachment and gingival recession.
- Dentine hypersensitivity.
- Root caries.

Due to the cumulative effects of periodontal diseases, both loss of attachment and recession are common in older patients and therefore the root surfaces are more susceptible to root caries. This is particularly so if the elderly adult lives alone and has frequent sucrose-containing snacks. Some lesions are very visible, whilst others are subgingival and located on approximal surfaces and are therefore difficult to diagnose. Tooth wear is also common.

By definition, older adults do not suffer from the classic forms of aggressive periodontitis. They may experience xerostomia due to the polypharmacy of drugs that many elderly people take. Physical disability (e.g. arthritis) often compromises tooth cleaning ability, whilst depression can make patients less inclined to engage in oral hygiene routines; infirmity can jeopardise attendance; and mental disability (e.g. Alzheimer's disease) can create confusion over advice given. Medical disorders including cardiovascular disease, stroke, diabetes, respiratory ailments and digestive problems become increasingly common with advancing years. A thorough history (particularly the medical and social history) and examination are important.

Periodontal management

Periodontal management follows the principles of initial, corrective and supportive therapy. It should use the skills of the dental surgeon, hygienist/therapist and oral health educator in the dental team, taking account of any special needs of the patient and that certain attributes may be enhanced or diminished with age (Figs 41.7, 41.8). Powered toothbrushes with their chunky handles provide a useful oral hygiene tool.

There are no conclusive data that age *per se* affects plaque build up, gingival inflammation, reduction in inflammation following treatment or response to surgical therapy. The treatment philosophy influences the treatment provided. Papapanou *et al.* (1990) and Wennstrom *et al.* (1990) proposed two approaches to treatment outcomes. To reach age 75 with one third of the root length, few patients would need treatment. To remove all signs of periodontal disease, 70% would need treatment for bleeding on probing, 28% for shallow pockets and less than 5% for deep pockets with bleeding on probing. Ultimately, the outcome of periodontal therapy needs to be realistic and agreed with the patient, and the patient should have similar expectations and choices as younger patients unless there are medical, physical or other risk factors or barriers.

Key points

- Biological age can vary from chronological age
- Periodontal diseases are age associated, not age related
- A favourable balance may exist
- Risk factors include tobacco smoking and education
- Clinical attachment loss and recession are common
- Medical history and polypharmacy will influence management
- Treatment goals need to be realistic and agreed with the patient

42 Team working in dental care

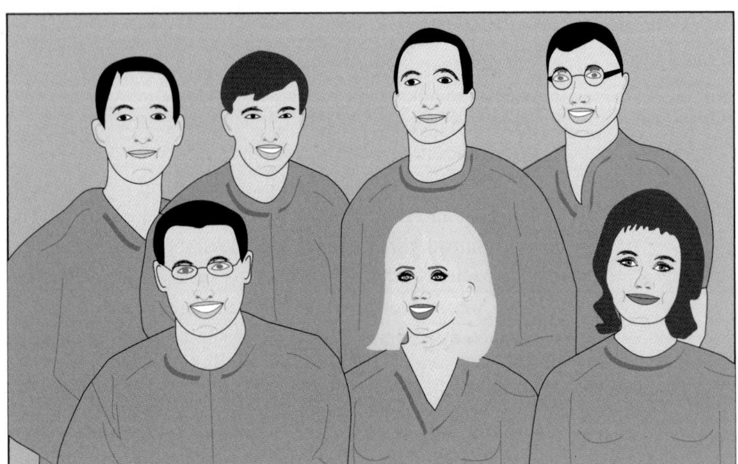

Individuals in the dental team will vary in different settings but will include many of the following:
- Dental nurse
- Oral health educator
- Dental hygienist or hygiene-therapist
- Dental technician
- Receptionist
- Practice manager
- General dental practitioner
- Specialist periodontist
- Medical practitioner and specialists
- Other dental specialists.

Figure 42.1 The dental team.

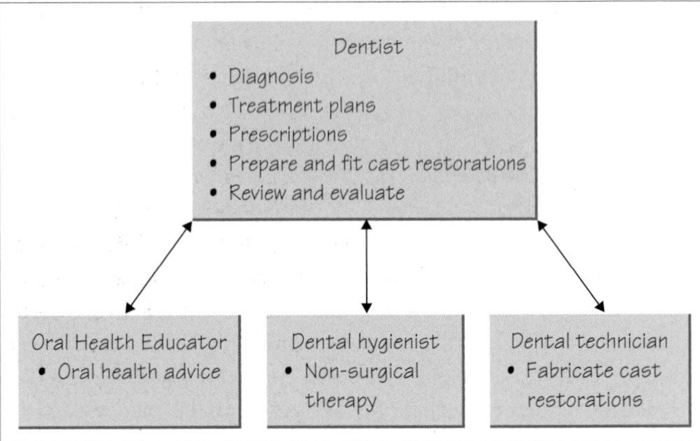

Figure 42.2 Example of working together in the dental team.

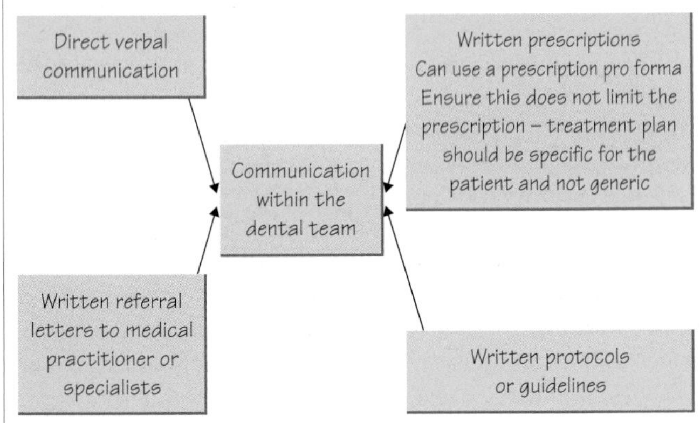

Figure 42.3 Communication within the dental team.

Periodontal therapy offers an excellent opportunity for the dental team to deliver patient care (Fig. 42.1). All members of the team need to be clear about their roles within the team and good communication is required so that health messages and practice policies are consistent (Figs. 42.2, 42.3). Additional training, duties that can be undertaken, and the registration of qualifications continue to change with time and differ across the world. Readers are referred to the websites of the appropriate country or state governing dental bodies for up-to-date information.

Team roles

Dentist

The dentist is the team leader and has the following responsibilities:
- The coordination and responsibility for the overall care of the patient and work of the team.
- Informing the patient of the diagnosis and prognosis.
- Discussing the options available to the patient.
- Drawing up a treatment plan.
- Identifying other members of the team who will play a part.
- Writing prescriptions for the oral health educator, dental hygienist, dental therapist and dental technician.
- Indicating the recall schedule.
- Assessing the response to treatment.
- Carrying out further treatment planning including:
  - developing an appropriate supportive regime;
  - determining if specialist input is required.

The dentist is in the best position to make clear to the team the sequence of appointments required and when the patient should be reviewed following periodontal treatment. Indicating the number of appointments required and the recall interval may be useful when delegating clinical work to other team members. The dentist will undertake extractions, removal of plaque retention factors and fixed and removable prosthodontics.

Professions complementary to dentistry

The development of professions complementary to dentistry (PCDs) has enabled periodontal care to be delivered efficiently across the dental team.

Dental hygienist

The dental hygienist:

• Provides oral health education.

• Can record the indices needed to plan treatment and monitor treatment response.

• Undertakes non-surgical periodontal treatment under local analgesia as prescribed by the dentist.

In the UK the hygienist can, with additional training, also take impressions, replace dislodged crowns with temporary cement and treat patients under conscious sedation.

Dental therapist

The dental therapist:

• Can take dental radiographs.

• Places direct restorations under local infiltration analgesia and fissure sealants.

• Extracts deciduous teeth under local infiltration analgesia.

A combined hygiene therapy course has now replaced separate hygiene and therapy courses in the UK. With further training a therapist can also undertake pulp treatment, place preformed crowns on deciduous teeth and do emergency temporary replacement of crowns and restorations. The exact remit of this PCD is likely to continue to develop and vary in different countries.

Dental nurse:

The dental nurse:

• Provides chairside assistance to the dentist.

• Is a bridge between the waiting area and dental surgery.

• Will assist in managing dental anxiety.

With additional training the nurse can provide oral health education as an oral health educator. Further post-certification courses are available in the UK.

Dental technician

The dental technician may be involved in care of the periodontal patient by:

• The production of study models.

• The fabrication of cast restorations, dentures or restorations for implants.

Specialist periodontist

The specialist periodontist:

• Accepts referrals of appropriate patients and carries out treatment planning (Chapter 43).

• Undertakes specialist forms of treatment such as periodontal surgery.

Receptionist

The receptionist:

• Is the first point of contact for the patient and is the public face of the practice.

• Provides administrative support and manages patient records.

The patient will begin to judge a practice on the telephone or face-to-face contact experienced when making an appointment and sitting in the waiting room. Ensuring that records are complete and available is essential to support the clinicians; for instance steps to minimise radiation exposure are redundant if a patient's radiographs are misfiled.

Communication within the dental team

Face-to-face communication between team members is valuable, though not always possible. In many countries PCDs also require a valid written prescription from the dentist before they can legally undertake treatment (Fig. 42.3).

Patients respond best to reinforcement of a consistent message such as oral hygiene advice. An effective way to achieve this is if all members of the dental team are engaged in the process. Everyone needs to know what the message is as it can be undermined if team members contradict each other. Regular practice meetings can keep everyone informed and allow different opinions to be discussed.

The dentist can facilitate the relationship between the PCDs and patients by explaining to the patient their role in the overall management. Patients may be unaware of the expanding role of PCDs and be unclear why the dentist is not doing all the treatment. Making available an overview of the planned treatment can also be valuable to other team members so that they can see how the treatment that they will provide fits into the holistic care for the patient.

Key points

• The dentist is the dental team leader

• Each member of the team has a valuable role in the team

• Clear communication is required for effective team working

• Communication within a team ensures that everyone feels that their contribution is valued and their views are heard

43 The decision to treat or refer periodontal patients

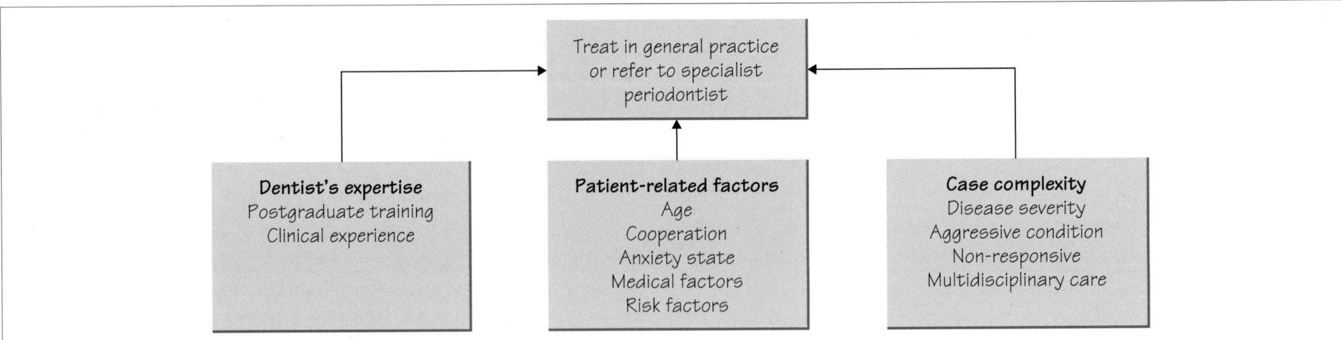

Figure 43.1 Making the decision to treat or refer.

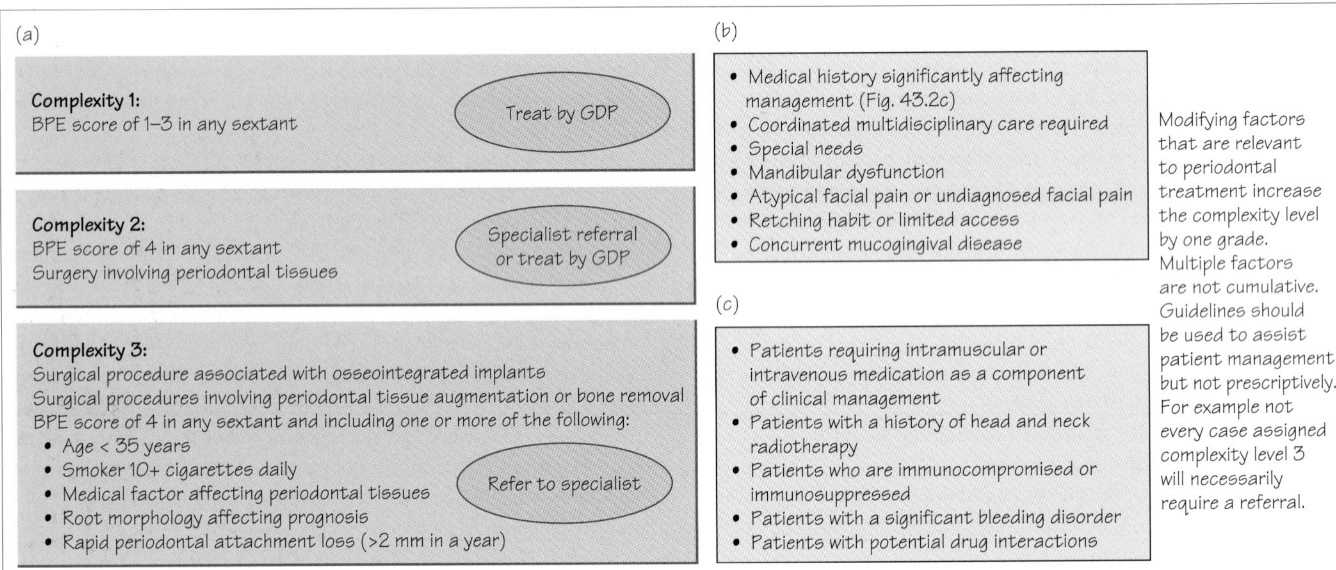

Figure 43.2 (a) Guidelines for referral based on complexity scores. (b) Modifying factors relevant to periodontal treatment for application to complexity scores. (c) Medical history that significantly affects clinical management. BPE, Basic Periodontal Examination; GDP, general dental practitioner.

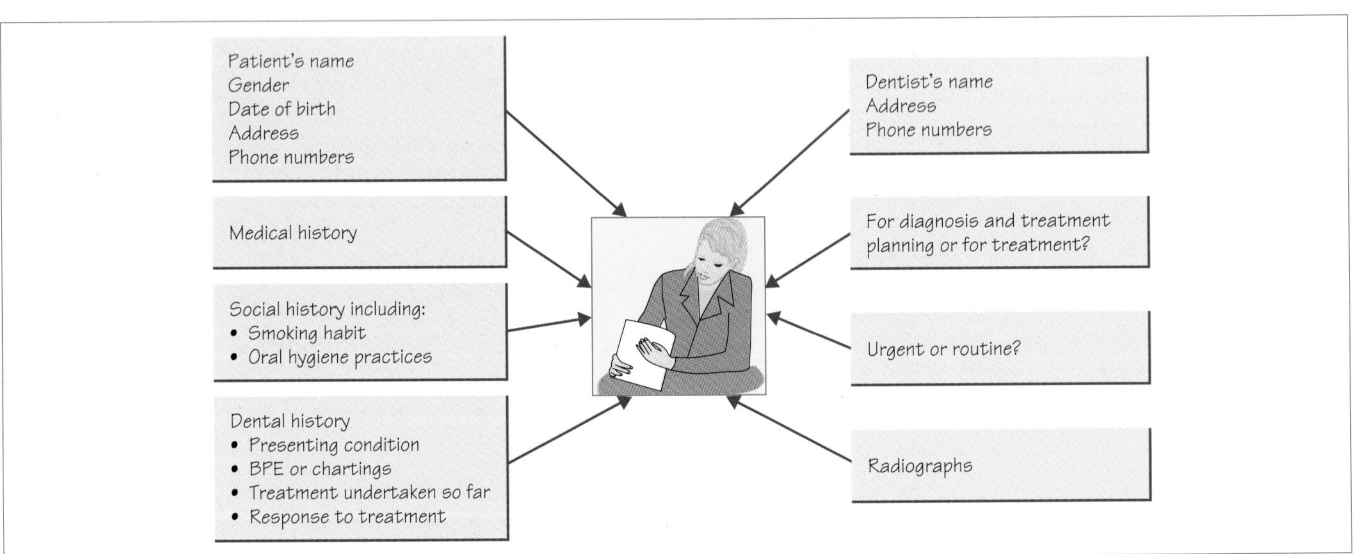

Figure 43.3 Key information to include in a referral letter.

For many patients the management of their periodontal condition can be solely carried out in general practice. However, for some patients referral to a specialist periodontist is appropriate. The treatment may be provided within the specialist referral centre or in combination with treatment in the general practice setting.

The decision to treat or refer a patient will be dependent on three broad issues (Fig. 43.1). Any decision is made on a case-specific basis, however it is useful to have guidelines to help inform that decision. One such set of guidelines (Clinical Effectiveness Committee of the Royal College of Surgeons of England, 2001) is based on using the Basic Periodontal Examination (BPE) (Chapter 17) index and taking into consideration modifying factors or medical factors that could impact on management to determine the complexity of a case (Fig. 43.2).

Role of the specialist periodontist

The specialist periodontist has the following responsibilities:

- To make diagnoses and plan the management of referred cases.
- Sometimes to provide the referring dentist with an expert opinion and treatment plan.
- To undertake the management of more complex cases.
- Sometimes to undertake periodontal surgery.

In many cases the general dental practitioner (GDP) may be willing and able to provide care in the primary care setting, but confirmation of a diagnosis or input in planning the management of the patient may be valuable. In most cases some part of the periodontal treatment plan of a referred patient will be carried out by the general dentist; usually the initial and supportive phases of therapy can be undertaken in practice and the corrective therapy by specialists.

The referral process

The referral letter

Most patients are referred to a specialist by a written referral letter. The quality of referral letters is variable but use of a pro forma or some form of template can prevent key pieces of information being left out. A checklist for information to include in a referral letter is shown in Fig. 43.3. The dentist should ensure that the patient understands why they are to be referred and consents to the referral.

Radiographs

Every attempt should be made to limit the radiation dose to the patient (Chapter 18) so it is good practice to have previous radiographs available when assessing a patient. The dentist should therefore send relevant radiographs to the specialist. Digital imaging enables the images to be sent without the radiographs leaving the practice. Sight of previous films may reduce the need for further films and help to assess the progress of the disease if sequential radiographs are available. Many specialists will have facilities for copying radiographs, enabling early return of the originals.

Starting periodontal therapy

For many patients it is appropriate for the dentist to start periodontal therapy and review the response to the initial phase of therapy before considering a referral. If the condition is thought to be aggressive the dentist may wish to start treatment and send a referral before evaluating response. The dentist should indicate the provisional diagnosis in the referral letter and flag up the urgency of the case. Some of the non-plaque-induced lesions (Chapter 31) will require an immediate referral for diagnosis and management in a specialist centre.

The specialist's reply

Following the patient's visit to the specialist, the dentist should receive a reply to the original referral letter. This will generally include:

- A summary of the clinical findings.
- A diagnosis and treatment plan.
- Clear indication of which parts of the treatment plan are to be carried out in the specialist centre and which in primary practice.

It is important that the patient, referring dentist and specialist are clear as to where the different parts of treatment will be delivered. Generally, routine dental care including treatment integral to the periodontal treatment plan, such as extractions or modification of plaque retention factors, and long-term periodontal management will fall to the referring practitioner. As periodontal therapy can extend over some time it is important that the patient understands that regular dental examinations should continue alongside any specialist periodontal provision.

Discharge from the specialist to referring dentist

On completion of the corrective phase of treatment at the specialist centre, the patient is evaluated and supportive therapy is planned. The periodontist may wish to review treatment response but then the patient will usually be discharged back into the referring practitioner's care. A letter of discharge should advise the dentist on the plan for supportive care, including sites requiring particular attention.

After an intensive period of treatment when the patient may have been very compliant it is easy for the patient to lapse into old habits and feel that the periodontal problem has been solved. It is therefore important in the supportive phase to be vigilant for any disease recurrence and review compliance with oral home care.

Key points

- The decision to refer may depend on:
  - the dentist's expertise
  - patient-related factors
  - the complexity of the case
- Specific categories of patients will be appropriate for specialist referral
- Patients may be referred for an opinion and treatment plan or for treatment
- Referral letters should contain key facts about the patient and condition
- Previous relevant radiographs should be made available to the specialist where possible
- The practitioner should be advised about the specialist's findings, treatment plan and eventual plan for care when the patient is discharged back

Appendix: References and further reading

Chapter 2

Armitage GC. Development of a classification system for periodontal diseases and conditions. *Annals of Periodontology* 1999; **4**: 1–6.

Chapter 3

Albandar JM, Rams TE. Global epidemiology of periodontal diseases: an overview. *Periodontology 2000* 2002; **29**: 7–10.

Barnes GP, Parker WA, Lyon TC, Fulz RP. Indices used to evaluate signs, symptoms and etiologic factors associated with diseases of the periodontium. *Journal of Periodontology* 1986; **56**: 643–51.

Borrell LN, Papapanou PN. Analytical epidemiology of periodontitis. *Journal of Clinical Periodontology* 2005; **32** (suppl 6): 132–58.

Brown LJ, Oliver RC, Loe H. Evaluating periodontal status of US employed adults. *Journal of the American Dental Association* 1990; **121**: 226–32.

Kelly M, Steele J, Nuttall N *et al. Adult Dental Health Survey. Oral Health in the United Kingdom, 1998*. The Stationery Office, London, 2000.

Last JM. *A Dictionary of Epidemiology*, 4th edn. International Epidemiological Association, Oxford University Press, New York, 2001.

Löe H, Silness J. The gingival index, the plaque index and the retention index systems. *Journal of Periodontology* 1967; **38**: 610–17.

Tu Y-K, Jackson M, Kellett M, Clerehugh V. Direct and indirect effects of interdental hygiene in a clinical trial. *Journal of Dental Research* 2008; **87**: 1037–42.

Chapter 4

Löe H, Theilade E, Jensen SB. Experimental gingivitis in man. *Journal of Periodontology* 1965; **36**: 177–87.

Loesche WJ. Chemotherapy of dental plaque infections. *Oral Science Reviews* 1976; **9**: 63–107.

Loesche WJ. Clinical and microbiological aspects of chemotherapeutic agents used according to the specific plaque hypothesis. *Journal of Dental Research* 1979; **58**: 2404–12.

Marsh PD. Sugar, fluoride, pH and microbial homeostasis in dental plaque. *Proceedings of the Finnish Dental Society* 1991; **87**: 515–25.

Marsh PD. Microbial ecology of dental plaque and its significance in health and disease. *Advances in Dental Research* 1994; **8**: 263–71.

Marsh PD. Dental plaque: biological significance of a biofilm and community life-style. *Journal of Clinical Periodontology* 2005; **32** (suppl 6): 7–15.

Theilade E. The non-specific theory in microbial etiology of inflammatory periodontal diseases. *Journal of Clinical Periodontology* 1986; **13**: 905–11.

Wood SR, Kirkham J, Shore RC, Brookes SJ, Robinson C. Changes in the structure and density of oral plaque biofilms with increasing plaque age. *FEMS Microbiology Ecology* 2002; **39**: 239–244.

Chapter 5

Socransky SS, Haffajee AD. Periodontal microbial ecology. *Periodontology 2000* 2005; **38**: 135–87.

Socransky SS, Haffajee AD. Periodontal infections. In: *Clinical Periodontology and Implant Dentistry*, 5th edn (Lindhe J, Lang NP, Karring T, eds), pp. 207–67. Blackwell Publishing, Oxford, 2008.

Socransky SS, Haffajee AD, Cugini MA, Smith C, Kent Jr RL. Microbial complexes in subgingival plaque. *Journal of Clinical Periodontology* 1998; **25**: 134–44.

Teles RP, Haffajee AD, Socransky SS. Microbiological goals of periodontal therapy. *Periodontology 2000* 2006; **39**: 180–218.

Chapter 6

Jin Y, Yip H-K. Supragingival calculus: formation and control. *Critical Reviews in Oral Biology and Medicine* 2002; **13**: 426–41.

Roberts-Harry EA, Clerehugh V. Subgingival calculus: where are we now? A comparative review. *Journal of Dentistry* 2000; **28**: 93–102.

Roberts-Harry EA, Clerehugh V, Shore RC, Kirkham J, Robinson C. Morphology and elemental composition of subgingival calculus in two ethnic groups. *Journal of Periodontology* 2000; **71**: 1401–11.

Chapter 8

Kinane DF, Berglundh T, Lindhe J. Pathogenesis of periodontitis. In: *Clinical Periodontology and Implant Dentistry*, 5th edn (Lindhe J, Lang NP, Karring T, eds), pp. 285–306. Wiley-Blackwell, Oxford, 2008.

Page RC, Schroeder HE. Pathogenesis of inflammatory periodontal disease. A summary of current work. *Laboratory Investigation* 1976; **33**: 235–49.

Chapter 9

DeRouen TA, Hujoel PP, Mancl LA. Statistical issues in periodontal research. *Journal of Dental Research* 1995; **74**: 1731–5.

Gilthorpe MS, Zamzuri AT, Griffiths GS, Maddick IH, Eaton KA, Johnson NW. Unification of the 'burst' and 'linear' theories of periodontal disease progression: a multilevel manifestation of the same phenomenon. *Journal of Dental Research* 2003; **82**: 200–5.

Socransky SS, Haffajee AD, Goodson JM, Lindhe J. New concepts of destructive periodontal disease. *Journal of Clinical Periodontology* 1984; **11**: 21–32.

Tonetti MS, Claffey N. Advances in the progression of periodontitis and proposal of definitions of a periodontitis case and disease progression for use in risk factor research. *Journal of Clinical Periodontology* 2005; **32** (suppl 6): 210–13.

Chapter 10

Beck JD. Risk revisited. *Community Dentistry and Oral Epidemiology* 1998; **26**: 220–5.

Last JM. *A Dictionary of Epidemiology*, 4th edn. International Epidemiological Association, Oxford University Press, New York, 2001.

Chapter 11

Genco RJ, Ho AW, Grossi SG, Dunford RG, Tedesco LA. Relationship of stress, distress, and inadequate coping behaviors to periodontal disease. *Journal of Periodontology* 1999; **70**: 711–23.

Genco RJ, Loe H. The role of systemic conditions and disorders in periodontal disease. *Periodontology 2000* 1993; **2**: 98–116.

Grossi SG, Genco RJ, Machtei EE *et al.* Assessment of risk for periodontal disease. II. Risk indicators for alveolar bone loss. *Journal of Periodontology* 1995; **66**: 23–9.

Grossi SG, Skrepcinski FB, DeCaro T *et al.* Treatment of periodontal disease in diabetics reduces glycated hemoglobin. *Journal of Periodontology* 1997; **68**: 713–19.

Heasman L, Stacey F, Preshaw PM, McCracken GI, Hepburn S, Heasman PA. The effect of smoking on periodontal treatment response: a review of clinical evidence. *Journal of Clinical Periodontology* 2006; **33**: 241–53.

Nishida M, Grossi SG, Dunford RG, Ho AW, Trevisan M, Genco RJ. Calcium and the risk for periodontal disease. *Journal of Periodontology* 2000; **71**: 1057–66.

Struch F, Dau M, Schwahn C, Biffar R, Kocher T, Meisel P. Interleukin-1 gene polymorphism, diabetes, and periodontitis: results from the Study of Health in Pomerania (SHIP). *Journal of Periodontology* 2008; **79**: 501–7.

Ylostalo P, Suominen-Taipale L, Reunanen A, Knuuttila M. Association between body weight and periodontal infection. *Journal of Clinical Periodontology* 2008; **35**: 297–304.

Chapter 12

Kuo LC, Polson AM, Kan T. Associations between periodontal diseases and systemic diseases: a review of the inter-relationships and interactions with diabetes, respiratory diseases, cardiovascular diseases and osteoporosis. *Public Health* 2008; **122**: 417–33.

Lopez R. Periodontal disease and adverse pregnancy outcomes. *Journal of Clinical Periodontology* 2008; **35**: 16–22.

Meyer MS, Joshipura K, Giovannucci E, Michaud DS. A review of the relationship between tooth loss, periodontal disease, and cancer. *Cancer Causes Control* 2008; **19**: 895–907.

Mustapha IZ, Debrey S, Oladubu M, Ugarte R. Markers of systemic bacterial exposure in periodontal disease and cardiovascular disease risk: a systematic review and meta-analysis. *Journal of Periodontology* 2007; **78**: 2289–302.

Taylor GW, Burt BA, Becker MP, Genco RJ, Shlossman M, Knowler WC, Pettitt DJ. Severe periodontitis and risk for poor glycemic control in patients with non-insulin-dependent diabetes mellitus. *Journal of Periodontology* 1996; **67**: 1085–93.

Chapter 13

Kaye EK. Bone health and oral health. *Journal of the American Dental Association* 2007; **138**: 616–19.

Merchant AT, Pitiphat W, Franz M, Joshipura KJ. Whole grain fiber intake and periodontitis risk in men. *American Journal of Clinical Nutrition* 2006; **83**: 1395–400.

Moynihan P. The interrelationship between diet and oral health. *Proceedings of the Nutrition Society* 2005; **64**: 571–80.

Nishida M, Grossi SG, Dunford RG, Ho AW, Trevisan M, Genco RJ. Calcium and the risk for periodontal disease. *Journal of Periodontology* 2000a; **71**: 1057–66.

Nishida M, Grossi SG, Dunford RG, Ho AW, Trevisan M, Genco RJ. Vitamin D and the risk for periodontal disease. *Journal of Periodontology* 2000b; **71**: 1215–23.

Nowjock-Raymer RE, Sheiham A. Numbers of natural teeth, diet, and nutritional status in US adults. *Journal of Dental Research* 2007; **86**: 1171–5.

Schifferle RE. Nutrition and periodontal disease. *Dental Clinics of North America* 2005; **49**: 595–610, vii.

Standing Committee on the Scientific Evaluation of Dietary Reference Intakes, Food and Nutrition Board, Institute of Medicine. *Dietary reference intakes for calcium, phosphorus, magnesium, vitamin D and fluoride*. National Academies Press, Washington, 1997.

Weaver CM, Proulx WR, Heaney RP. Choices for achieving adequate dietary calcium with a vegetarian diet. *American Journal of Clinical Nutrition* 1999; **70**: S543–8.

Chapter 14

Armitage GC. Development of a classification system for periodontal diseases and conditions. *Annals of Periodontology* 1999; **4**: 1–6.

Chapter 15

Lindhe J, Ericsson I. The effect of elimination of jiggling forces on periodontally exposed teeth in the dog. *Journal of Periodontology* 1982; **53**: 562–7.

Lindhe J, Nyman S. A longitudinal study of combined periodontal and prosthetic treatment of patients with advanced periodontal disease. *Journal of Periodontology* 1979; **50**: 163–9.

Lindhe J, Nyman S, Ericsson I. Trauma from occlusion: periodontal tissues. In: *Clinical Periodontology and Implant Dentistry*, 5th edn (Lindhe J, Lang NP, Karring T, eds), pp. 349–62. Wiley-Blackwell, Oxford, 2008.

Polson AM, Zander HA. Effect of periodontal trauma upon infrabony pockets. *Journal of Periodontology* 1983; **54**: 586–91.

Chapter 17

British Society of Periodontology. Periodontology in General Dental Practice in the United Kingdom. A policy statement, 2001. www.bsperio.org.uk, accessed 30 June 2009.

Clerehugh V. Periodontal diseases in children and adolescents. *British Dental Journal* 2008; **204**; 469–71.

Chapter 19

Armitage GC. Development of a classification system for periodontal diseases and conditions. *Annals of Periodontology* 1999; **4**: 1–6.

Chapter 20

Badersten A, Nilveus R, Egelberg J. Effect of non-surgical periodontal therapy II. Severely advanced periodontitis. *Journal of Clinical Periodontology* 1984; **11**: 63–76.

Cullinan MP, Westerman B, Hamlet SM, Palmer JE, Faddy MJ, Seymour GJ. The effect of a triclosan-containing dentifrice on the progression of periodontal disease in an adult population. *Journal of Clinical Periodontology* 2003; **30**: 414–19.

Drisko C. Sonic and ultrasonic scalers in periodontics. Position Paper of the American Academy of Periodontology. *Journal of Periodontology* 2000; **71**: 1792–801.

Ellwood RP, Worthington HV, Blinkhorn AS, Volpe AR, Davies RM. Effect of a triclosan/copolymer dentifrice on the incidence of periodontal attachment loss in adolescents. *Journal of Clinical Periodontology* 1998; **25**: 363–7.

Greenstein G. Nonsurgical periodontal therapy in 2000: a literature review. *Journal of American Dental Association* 2000; **131**: 1580–92.

Gunsolley JG. A meta-analysis of six-month studies of antiplaque and antigingivitis agents. *Journal of American Dental Association* 2006; **137**: 1649–57.

Jackson MA, Kellett M, Worthington HV, Clerehugh V. Comparison of interdental cleaning methods: a randomized controlled trial. *Journal of Periodontology* 2006; **77**: 1421–9.

Lovdal A, Arno A, Schei O, Waehaug J. Combined effect of subgingival scaling and controlled oral hygiene on the incidence of gingivitis. *Acta Odontologica Scandinavica* 1961; **19**: 537–55.

Mongardini C, van Steenberghe D, Dekeyser C, Quirynen M. One stage full- versus partial-mouth disinfection in the treatment of chronic adult or generalized early-onset periodontitis. I. Long-term clinical observations. *Journal of Periodontology* 1999; **70**: 632–45.

Robinson P, Deacon SA, Deery C *et al.* Manual versus powered toothbrushing for oral health. *Cochrane Database of Systematic Reviews* 2005, Issue 2. Art. No.: CD002281. DOI: 10.1002/14651858.CD002281.pub2.

Rosling B, Wannfors B, Volpe AR, Furuichi Y, Ramberg P, Lindhe J. The use of a triclosan/copolymer dentifrice may retard the progression of periodontitis. *Journal of Clinical Periodontology* 1997; **24**: 873–80.

Tu Y-K, Jackson M, Kellett M, Clerehugh V. Direct and indirect effects of interdental hygiene in a clinical trial. *Journal of Dental Research* 2008; **87**: 1037–42.

Chapter 31

Armitage GC. Development of a classification system for periodontal diseases and conditions. *Annals of Periodontology* 1999; **4**: 1–6.

Chapple ILC, Hamburger JH. *Periodontal Medicine*. Quintessence, London, 2006.

Chapter 33

Chapple ILC, Hamburger JH. *Periodontal Medicine*. Quintessence, London, 2006.

Chapter 40

Ainamo J, Nordblad A, Kallio P. Use of the CPITN in populations under 20 years of age. *International Dental Journal* 1984; **34**: 285–91.

Armitage GC. Development of a classification system for periodontal diseases and conditions. *Annals of Periodontology* 1999; **4**: 1–6.

Clerehugh V. Periodontal diseases in children and adolescents. *British Dental Journal* 2008; **204**; 469–71.

Clerehugh V, Lennon MA, Worthington HV. Five-year results of a longitudinal study of early periodontis in 14 to 19-year-old adolescents. *Journal of Clinical Periodontology* 1990; **17**: 702–8.

Clerehugh V, Seymour GJ, Bird PS, Cullinan M, Drucker DB, Worthington HV. The detection of *Actinobacillus actinomycetemcomitans*, *Porphyromonas gingivalis* and *Prevotella intermedia* using an ELISA in an adolescent population with early periodontitis. *Journal of Clinical Periodontology* 1997; **24**: 57–64.

Clerehugh V, Tugnait A, Chapple ILC. *Periodontal Management of Children, Adolescents and Young Adults*. Quintessence, London, 2004.

Hamlet S, Ellwood R, Cullinan M *et al.* Persistent colonisation with *Tannerella forsythensis* and loss of attachment in adolescents. *Journal of Dental Research* 2004; **83**: 232–5.

Pendry L, Lashkari G, Bewley H. *Technical Report: 2003 Children's Dental Health Survey*. Office for National Statistics, London, 2004.

White DA, Chadwick BL, Nuttall NM, Steele JG. Oral health habits amongst children in the United Kingdom in 2003. *British Dental Journal* 2006; **200**: 487–91.

Chapter 41

Beck JD. Periodontal implications: older adults. *Annals of Periodontology* 1996; **1**: 322–57.

Dolan TA, Atchison K, Huynh TN. Access to dental care among older adults in the United States. *Journal of Dental Education* 2005; **69**: 961–74.

Jones JA, Wehler CJ. The Elders' Oral Health Summit: introduction and recommendations. *Journal of Dental Education* 2005; **69**: 957–60.

Kelly M, Steele J, Nuttall N *et al. Adult Dental Health Survey. Oral Health in the United Kingdom 1998*. The Stationery Office, London, 2000.

Klinge B, Norlund A. A socio-economic perspective on periodontal diseases: a systematic review. *Journal of Clinical Periodontology* 2005; **32** (suppl 6): 314–25.

Papapanou PN, Wennstrom JL, Sellen A, Hirooka H, Grondahl K, Johnsson T. Periodontal treatment needs assessed by the use of clinical and radiographic criteria. *Community Dentistry and Oral Epidemiology* 1990; **18**: 113–19.

Wennstrom JL, Papapanou PN, Grondahl K. A model for decision making regarding periodontal treatment needs. *Journal of Clinical Periodontology* 1990; **17**: 217–22.

Chapter 43

Clinical Effectiveness Committee of the Royal College of Surgeons of England. *Restorative Dentistry Index of Treatment Need Complexity Assessment*. 2001. http://www.rcseng.ac.uk/fds/clinical_guidelines/documents/complexityassessment.pdf (accessed 25 February 2009).

Index

Note: Page numbers in *italics* refer to Figures, page numbers in **bold** refer to Tables.